ADOLESCENT HEALTH

This book is dedicated to my twin children,
Richard and Carina, who safely navigated their adolescence
to become competent, caring, and compassionate young adults.

ADOLESCENT HEALTH

A Multidisciplinary

Approach to

Theory,

Research, and

Intervention

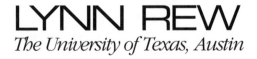

LYNN REW

The University of Texas, Austin

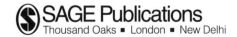

SAGE Publications
Thousand Oaks ▪ London ▪ New Delhi

For information:

Sage Publications, Inc.
2455 Teller Road
Thousand Oaks, California 91320
E-mail: order@sagepub.com

Sage Publications Ltd.
1 Oliver's Yard
55 City Road
London EC1Y 1SP
United Kingdom

Sage Publications India Pvt. Ltd.
B-42, Panchsheel Enclave
Post Box 4109
New Delhi 110 017 India

Printed in the United States of America

Library of Congress Cataloging-in-Publication Data

Rew, Lynn.
Adolescent health: a multidisciplinary approach to theory, research,
and intervention / by Lynn Rew.
        p. cm.
Includes bibliographical references and index.
ISBN 0–7619–2911–8 (cloth: acid free paper)
    1. Youth—Health and hygiene—United states. 2. Teengers—Health and hygiene—United States. 3. Health behavior in adolescence—United States. I. Title.
RJ102. R49 2005
613′. 0433—dc22

                                        2004010261

This book is printed on acid-free paper.

04   05   06   07   08   10   9   8   7   6   5   4   3   2   1

Acquisitions Editor:	Jim Brace-Thompson
Editorial Assistant:	Karen Ehrmann
Copy Editor:	Catherine Chilton
Production Editor:	Kristen Gibson
Typesetter:	C&M Digitals (P) Ltd.
Proofreader:	Kristin Berystad
Cover Designer:	Michelle Lee Kenny

Contents

List of Figures _____

List of Tables

Foreword _____

How refreshing to find a single volume that not only tells us where we've been, but clearly illuminates the critical pathways we must travel for the foreseeable future of interdisciplinary adolescent health research. A generation of insights has led us to some inescapable truths: No one discipline has a monopoly on the theories, methods, and skills needed to adequately describe and understand the health, behaviors, and social contexts of youth. Breadth of perspective is a necessary ingredient for scholars and practitioners alike who are engaged in the science and skills of adolescent health. And our learners, more diverse than ever before, are in need of accessible yet sophisticated material that grounds them in a field characterized by rapidly expanding boundaries and a dazzling array of theory and methods to guide and propel their research.

It would have been so much easier to write a book like this one 20 years ago—but even then, it would have been a daunting task. Instead, Dr. Lynn Rew, with the insights of a clinician and the imagination of an adolescent health researcher unfettered by disciplinary parochialism, has provided us with a thoughtful and comprehensive work that will, at once, accomplish two things: It will guide and inspire learners at multiple levels, and it will provide well-organized and richly articulated material for the teachers of that interdisciplinary audience.

In this last generation, we have nurtured a group of adolescent health investigators who often lack formal schooling in relevant theory and the skills and logic of theory testing. For many, that lack of formal preparation is offset to a large extent by a substantial dose of practical wisdom arising from clinical and programmatic interactions with young people. However, the transition to scholarly sensitivities requires deliberate instruction that is often lacking among those who have not grown up through the mechanisms of classic academic research training. This volume does an extraordinary job of helping such learners understand theory as a guide to and framer of their understanding. Rew also thoroughly grounds the reader in contemporary threats to the health of young people, the principles of adolescent development, and the organized response to those health threats as reflected in national objectives to improve the health of young people.

Through a well-orchestrated and thoughtful progression, this book provides us with the theories to frame our questions and the language to give those questions real substance and application. This work helps us to reach across the divides of discipline-specific thinking and methods and leaves us enriched, ultimately, and better able to collaborate with each other. Our field, and the needs of young people, deserve no less.

Michael D. Resnick, Ph.D.
Professor and Director of Research
Division of General Pediatrics and Adolescent Health
Director, Healthy Youth Development
Prevention Research Center
University of Minnesota

Acknowledgments _____

I am grateful to many professional colleagues, friends, and family members for their support while I was writing this book. Dr. Lorraine Walker, professor in the School of Nursing at The University of Texas at Austin, is not only the author of the theory construction book on which most of Chapter 2 of this book is based, but provided encouragement and review as I began to put my ideas into words. She is a wonderful role model and friend. Dr. Kay Avant also reviewed chapter 2 and provided helpful comments. Dr. Sharon Horner is another colleague who consistently provided "reality checks" for me, and I appreciate her thoughtful critique and support throughout this writing process.

Not only did I receive critiques and support from my peers, I also received these gifts from my doctoral student, Jane Kass-Wolff, and three of my research assistants, Dann Coakwell, Kate Jackson, and Lou Riesch. They all completed their work in such a way that I was freed up many afternoons to go home and write. I had also learned that Dann Coakwell had great computer skills in drawing figures, so I hired him to work on the weekends, drawing some of the original figures that are in this text. Then there is Margaret Hill, Assistant Dean for Administration at the School of Nursing: I learned that she was also interested in my writing project and was willing to be employed part-time on weekends to proofread the first drafts of chapters. Her eagle eye and gracious support were a great help.

A book like this does not happen without significant guidance and wisdom from the publisher. I must take this opportunity to thank Dan Ruth at Sage for his assistance in introducing me to Jim Brace-Thompson and Karen Ehrmann. I had worked with Dan for about 6 years as editor of the *Journal of Holistic Nursing* when I told him about my idea for this book. He immediately put me in contact with Jim, and the ensuing association with these folks has been wonderful.

None of this would have happened without the mentorship of Michael Resnick from the University of Minnesota and my husband, dick (yes, he prefers the lower case spelling of his name—something left over from late adolescence, being a math major in college, and differential equations).

These two men have nurtured me in phenomenal ways, each providing just the right balance between challenge and opportunity. They believed in my vision, my creativity, and my ability to produce.

Finally, I especially want to acknowledge a family friend, John Langford, who provided a sincere and thoughtful blessing when the book was completed.

All of these individuals placed their fingerprints on early drafts of this book, but, more important, each made an indelible print on my heart. We rarely take the opportunities we have to thank the important people in our lives. So my last words of thanks must go to my parents, Charles and Clara Cannon. I am thankful that they did not abandon me when I went through my adolescence and that, at 88 years of age, my mom still has the patience to listen to me and to care about my work.

Introduction _____

The 1995-1996 academic year was a defining time period in my professional development. Metaphorically speaking, you could say it was the adolescent phase of my professional development. With funding for a Faculty Research Award from The University of Texas at Austin and a senior fellowship award (1 F33 NR07126–01) from the National Institute of Nursing Research, National Institutes of Health, I participated in a multidisciplinary postdoctoral program at the University of Minnesota School of Medicine. Working with internationally known and caring mentors such as Robert W. Blum, Michael D. Resnick, Lyn H. Bearinger, and Cheryl Perry, I was able to redirect my identity as a researcher and focus my research program on adolescent health-risk behaviors. Not only did I improve and increase my research skills, I also began to connect with an incredible network of researchers, educators, and practitioners in this fascinating field. Through this network I have fielded many questions about the existence of a comprehensive textbook of theories about adolescent health and health-risk behaviors suitable for graduate students in various disciplines. At last, I decided to submit a prospectus to Sage Publications, Inc., for such a book. Their reviewers really liked the idea; thus I've done my best to turn that dream into a reality.

Writing a book for readers from a variety of disciplines has been a great challenge. The size limitations of the book meant that I had to make critical choices in determining which theories to include and which to leave out. Also, although I am clearly not an expert on all the theoretical perspectives and models that are found in this text, I hope I have given enough details to motivate students and their mentors to think more broadly and deeply about the science of adolescent health.

1

Adolescent Health and Health-Risk Behaviors

A dolescent health is a topic of great interest to members of several professions. In fact, it is probably of greater interest to us than it is to adolescents themselves. Compared to their parents, who may exchange information with friends and coworkers about how to avoid specific diseases such as cancer or how to reduce complications of chronic illnesses such as diabetes mellitus or hypertension, adolescents spend little time discussing their health with one another. Yet adolescents engage in activities on a daily, sometimes hourly, basis that may threaten their immediate safety or their long-term health and well-being. Patterns of health-risk behaviors established in this critical stage of development such as overeating, smoking, and minimal physical activity can have long-term health consequences. What is the health status of adolescents in America at the dawn of the 21st century?

Overview of Adolescent Health Status

The current health status of America's youth may be assessed in several ways. *Morbidity* refers to those conditions that are considered to be pathological or threatening to a person's health; *mortality* refers to conditions that cause a person's death. Morbidities include both acute and chronic conditions, such as upper respiratory infections (acute), which are common among all adolescents, and asthma (chronic), which is not common among most adolescents.

Another way to assess the health status of adolescents is to identify their access to and use of health-care services and institutions (Ozer, Park, Paul, Brindis, & Irwin, 2003). Remaining healthy over time may be related to periodic examinations by a health professional; routine prophylaxis, such as dental cleaning or immunizations; and judicious application of technology, as in the use of x-rays and surgical techniques to detect and set broken bones. Access to these resources, however, depends on the adolescent's knowledge of them and familiarity with how to use them. Access also depends on the ability to pay for services, either with cash or through health insurance. For millions of American adolescents, neither of these options is available.

Still another way of viewing the health status of adolescents is to examine those behaviors that increase the risk for morbidities or mortalities. These behaviors have been identified by many different terms, including *problem behaviors, risk-taking behaviors, deviant behaviors, risky behaviors,* and *health-risk behaviors.* This group of behaviors is related, either directly or indirectly, to the major mortalities of youth. And many of these behaviors lead directly or indirectly to chronic health problems. Finally, the overall health of adolescents may be assessed by examining indicators of well-being as reported by the Federal Interagency Forum on Child and Family Statistics (2002). According to this report, indicators of adolescents' well-being include economic security, mortality rates, birth rates for adolescents, cigarette use, and violent crime victimization and offending.

Health Status

Health status refers to the meaning that individuals and groups ascribe to their personal experiences of health. With respect to adolescent health, various groups may ascribe very different meanings to similar experiences. In general, adults, particularly parents, may be more concerned than their adolescent children are about developing good health habits or a healthy lifestyle. Parents may also underestimate their adolescent children's involvement in health-risk behaviors (Stanton et al., 2000). Similarly, adult professionals, such as teachers, psychologists, nurses, and physicians, may attach still other meanings to health status. The teacher may be concerned about how an adolescent's chronic illness interferes with his or her cognitive development and academic progress. The psychologist may focus on the way stress is expressed as somatic complaints. Nurses and physicians may anticipate health problems before they occur and provide guidance to parents and youth to help them avoid predictable threats to health and well-being.

Adolescents themselves have their own view of how healthy they are, which is often not congruent with the views held by the adults in their lives. Their concerns about health are unique to their developmental stage. Other variations are related to gender, ethnicity, and socioeconomic status. Perceptions of health status among adolescents are also related to their beliefs and knowledge about health and their feelings of invulnerability to adverse health outcomes (Millstein, 1993). In this chapter, recent research about adolescent health status and associated health-risk behaviors is presented to provide the context for the remainder of the book, which focuses on the role of theories and conceptual frameworks to guide further scholarship and intervention development in multiple adolescent health disciplines.

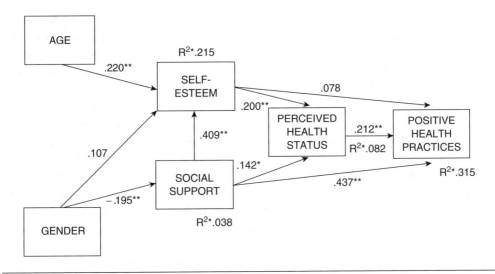

Figure 1.1   A Model of Positive Health Practices in Adolescents

$* p < .05; ** p < .01$.

SOURCE: Yarcheski et al. (1997). Reprinted with permission.

Perceived Health Status in Adolescents

Perceived health status has been hypothesized as a factor that influences positive health practices among adolescents. Yarcheski, Mahon, and Yarcheski (1997) tested two alternate causal models to test this hypothesis. With data from a sample of 202 adolescents (91 males and 111 females) who were between 15 and 21 years old ($M = 18.65 + 2.24$), they tested the models through structural equation modeling, using the LISREL 7 program. The goodness-of-fit index and the adjusted goodness-of-fit index were 0.99 and 0.98, respectively, indicating good fit with the data. Results of testing the first model did not support the proposed direct and indirect effects among theoretical variables. However, the second model, shown in Figure 1.1, showed significant direct effects of self-esteem and social support on perceived health status and significant direct effects of perceived health status and social support on positive health practices.

Meaning of Health to Adolescents

Adolescence, roughly defined as the second decade of life, is a time of transition and experimentation. It is a time when children undergo multiple physical, social, psychological, and cognitive changes that propel them toward physical maturity and an adult lifestyle. Adolescence is viewed as consisting of three general developmental stages: (a) early adolescence, from 10 to 13 years old; (b) middle adolescence, from 14 to 17 years old; and

(c) late adolescence, from 18 to 21 years old (Radzik, Sherer, & Neinstein, 2002). On the whole, adolescents enjoy relatively good health. In the 21st century, they can reap the benefits of scientific technology that protects them from the ravages of deadly communicable diseases, such as polio, smallpox, and scarlet fever. Nonetheless, some have been born with conditions that create chronic health problems, such as those associated with spina bifida or cerebral palsy. But these are the exceptions rather than the rule.

The concept of health is evolving and has been defined in a number of ways by members of various disciplines. The World Health Organization (WHO, 1946) emphasizes wholeness in its definition: "Health is a state of complete physical, mental, and social well-being and not merely the absence of disease or infirmity" (p. 100). Another definition of health is "the state of being sound, or freedom from defect or separation" (Smith, 2002, p. 6). Other definitions include the biological model, with its focus on the absence of disease or injury, and broader definitions, such as the biopsychosocial model, which focuses on a person's individual experiences of well-being (Millstein, Petersen, & Nightingale, 1993). Health has also been described as an expansion of consciousness that encompasses all life processes (Newman, 1994).

Perry (1999) notes that health is more than absence of disease or prevention of an untimely death. She describes health as a dynamic state of well-being, with physical, social, psychological, and spiritual dimensions. Perry maintains that a broad view of health that includes all these dimensions is very important when considering the health behaviors of adolescents, because the outcomes of health-risk behaviors may occur in more than one dimension of a young person's life. Researchers have used these various definitions of health to develop scales to enable them to study health status in adolescents and adults. However, a single self-rated item in which a person is asked to rate her or his health as poor, fair, good, or excellent compared to others is the most widely used measure of this phenomenon (Ratner, Johnson, & Jeffery, 1998).

How do adolescents view the concept of health? Millstein (1993) notes that adolescents and adults apply similar criteria to define health. That is, health is associated with positive affective states; living up to one's potential; and functioning in physical, psychological, and social domains. Millstein asserts that through the process of maturation, adolescents conceptualize health in more abstract and inclusive terms than they did at younger ages. This means that they are more able to recognize their personal responsibility for health as they mature.

Weiler (1997) conducted a study of 419 high school students who lived in a rural area of the Midwest. From this convenience sample, he collected data about the participants' health concerns and those of their peers. He found that the top 10 health concerns of the adolescent participants were centered primarily around their future and their relationships (see Table 1.1).

Other concerns of these adolescents were related to personal health, such as acne, body shape, weight, fitness, and personal attractiveness. Human sexuality concerns were related to having sexual intercourse, using contraceptives,

Table 1.1   Top Ten Concerns of a Sample of Rural Adolescents

The Future	Relationships
1. Being successful	5. Getting along with friends
2. Selecting a career	6. Dating
3. Getting good grades	7. Attending college
4. How I want to be in 10 years	8. Having a romantic partner
	9. Having my own family
	10. Getting along with parents

SOURCE: Based on study by Weiler (1997).

and teenage pregnancy. Substance use and abuse, including driving under the influence of alcohol, and personal safety were also expressed as concerns. In comparing themselves to their peers, participants reported that their best friends and other adolescents had greater concerns about substance use and abuse; they also thought these other two groups were less concerned about the future.

Using data from the 1997 Commonwealth Fund Survey of the Health of Adolescent Girls and Boys, Ackard and Neumark-Sztainer (2001) examined adolescents' sources of information about health and their beliefs about what information health providers should share with them. From a representative national sample of 3153 males and 3575 females, they found that these adolescents received most of their information about health from their mothers. They identified five topics that adolescents wanted information about from health providers. In order of frequency of identified topics, they wanted more information about (a) drugs, (b) sexually transmitted diseases, (c) smoking, (d) good eating habits, and (e) alcohol use.

Health and Behavior

Recently, the Institute of Medicine's (2001) Committee on Health and Behavior defined positive health as comprising the following constructs: "a healthy body; high-quality personal relationships; a sense of purpose in life; self-regarded mastery of life's tasks; and resilience to stress, trauma, and change" (p. 23). From this definition, it can be seen that the concept of health encompasses more than having a body free from disease or dysfunction. Personal relationships, mastery of tasks, and resilience to stress and change suggest action or behavior. The institute's report proposed a model of the intersection of health and behavior based on two assumptions: (a) a variety of factors that are genetic, behavioral, and social interact reciprocally to influence health over time, and (b) because health is a function of biological, social, and psychological variables, many factors previously considered as irrelevant to health status may be critical to individuals and specific populations (p. 27).

Health behavior can be broadly defined as those actions taken by individuals, groups, and organizations to improve quality of life (Glanz, Lewis, & Rimer, 1997). Behavior directed toward promoting, maintaining, or restoring health may be motivated by beliefs, needs, and desires. Health behavior encompasses related terms, such as *health protection* and *health promotion*. Health-protecting behavior is generally directed at prevention. The individual who engages in health-protecting behaviors is motivated to protect health by preventing disease or injury or by decreasing the disability and discomfort associated with such health conditions. Health-protecting behaviors include active measures such as obtaining immunization against hepatitis B or participating in regular screening for cervical, breast, or testicular cancers. The focus of health protection is the avoidance of the negative states of disease, injury, or disability. In contrast, health-promoting behaviors focus on the positive states of well-being and self-actualization. Health-promoting behavior is associated with a lifestyle for which high quality of life is a highly probable outcome (Pender, Murdaugh, & Parsons, 2002).

Variations in Health and Health Behaviors

Some children come from backgrounds that place them at high risk for health problems in adolescence and beyond. Children living at or near poverty levels, in families with no health insurance, may not have the knowledge or opportunity to engage in either health-protecting or health-promoting behaviors. These children approach adolescence with compromised physical and mental health statuses. They may have inadequate immunizations against the usual childhood diseases, and their nutritional status may have contributed to physical and mental development that means they are functioning at less than their full potential. Other children come from backgrounds that place them at low risk for health problems. These children approach adolescence with complete immunizations, a regular pattern of routine physical examinations, and health-promoting diets and activity levels. Some of the children who come from disadvantaged backgrounds (i.e., those that place them at high risk) do very well in spite of their levels of risk. Similarly, some children who come from advantaged backgrounds, placing them at low risk for adverse health outcomes, end up engaging in behaviors that threaten their health and safety.

Professionals in health fields such as nursing and medicine have a great stake in understanding health and health-risk behaviors of these youngsters because their daily work brings them face to face with adolescents' health problems. Adolescence is a time when major morbidities are not generally related to diseases such as heart disease and cancer, which strike disproportionately at older adults. Rather, the morbidities and mortalities of adolescence are usually related to adolescents' social behaviors. Today's adolescents face incredible challenges related to the economy, education, crime, and changing family structure (Bronfenbrenner, McClelland,

Wethington, Macu, & Ceci, 1996). Most of the social morbidities and mortalities that account for illness, injury, and death in adolescents are behavioral responses to these challenges. Whether we are talking about physical, emotional, spiritual, or social health, it is the behavior of adolescents, how they act and interact from day to day, that puts them at risk for adverse outcomes in any of these dimensions. Given the complexity of health issues facing today's youth, understanding what accounts for differences in those who engage in behaviors that increase or decrease their risk for poor health outcomes during adolescence is the focus of professionals in a variety of disciplines. As social scientists from many disciplines, it is our responsibility to create the knowledge that can help our youth face these challenges in healthier ways. Researchers have shown that adolescents are concerned about their health and about how their behavior can adversely affect their health (Halpern-Felsher & Cauffman, 2001).

Adolescent Mortalities

There has been a gradual decline in the mortality rates for adolescents since the early 1980s. At present, unintentional injuries account for the largest number of deaths in persons 10 to 24 years old, both in the United States and in many other countries of the world (Call et al., 2002). Preliminary findings for 2001 were that unintentional injuries were still the leading cause of death in Americans between 5 and 24 years old. This represented a rate of 6.8 deaths per 100,000 among 5- to 14-year-olds and 34.7 deaths per 100,000 population among 15- to 24-year-olds. Homicide accounted for 12.8 deaths per 100,000 and suicide for 9.6 deaths per 100,000 among 15- to 24-year-olds (Arias & Smith, 2003). More specifically, 78% of deaths among persons aged 15–19 years were from motor vehicle accidents and claimed the lives of almost two males for every female. Compared with other racial/ethnic groups, non-Hispanic Alaskan Natives and American Indians had the highest mortality rate from motor vehicle accidents (Ozer et al., 2003). From 2001 to 2002, the number of crashes involving drivers between the ages of 16 and 20 years decreased from 1,666,000 to 1,638,000, but fatalities increased from 7,627 to 7,738 (National Highway Traffic Safety Administration [NHTSA], 2003). The NHTSA noted that more than one in four fatalities was related to drinking and driving. Other deaths resulted from the failure to use seat belts in cars and helmets while riding bicycles (NHTSA, 2001; Ozer et al., 2003).

Unintentional Injury

According to the Centers for Disease Control and Prevention (CDC, 2003a), the leading causes of death for persons 10 to 24 years old were (a) motor vehicle crashes (31%), (b) homicide (15%), (c) suicide (12%), (d) other injuries (12%), (e) HIV infection (1%), and (f) other causes (29%). Data from the total United States sample of the 2001 Youth Risk Behavior Surveillance (CDC, 2003a) suggested that these deaths resulted from the prevalence of the following listed behaviors. Of the adolescents surveyed:

- 47% had drunk alcohol in the past month
- 33% had been in a physical fight within the past year
- 31% had, in the past month, ridden with a driver who was drinking
- 30% reported episodic heavy drinking in the past month
- 17% had carried a weapon during the past month
- 14% rarely or never used seat belts

Adolescents between 15 and 19 years old are more likely than younger children to die from injuries from firearms or motor vehicle accidents. Both of these mortalities were greater among males than females. Both Hispanic and African American males were more likely than other adolescents to die from firearm injuries, and African American males were much more likely to die from a firearm injury than from one sustained in a motor vehicle accident (CDC, 2003b).

Homicide

Overall, among 10- to 24-year-olds, homicide is the second leading cause of death and is the leading cause among non-Hispanic African American males of the same ages. Homicide rates among 15- to 19-year-olds peaked in the 1990s and have continued to decline steadily since 1994 (Ozer et al., 2003).

Suicide

In the year 2000, 4294 adolescents between the ages of 10 and 24 years succeeded in committing suicide. Females commit suicide at rates much lower than that of males, and Alaskan Native and Native American males have the highest rates of all adolescents. Although males are more likely to succeed in committing suicide, adolescent females are more likely to attempt suicide than their male peers (Ozer et al., 2003).

Adolescent Morbidities

Adolescents growing up in the 21st century are not likely to experience many of the common childhood diseases that often resulted in health complications during adolescence in their parents' and grandparents' time. For example, antibiotics and sophisticated diagnostic tests have reduced the threats of death and permanent disability from diseases such as polio and scarlet fever that took their toll on previous generations of children and adolescents.

Many of the causes of adolescent mortalities result in injuries rather than death. For example, many unintentional and intentional injuries, as well as suicide attempts, fortunately do not result in death. Nevertheless, adolescents experience serious and sometimes disabling injuries in addition to various acute and chronic diseases and illnesses.

Unintentional and Intentional Injuries

A study of injuries occurring in the Los Angeles Unified School District, the second largest school district in the United States, was done to determine the incidence of injuries related to violent behaviors among the nearly 700,000 students enrolled. In 1997, the rate of injuries that occurred and were reported at school for elementary, middle, and high school students was 1.74 injuries per 100 students per year. Of these, 77.2% were unintentional and 16.8% were intentional. The final 6.0% of injuries were of unknown intent. Students in elementary schools reported the most injuries, but the highest rate of 2.22 per 100 students was among those in high school. Among all grade levels, males were more likely than females to sustain both unintentional and intentional injuries. Again, the highest rate was among males in high school, with a rate of 2.8 per 100 students. The most common cause of injury was falls, which accounted for more than 40% of unintentional injuries in all grades. Many of these falls were related to sports activities. The second most common type of injury was collision or being struck by an object (Limbos & Peek-Asa, 2003).

Attempted Suicide

In addition to the alarming number of adolescents who successfully commit suicide, an untold number attempt suicide each year. Surveys of students enrolled in public high schools indicate attempted suicide rates ranging from 7.3% (Thatcher, Reininger, & Drance, 2002) to 19.3% (CDC, 2000).

Significant risk factors include being female (DuRant & Smith, 2002), feeling intimidated, using cocaine and alcohol, dieting and bulimic behaviors, and experiences of sexual and physical abuse (Thatcher et al., 2002).

Sexually Transmitted Infections and Diseases

The prevalence of sexually transmitted infections and diseases among adolescents is staggering. Inconsistent use of condoms and high-risk social

Table 1.2   Sexually Transmitted Diseases Prevalent Among Adolescents

Disease	Prevalence in Adolescents	Complications
Chlamydia trachomatis	Highest among 12- to 19-year-old females	Cervicitis and PID in women; torsion of spermatic cord in males
Gonorrhea	Highest in 15- to 24-year-olds	PID and infected Bartholin's gland in women; prostatitis in males
Hepatitis B	15% of cases are in 15- to 19-year-olds	Chronic liver disease and hepatocellular carcinoma
Herpes genitalis	Highest among 30-year-olds 6% of 12- to 19-year-olds	Encephalitis, meningitis, neonatal infections, psychological distress
Human immunodeficiency virus	20% of cases in 20- to 29-year-olds, contracted 7-10 years earlier	Pulmonary tuberculosis, bacterial pneumonia, cervical cancer, AIDS
Human papillomavirus	15%–20% female adolescents	Cancer of vulva and cervix
Syphilis	Highest rate in 20- to 30-year-olds	Meningitis, congenital syphilis

SOURCE: Data taken from Neinstein (2002).

NOTE: PID indicates pelvic inflammatory disease.

environments increase the probability of developing a sexually transmitted disease (STD) (Capaldi, Stoolmiller, Clark, & Owen, 2002; Niccolai, Ethier, Kershaw, Lewis, & Ickovics, 2003). Seven of the most common STDs are summarized in Table 1.2.

Chronic Diseases

Chronic health conditions are defined as having three characteristics: (a) they have a biological, psychological, or cognitive basis; (b) the condition has lasted or is expected to last at least 12 months; and (3) the individual with the condition experiences functional limitations that require reliance on compensatory assistance, such as medication, diet, personal assistance, and medical technology. Using these criteria, it is estimated that 14.8% to 18% of children up to 17 years old have a chronic health condition or disease. The most common chronic diseases of adolescents are arthritis, asthma, diabetes mellitus, epilepsy, and heart disease (Coupey, Neinstein, & Zeltzer, 2002). Other prevalent chronic diseases include cystic fibrosis, disabling conditions associated with congenital anomalies, eating disorders, and mental illness. Many adolescents who have such conditions experience stigma and marginalization, making the transitions of this developmental stage more challenging. As a consequence of these experiences, these youth are at risk for depression and other psychosocial problems (DiNapoli & Murphy, 2002). Although some children outgrow some of these conditions, others experience sleep disturbances, school absences, and restrictions in physical and social activity (Yeatts & Shy, 2001) as well as long-term complications (Donaghue et al., 2003).

Disabling Conditions

A number of physical, cognitive, and psychological conditions render adolescents unable to fully participate in activities that are normative for their peers. Congenital anomalies such as spina bifida, a defect of the spinal membranes and nerves, may be accompanied by limited mobility, severe orthopedic problems, or paralysis (Sawin, Brei, Buran, & Fastenau, 2002). Certain genetic anomalies, such as Turner syndrome, an abnormality with 45 chromosomes and one X chromosome, are accompanied by stigmata and sexual infantilism that may be socially and psychologically disabling to some adolescents.

Eating Disorders

The incidence of eating disorders is greatest among female adolescents between the ages of 13 and 18 years. Both males and females are influenced by media exposure to dieting and thin role models (Labre, 2002; Utter, Neumark-Sztainer, Wall, & Story, 2003). Males and females across various races and ethnicities engage in smoking cigarettes to control or lose weight (Fulkerson & French, 2003). Long-term consequences of smoking include stunted growth (Lantzouni, Frank, Golden, & Shenker, 2002), cardiac arrhythmias (Eidem, Cetta, Webb, Graham, & Jay, 2001; Galetta et al., 2003), osteopenia, menstrual irregularities, infertility, and high-risk pregnancies (Elford & Spence, 2002). Obesity is fast becoming a chronic disease among youth and is strongly related to the development of cardiovascular disorders in adulthood (Sinaiko, Donahue, Jacobs, & Prineas, 1999).

Mental Illness and Psychosocial Distress

Mental illness and psychosocial distress are significant problems for many adolescents. The stress associated with multiple changes that occur in adolescence, complications of chronic diseases, and anxiety about performance expectations in school and social arenas are but a few of the factors that contribute to this situation. Children who have experienced behavioral and learning problems, such as those typical of attention deficit hyperactivity disorder (ADHD), may continue to experience these problems in adolescence. Mood disorders such as major depression, substance-induced mood disorder, and manic episodes may manifest first in adolescence (American Psychiatric Association, 1994). Symptoms of mental illness such as anxiety and depression are often found associated with eating disorders and engaging in health-risk behaviors such as having multiple sexual partners, using substances such as alcohol and illicit drugs, and frequent fighting. Researchers have shown that children and adolescents who are exposed to violence are prone to post-traumatic stress disorder, depression, and behavioral problems, as well as desensitization to violence (Garbarino, Bradshaw, & Vorrasi, 2002).

Many youth who show signs of mental illness or psychosocial distress are at risk for school drop-out and attempted suicide (Brooks, Harris, Thrall, & Woods, 2002; Eggert, Thompson, Randell, & Pike, 2002). Expanded school programs to provide a full array of mental health prevention and intervention programs are being developed to meet a growing demand for services for the nation's adolescents (Weist et al., 2003).

Skin Disorders

A large number of adolescents experience skin disorders that affect their health and well-being. Acne vulgaris occurs to some degree in approximately 85% of all adolescents. The condition results from increased oil production in the glands of the face, shoulders, chest, upper arms, and neck. The oil glands become plugged with oils and bacteria grow, forming papules of inflammation, better known as pimples. Scarring can occur. Males tend to have a more severe condition than females (Pakula & Neinstein, 2002). In addition to this common skin disorder, about 30% of adolescents spend numerous hours in the sun without protection from ultraviolet rays. Another 10% use indoor tanning sun lamps or beds (Cokkinides, O'Connell, Thun, & Weinstock, 2002). Consequently, a substantial number experience sunburns that may be the precursors of neoplasms in adulthood (Cokkinides et al., 2001).

Adolescent Access to and Use of Health-Care Resources

Although adolescents in general are healthy, they still have multiple needs for health-care resources. They need preventive services, such as those associated with preventing unplanned pregnancy and sexually transmitted diseases. They also need the preventive resources of immunizations against infectious diseases. Many could benefit from screening for physical and mental health problems, such as depression and substance abuse (Brindis, Park, Ozer, & Irwin, 2002). Adolescents also need treatment for any number of illnesses, diseases, and injuries.

The Medical Expenditure Panel Survey collects data on health-care use and expenditures from a nationally representative sample (Elixhauser et al., 2002). In the first 6 months of 2000, more children in the 15- to 17-year-old age range were uninsured than children under the age of 4 years. Among 10- to 14-year-olds, 67.7% had private insurance, 17.9% had public insurance, and 14.4% had no insurance at all. In this age group, 62.6% had visited a physician's office, 5.5% had had outpatient visits at a hospital, 8.9% had visited the emergency department of a hospital, and 53% had had dental visits. For these early adolescents, hospitalizations occurred primarily for injury and poisoning. Mental disorders accounted for 15.5% of hospital stays among this age group. Among the 15- to 17-year-olds, 68.4% had private insurance, 15% had public insurance, and 16.6% had no insurance at all. In this age group, 60.6% had visited a physician's office, 5.7% had had outpatient visits at a hospital, 11.1% had visited the emergency department of a hospital, and 49.9% had had dental visits. Among these older adolescents, 36.6% of hospitalizations were related to pregnancy and childbirth, 13.9% were due to injury and poisoning, and 14.5% were for mental disorders (Elixhauser et al., 2002). In terms of cost, health care for adolescents was lower than that for adults. However, expenditures for adolescents with disabilities and functional impairments were disproportionately high, whereas expenditures for adolescents living in poverty and those who were African American were disproportionately low (Newacheck, Wong, Galbraith, & Hung, 2003).

For adolescents, two major constraints of the external environment are socioeconomic status and health-care providers and services that are not adolescent-friendly. Those living at or near the 100% poverty line have few resources to exchange for regular health care, including insurance. In 2001, the mean age of children living in families with incomes below 200% of poverty was 9.4 years (±5.4). Of these, 48.3% were male, 24.9% were African American, and 24.3% were Hispanic. Of these children and adolescents, 74.4% perceived themselves to be in excellent or very good health, whereas only 6% considered themselves to be in fair health. For children under 19 years old, 16.1% of those living below 200% of poverty were uninsured, compared to 20.0% of those living below 100% of poverty (Cunningham, Hadley, & Reschovsky, 2002).

A secondary analysis of three national data sets (National Ambulatory Medical Care Survey, Comprehensive Adolescent Health Services Survey, and National Hospital Ambulatory Medical Care Survey) was done to identify health-care use by adolescent males. In sites for specialized adolescent care, such as school-based health centers and community or health department programs, males made fewer visits than females. In other sites, however, younger males (i.e., those younger than 16 years old) made visits in almost equal proportions to those made by females (Marcell, Klein, Fischer, Allan, & Kokotailo, 2002).

Seeking routine health-care services may not be viewed as an important use of time by adolescents, who may see themselves as invulnerable to the threat of disease or injury. As they gain increased independence from their parents, adolescents are less likely to be taken for routine health-care examinations than they were at younger ages. In addition to a general reluctance to seek routine health-care services, an expanding number of adolescents are without health-care insurance, making visits for acute health problems even more challenging.

Many adolescents experience financial and other environmental barriers to health care. Many adolescents fail to seek care not because they have no insurance but because they cannot pay the copayment requirements. Moreover, many preventive services are not fully covered by private insurance plans. Environmental barriers include laws common in many states that require notification of parents and lack of confidentiality when parents are notified of an adolescent's visit or when a youth is afraid to file an insurance claim because his or her parents will learn about the visit. Other barriers are structural and include the location of clinics at an inconvenient distance or location, business hours that coincide with school, lack of transportation, and the lack of an appealing waiting area. Adolescents also find that many health-care providers lack sensitivity to the culture of adolescence (Oberg, Hogan, Bertrand, & Juve, 2002) and to the cultures of racial and ethnic minority groups (Villarruel & Rodriguez, 2003). In a study of 847 male and 1126 female adolescents, Fortenberry and colleagues (2002) found that stigma and shame were barriers to seeking care for suspected STDs.

In an exploratory study of 18 female Mexican American adolescents 10 to 16 years old, Rew (1997) found two themes in seeking care for prevention of illness and in managing health-care problems. Themes derived from focus groups were primarily differences in using formal versus informal resources for health information and health care. More specifically, these adolescent females described seeking formal help from physicians and health clinics for problems such as respiratory infections and gastrointestinal problems. They also described using informal resources such as mothers, friends, or other female relatives for information and help with their concerns related to pubertal development and reproduction. In another study of 693 female adolescents (12 to 20 years old, mean age = 14.96 ± 1.83), the majority of participants reported using informal sources more frequently than formal sources of care. Hispanic and European American participants were more likely than African American, Asian American, or Native American participants to seek help from peers [$F(4) = 5.52$, $p < .0001$], whereas African American females were more likely to seek help from parents (Rew, Resnick, & Blum, 1997).

Access to Reproductive Health Services. American adolescents are less able to access convenient and youth-friendly reproductive health services than their peers in other countries. Some of the limitations are related to adolescents' lack of insurance. Other barriers are structural, such as lack of confidentiality and the need for parental consent. Of the 50 states, only 27 and the District of Columbia have statutes or policies that allow adolescents to give their own consent to obtain contraceptives (Hock-Long, Herceg-Baron, Cassidy, & Whittaker, 2003).

Access to Mental Health Services. It is estimated that more than 50% of adolescents will need mental health services during the transition to adulthood. Schools provide the primary entry point to these services because of students' learning and behavioral problems or substance use (Farmer, Burns, Phillips, Angold, & Costello, 2003). However, schools are not adequately equipped with specialized personnel to address the multiple mental health needs of today's youth.

Access to Health Resources by Gender and Ethnicity. There is mounting evidence of health disparities in America that are related to both gender and ethnicity. Using data from the 1987 National Medical Expenditure Survey (NMES), Bartman, Moy, and D'Angelo (1997) studied access to ambulatory care in a sample of 3102 adolescents between the ages of 11 and 17 years. They found that compared to Whites, African Americans and Hispanics were significantly less likely to have received care in a physician's office ($p < .001$). Similarly, Lieu, Newacheck, and McManus (1993) analyzed data from the 1988 National Health Interview Survey of adolescents ($N = 7465$) and found that Hispanics were less likely to seek care for routine and acute care than Whites and African Americans.

The health status of adolescents is closely related to behaviors. As noted earlier, these behaviors have been identified by many different terms, including problem behaviors, risk-taking behaviors, deviant behaviors, risky behaviors, and health-risk behaviors. Research findings are often difficult to compare because of the variation in terms used. Whenever possible in this book, behaviors that are associated with increasing an adolescent's chances of experiencing an adverse health outcome (morbidity or mortality) will be referred to as health-risk behaviors unless a study using a different term is being cited.

Adolescent Health-Risk Behavior

The concept of *risk* is central to our understanding of adolescent health behaviors. The term comes from the discipline of epidemiology, where it refers to the probability of loss, injury, illness, or disability (Lescohier & Gallagher, 1996). Risk-taking behavior is considered by some to be a normal part of adolescent development. Experimentation with breaking the rules (e.g., skipping school without parental permission, coming home later than one's curfew) represents an adolescent's willful decision to engage in an activity with a degree of risk of being caught and being punished. Experimentation with sexual behavior, smoking, and alcohol use, however, represents an adolescent's willful decision to engage in activities with associated risks of health- or life-threatening outcomes. These latter behaviors are designated as health-risk behaviors because they threaten the development, health, and well-being of adolescents. As adolescents gain more independence and begin to experiment with new behaviors, some of these behaviors place them at risk for potentially negative health consequences (Green, 1999), whereas other health-risk behaviors may improve their healthy growth and development. In general, health-risk behaviors in youth increase the likelihood that an adolescent will experience one or more of the major morbidities or mortalities, because such behaviors have been found to cluster or covary, and these associations increase with age (Lytle, Kelder, Perry, & Klepp, 1995).

Brindis et al. (2002) note that 70% of adolescent mortalities can be accounted for by six categories of risk-taking behaviors. Those categories are (a) unsafe sexual activity, (b) violence, (c) minimal physical activity, (d) poor nutritional habits, (e) alcohol and other drug use, and (f) use of tobacco products. The risk of adverse health outcomes associated with these behaviors increases for those youth who also have chronic physical or mental health problems or disabilities, who are incarcerated, or who are homeless. In fact, many of the national health objectives identified in *Healthy People 2010* specifically target changes in these behaviors for adolescents (U.S. Department of Health and Human Services [USDHHS], 2000).

Adolescents with chronic health conditions increase their vulnerability to adverse health outcomes by engaging in health-risk behaviors. For example, smoking is a stimulus that can trigger asthma, yet adolescents with asthma begin smoking as often as those without this condition (Zbikowski, Klesges, Robinson, & Alfano, 2002). Compared with 16,262 students in regular high schools, youth attending alternative schools ($n = 8918$) were found to have significantly more health-risk behaviors, including unintentional injuries; sexual activity; poor nutritional habits; physical inactivity; and tobacco, alcohol, and other drug use (Grunbaum, Lowry, & Kann, 2001).

Millstein and Halpern-Felsher (2002) distinguish between the terms *risk judgment* and *risk identification*. Risk judgment is an assessment of the magnitude of risk (e.g., how likely is it that I will die from lung cancer if I smoke cigarettes?), whereas risk identification is not an assessment of the magnitude of the risk but rather an acknowledgment that a specific behavior is associated with some risk for adverse outcomes (e.g., what might happen if I smoke cigarettes?). The related concept of vulnerability focuses on how concerned or anxious the individual is about being at risk for an adverse outcome (e.g., how worried are you that your smoking might lead to a serious health problem such as lung cancer?).

There is some evidence that risk identification increases with age in adolescents (Beyth-Marom, Austin, Fischhoff, Palmgren, & Jacobs-Quadrel, 1993). There is limited evidence that risk judgment also varies inversely with age (Millstein & Halpern-Felsher, 2002). Moreover, researchers have found that an adolescent's perception that a particular behavior carries a risk for unpleasant consequences plays an important part in influencing the youth's behavior. Other factors that influence an adolescent's behavior include the perceived benefits of engaging in that behavior. Adolescents often initiate or continue a specific behavior that is associated with increased risk for adverse health outcomes (e.g., smoking cigarettes) because that behavior is perceived as having great social benefit. In other words, a person may acknowledge that smoking cigarettes will increase the risk of developing lung cancer, but will be willing to start smoking and continue to smoke because she or he perceives that the behavior will make her or him more well liked by peers (Millstein & Halpern-Felsher, 2002).

The ways in which adolescents think about their own vulnerability to specific adverse outcomes are addressed by many theories of health. Theories such as the Health Belief Model (Rosenstock, 1974a, 1974c), social cognitive and self-efficacy theories (Bandura, 1986, 1997), self-regulation theory, the theory of reasoned action (Fishbein & Ajzen, 1975), and the theory of planned behavior (Ajzen, 1985) all contain propositions concerning how individuals' beliefs about consequences and their vulnerability to those consequences affect their behavior (Millstein & Halpern-Felsher, 2002, p. 415).

National Objectives to Improve Adolescent Health

The nation's objectives to improve the health status of the American people are outlined in *Healthy People 2010* (U.S. Department of Health and Human Services, 2000). In addition to the several global goals identified for all citizens (e.g., increasing quality and years of healthy life), many objectives are targeted primarily at adolescents. They include the following:

- Reduce deaths from accidents
- Increase use of safety belts
- Reduce substance abuse and binge drinking
- Reduce marijuana use
- Increase disapproval of smoking
- Increase use of contraceptives that protect against STDs and pregnancy
- Reduce rates of *Chlamydia trachomatis* infections
- Reduce weapon carrying on school properties
- Reduce proportion of those with disabilities who are sad, unhappy, or depressed
- Improve mental health and access to appropriate services
- Promote health associated with diet and weight
- Reduce dental caries
- Increase proportion who receive all vaccinations

These objectives address the major morbidities and mortalities of adolescents. Moreover, they suggest that those concerned about adolescent health should address health promotion activities such as increasing use of safety belts, promoting proper diet and weight, and increasing the number of youth who are immunized against preventable, communicable diseases, as well as focusing on only the more obvious health-risk behaviors.

Organization of the Book

Theories selected for this book are those that are applicable to the current state of actual and potential health concerns for adolescents. They are arranged in a sequence that proceeds from outlining the context of adolescence as a distinct phase of human development to specific models of behavior change that can guide interventions. Chapter 2 begins with an introduction to the purpose of theory and its relationship to scientific inquiry. In this chapter, several strategies for developing and evaluating theories are described. In subsequent chapters, theories about a particular theme or phenomenon of concern are presented. Each of the theories and conceptual models presented is relevant to the six major types of adolescent health-risk behaviors: nutrition, physical activity, sexual activity, alcohol and other drug use, tobacco use, and violence. Every chapter begins with an introductory section, followed by a critical analysis of two or more theories or conceptual models. Each theory or model is presented in terms of criteria for evaluating theory: (a) origins; (b) purpose; (c) meaning; (d) scope, parsimony, and generalizability; (e) logical adequacy; (f) usefulness; and (g) testability. Whenever possible, empirical referents for major constructs of each theory or model are also presented, along with psychometric properties of these referents. Each chapter includes examples of related research on adolescent health and health-risk behavior. Each chapter concludes with implications for further study and a chapter summary. At the end of each chapter are two lists: selected Web sites, to be used as a resource for gaining further information about the topic presented in that chapter, and suggestions for additional reading.

Chapter 3 contains an overview of selected developmental theories. Adolescence is conceptualized as a specific phase in the life-span development of the human being. The theories and models presented in this chapter provide the context for understanding the adolescent person and how adolescents change in physical, cognitive, emotional, social, and spiritual dimensions in response to their environment. Developmental theories explain the various ways in which adolescents, over time, are capable of engaging in more complex behaviors that carry an increasing risk for short- and long-term health consequences. Lerner's model of developmental contextualism provides additional insight into the reciprocal nature of human development as a response to the environment in which that development takes place. The chapter concludes with a presentation of the Youth Development Model. Although this model does not have the attributes of a scientific theory, it has been found to be extremely useful in planning and implementing successful programs that address the unique developmental needs of adolescents.

Chapter 4 augments the developmental approach taken in Chapter 3. The focus of this chapter is the development of a sense of self or personal identity. Beginning with William James's differentiation of the subjective from the objective sense of self, the works of Erik Erikson are analyzed with his assertion that development of self-identity was the primary and essential developmental task of adolescence. The work of Erikson's followers, primarily James Marcia, who elaborated on ego-identity status, provides a broader and deeper context for understanding the health and health-risk behaviors of adolescents. Theories that address the development of a sense of self or personal identity relate to the six types of health-risk behaviors because each of these behaviors may become the focus of an identity formation. That is (for example), a female adolescent may form part of her self-image or identity as a smoker from the use of tobacco products, or she may alter her sense of being female owing to her participation in sexual activities.

Chapter 5 addresses theories of stress and coping. The General Adaptation Syndrome described by Hans Selye forms the backdrop against which more recent models of stress and coping are presented. Many of the health-risk behaviors found among adolescents may be conceptualized as adaptive or maladaptive coping responses to perceived stressors. Chapter 6 covers concepts of risk and vulnerability that arise from the intersection of stress and adolescent development. The problem-behavior theory of Jessor and Jessor is presented as a model for assessing specific health-risk behaviors in this developmental phase of life. This theory and its recent extensions address the health-risk behaviors directly. Chapter 7 consists of conceptualizations of protection and resilience. Viewed as a response to stress, resilience is central to our understanding of health-risk behaviors in young people.

The next three chapters focus specifically on adolescent behaviors and theories of cognitive and behavioral change. Chapter 8 begins with social cognitive theory and addresses the connection between the adolescent's cognitive development and social interactions within the environment. Theories of reasoned action and planned behavior are also included, along with examples of their application in helping adolescents change health-compromising behaviors. Chapter 9 includes a discussion of the Health Belief Model and Pender's Health Promotion Model. These formulations focus specifically on attitudes, beliefs, and behaviors that directly influence health. Moreover, they include strategies to motivate adolescents to engage in behaviors that promote or enhance health status. Chapter 10 addresses theories of decision making and stages of behavioral change. To promote and maintain the health of adolescents, these models contain specific guidelines for developing age- and behavior-appropriate interventions. In particular, the Transtheoretical Model of Behavior Change identifies various stages in the process of making a decision to change a behavior and includes strategies for helping a person sustain the behavioral change.

The final chapter, Chapter 11, contains a description of a variety of qualitative approaches to developing theories of adolescent health and health-risk behavior. Specifically, this chapter includes a description of content analysis and case studies, grounded theory, focus groups, narrative analysis, and participatory action research methodologies. These descriptions are then followed with examples directly related to adolescent health and health-risk behaviors.

Chapter Summary

The current health status of American adolescents is excellent in many ways. However, adolescents are at risk for a variety of social morbidities and mortalities related to health-risk behaviors. A substantial number of adolescents are uninsured and experience financial and environmental barriers to health-care services. Health disparities exist for adolescents who are racial minorities and who live in conditions of poverty. Mental health and physical health services associated with school health clinics may increase access to and use of health care by many adolescents, but there remains a lack of coordinated care for those who drop out of school or who are marginalized for any number of reasons. The national health objectives provide direction for adolescent health providers and researchers through which they may focus intervention efforts on the major morbidities and mortalities encountered in the second decade of life.

Related Web Sites

American Cancer Society: http://www.cancer.org

American Diabetes Foundation: http://www.diabetes.org

Asthma and Allergy Foundation of America: http://www.aafa.org

Congenital Heart Defects in Children and Adolescents: http://pediatrics. about.com/library/weekly/aa021200.htm

Cystic Fibrosis Foundation: http://www.cff.org

Epilepsy Foundation of America: http://www.efa.org

Federal Interagency Forum on Child and Family Statistics: http://childstats. gov/americaschildren

Future of Children: http://www.futureofchildren.org

Health, United States, 2000, with Adolescent Health Chartbook (Centers for Disease Control and Prevention [CDC]): http://www.cdc.gov/nchs/ data/hus/hus00.pdf

Healthy People 2010: http://www.healthypeople.gov

Monitoring the Future Study (Institute for Social Research, University of Michigan): http://monitoringthefuture.org/

National Adolescent Health Information Center: http://youth.ucsf.edu/nahic

National Center for Chronic Disease Prevention and Health Promotion: http://www.cdc.gov/nccdphp

National Health and Nutrition Examination Survey (National Center for Health Statistics, CDC): http://www.cdc.gov/nchs/nhanes/nhanes.htm

National Longitudinal Study of Adolescent Health (Add Health): http://www.arhp.org/rap/

Planned Parenthood® Federation of America online magazine: http://www.teenwire.com (in Spanish and in English; winner of 2002 Webby Award for Best Health Web Site for adolescents)

Sexually Transmitted Disease Surveillance (CDC): http://www.cdc.gov/std/stats/ TOC2000.htm

Statistics from the Insurance Institute for Highway Safety: http://www.iihs.org

United Cerebral Palsy Association: http://www.ucpa.org

Vital and Health Statistics (CDC): http://www.cdc.gov/nchs/nsfg.htm

World Health Organization: http://www.who.int/about/definition/en/

Youth Risk Behavior Survey (CDC): http://www.cdc.gov/nccdphp/dash/yrbs/

Suggestions for Further Reading

American Academy of Pediatrics, Committee on Adolescence. (2000). Suicide and suicide attempts in adolescents. *Pediatrics, 105,* 871-874.

Archibald, A. B., Linver, M. R., Graber, J. A., & Brooks-Gunn, J. (2002). Parent-adolescent relationships and girls' unhealthy eating: Testing reciprocal effects. *Journal of Research on Adolescence, 12,* 451-461.

Azzopardi, K., & Lowes, L. (2003). Management of cystic fibrosis-related diabetes in adolescence. *British Journal of Nursing, 12,* 359-363.

Betts, P. R., Jefferson, I. G., & Swift, P. G. F. (2002). Diabetes care in childhood and adolescence. *Diabetic Medicine, 19*(Suppl. 4), 61-65.

Brackis-Cott, E., Mellins, C. A., & Block, M. (2003). Current life concerns of early adolescents and their mothers: Influence of maternal HIV. *Journal of Early Adolescence, 23,* 51-77.

Brown, J. D., Steele, J. R., & Walsh-Childers, K. (Eds.). (2002). *Sexual teens, sexual media: Investigating media's influence on adolescent sexuality.* Mahwah, NJ: Lawrence Erlbaum.

Canobbio, M. M. (2001). Health care issues facing adolescents with congenital heart disease. *Journal of Pediatric Nursing, 16*, 363-370.

Cook, R. L., Pollock, N. K., Rao, A. K., & Clark, D. B. (2002). Increased prevalence of herpes simplex virus type 2 among adolescent women with alcohol use disorders. *Journal of Adolescent Health, 30*, 169-174.

Dwyer, J. M. (2001). High-risk sexual behaviours and genital infections during pregnancy. *International Nursing Review, 48*, 233-240.

Giuliano, A. R., Harris, R., Sedjo, R. L., Baldwin, S., Roe, D., Papenfuss, M. R., et al. (2002). Incidence, prevalence, and clearance of type-specific human papillomavirus infections: The young women's health study. *Journal of Infectious Diseases, 186*, 462-469.

Irwin, C. E., Burg, S. J., & Cart, C. U. (2002). America's adolescents: Where have we been, where are we going? *Journal of Adolescent Health, 31*, 91-121.

Kanner, S., Hamrin, V., & Grey, M. (2003). Depression in adolescents with diabetes. *Journal of Child and Adolescent Psychiatric Nursing, 16*(1), 15-24.

Madsen, S. D., Roisman, G. I., & Collins, W. A. (2002). The intersection of adolescent development and intensive intervention: Age-related psychosocial correlates of treatment regimens in the diabetes control and complication trial. *Journal of Pediatric Psychology, 27*, 451-459.

Mannino, D. M., Homa, D. M., Akinbami, L. J., Moorman, J. E., Gwynn, C., & Redd, S. C. (2002). Surveillance for asthma: United States, 1980-1999. *Morbidity and Mortality Weekly Report, 51*(SS-1), 1-13.

Nixon, G. M., Glazner, J. A., Martin, J. M., & Sawyer, S. M. (2002). Urinary incontinence in female adolescents with cystic fibrosis [Abstract]. *Pediatrics, 110*, 397.

Rich, M., Patashnick, J., & Chalfen, R. (2002). Visual illness narratives of asthma: Explanatory models and health-related behavior. *American Journal of Health Behavior, 26*, 442-453.

Ritchie, M. A. (2001). Self-esteem and hopefulness in adolescents with cancer. *Journal of Pediatric Nursing, 16*(1), 35-42.

Sawyer, S. M., Tully, M. A., & Colin, A. A. (2001). Reproductive and sexual health in males with cystic fibrosis: A case for health professional education and training. *Journal of Adolescent Health, 28*, 36-40.

Van Devanter, N., Gonzales, V., Merzel, C., Parikh, N. S., Celantano, D., & Greenberg, J. (2002). Effect of an STD/HIV behavioral intervention on women's use of the female condom. *American Journal of Public Health, 92*, 109-115.

Theoretical Approaches to Adolescent Health and Health-Risk Behavior

Much of what we know about early adolescent health-risk behavior is based on atheoretical studies of middle or high school students. For example, the Youth Risk Behavior Surveillance System (YRBSS) is a national, school-based survey conducted by the Centers for Disease Control and Prevention (CDC). The YRBSS monitors six categories of health-risk behaviors among American youth: tobacco use, alcohol and other drug use, sexual behaviors, dietary behaviors, physical activity, and behaviors contributing to intentional and unintentional injuries; however, the survey has been limited largely to youth in high school (Kann et al., 1995). The Indiana Student Health Survey, similar in design to the YRBSS, was administered to a random sample of 2037 9th- and 12th-grade students. The survey found that males reported higher prevalence of health-risk behaviors, substance abuse, sexual intercourse, and fat-food consumption than females (Ellis & Torabi, 1994). Other studies have shown that many health-risk behaviors such as drug use, failure to wear seat belts, school truancy, and unprotected sexual intercourse tend to cluster in certain groups of adolescents (Neumark-Sztainer et al., 1996; Schuster, Bell, & Kanouse, 1996). Studies based on the YRBSS and similar surveys provide facts about prevalence, gender, distribution, and clustering of health-risk behaviors. Because they lack a theoretical base, however, they contribute little to the development of a science of adolescent health.

Adolescent health is a phenomenon of concern to members of many disciplines. Scholars and practitioners in education, sociology, psychology, nursing, nutrition, medicine, social work, health education, and other fields share a common interest in the healthy growth and development of youth in the second decade of life. Despite our common interest, however, we may have different perspectives, and we may use different jargon to communicate our concern and to improve our understanding and practice. Because we come from a variety of academic disciplines and practice settings, we see the health behavior of adolescents in a slightly different light. Our ideas about why adolescents behave as they do are described using different terms. Some of our disciplines are more fully developed than others, yielding more formalized theories that explain and predict adolescent health behavior. Theory, which is a primary goal of science, offers a vehicle for making a network of connections between various disciplines. By understanding why and how theories are constructed, tested, and validated, we can establish a communication network to facilitate knowledge development about the important phenomena of adolescent health and adolescent health-risk behavior.

Theory as the Aim of Science

Kerlinger (1973) claims that "the basic aim of science is theory" (p. 8). A theory, by definition, is an abstraction of something that exists in the real world, but it is not the thing itself. The process of observation, explanation, experimentation, and prediction that results in a systematized body of knowledge about a particular phenomenon or group of phenomena is known as a science. A scientific body of knowledge provides a method for categorizing concepts, resulting in a typology of the phenomena of interest to a particular discipline. This body of knowledge allows us to explain past events or situations and predict future events or situations. It also allows for some understanding of what causes events or situations to occur, as well as some control over outcomes related to these events or situations. The set of concepts and statements linking the concepts together comprise a theory about the phenomenon of interest (Reynolds, 1971).

Simply put, a theory is an organized set of concepts and statements related to significant questions about a particular domain of knowledge. Theory is an abstraction of reality. It is a systematic group of concepts, descriptive statements, and propositions constructed for some purpose. Theory is symbolic and is invented to describe, explain, predict, prescribe, or control events or situations. Use of the term *theory* by nonscientists leads to erosion of its scientific meaning. Vague hunches or descriptions of events or situations that have not been tested rigorously do not qualify as theory. The scientific approach or method allows us to systematically and critically investigate proposed relationships among natural phenomena. Beginning with an idea or a problem to solve, the scientist proposes a hypothetical outcome or solution, which is then subjected to observation or experimentation (Kerlinger, 1973). As a result, new knowledge is formed. Other methods for developing theory arise from an inductive process originating in a naturalistic setting. Grounded theory, for example, is a method for developing theory that begins with data from practice or some other naturalistic setting.

As already noted, the phenomena of adolescent health and health behavior are not restricted to the domain of any one scientific discipline. This makes locating theories capable of guiding research and practice somewhat difficult. Unlike concepts pertaining to the natural sciences, concepts related to adolescent health and health behavior do not *belong* to any one theoretical tradition or practice discipline. Psychologists may focus on the development of an adolescent's identity and its relationship to health and health-risk behavior, nurses may focus on the adolescent's ability to provide self-care to promote overall health, and sociologists may focus on the impact of the environment on the adolescent's health and health-risk behavior. This multiple approach to understanding and providing services to adolescents to promote and maintain their health is one good reason why it is important to understand the theoretical perspectives that may help us meet our mutual goals.

The Purpose of Theory

The primary purpose of theory is to guide research. Theory provides the framework and content for a specific branch of science. From theories and conceptual models, the researcher can generate hypotheses that can be tested or verified. Theoretical hypotheses are statements of how specific phenomena or concepts are related to one another. Statistical hypotheses test the possibility that the proposed relationship exists in the real world merely by chance (Lum, 2002).

The secondary purpose of theory is to guide practice or intervention. More to the point, theory guides the research conducted by scientists that is then disseminated and translated into information that can be used in practice. In the case of adolescents, practice may refer to services provided by health-care professionals, such as physicians, nurses, dieticians, physical therapists, social workers, psychologists, and pharmacists, or by parents and other community leaders, such as teachers, coaches, and health educators, who work with these young people. Theories provide a framework for organizing observations about adolescents and their behaviors. They help us arrange and order our observations to establish a body of knowledge and are useful for retrieving and using "generated and stored knowledge" of interest (Ellis, 1968, p. 218).

A very practical purpose of theory is to organize observations and findings that may appear inconsistent or chaotic (Rogers, 1970). This purpose is particularly germane to the study of adolescent health and health-risk behaviors because much of our research is organized around concepts or variables with similar names but, often, very different operational definitions. Moreover, much of what we know about these phenomena is atheoretical, meaning that it is not organized into a coherent abstraction of reality.

Perhaps one of the most important purposes of theory is that it facilitates communication. Theory provides a common language that enables members of one or several disciplines to talk about common problems and concerns. Theory consists of a set of concepts or variables that are defined explicitly for their meaning within a topic of concern. Theory may be viewed as a

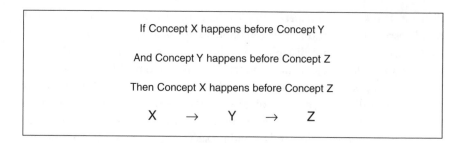

Figure 2.1   Diagramming Relationships Among Concepts in a Theory to
Determine Logical Adequacy

language, with various structural components, including syntax and semantics. Syntax refers here to the concepts of the theory that are evident in statements that are made in the form of axioms, postulates, or hypotheses. Syntax also refers to the relationships among these statements. Semantics, in this sense, refers to the specific meaning of the concepts. Primitive terms that appear in the theory are not defined. Derived terms, in contrast, are defined specifically for the theory. When a theory is made explicit, relationships among concepts can be examined for logical adequacy (Hardy, 1997). Symbols may be substituted for concepts and diagrammed by using a matrix to illustrate their interrelationships (see Figure 2.1).

Most theories are provisional or evolving because conceptualizations of phenomena and problems change over time. Evidence to support or refute hypotheses also may change over time (Hardy, 1997). Of particular concern to those studying adolescent health in the 21st century are the social morbidities and mortalities that change in response to an ever-changing environment. Thus, theories change as the context for understanding adolescence changes. Theories permit us to "formulate a minimum set of generalizations that allow one to explain a maximum number of observable relationships among the variables" (Meleis, 1997, p. 20). Theories, thus, provide the structure and content of science.

Types and Levels of Theory

Theory consists of a set of interrelated concepts and statements constructed for some purpose (Walker & Avant, 2005). The set of concepts and statements comprising a theory often are based on assumptions, which are statements accepted as truths about the concepts and the relationships among them. These assumptions often represent values and philosophical beliefs about the phenomena or the discipline for which the theory is developed (Meleis, 1997). Concepts represent the phenomena of concern, the topics about which we want to know more. Naming these phenomena allows us to observe, describe, classify, make predictions, and control them in a systematic way. Statements give definitions to concepts and provide the language for making connections or associations between concepts. Statements may simply acknowledge that a phenomenon exists, or they may provide detailed explanations of how the concept will be used within a specific theoretical formulation. Finally, statements allow us to hypothesize relationships that improve our understanding of how things operate in the world. Theories, as systematic groups of concepts and statements, permit us to identify an area where knowledge is needed and then give us the tools for creating or discovering that knowledge.

Science is recognized as the hallmark of knowledge, particularly in the physical sciences, where theory often takes the form of a *set of laws* or *set of causal process* (Reynolds, 1971). Such types of theories have little application to social phenomena. As Phillips (1987) claimed,

> The physical sciences, with their emphasis on uncovering the causes that produce effects, are not a relevant model for the social sciences for a simple reason: people act because they are swayed by reasons, or because they decide to follow rules, *not* because their actions are causally determined by forces. (p. 105)

The social or human sciences have developed a number of approaches to develop or establish theories that describe, explain, and predict human behavior. For example, the methodology of grounded theory allows us to generate theory through a process of simultaneous data collection and analysis known as the *constant comparative* method. As in other forms of scientific research leading to theory, grounded theory methods produce multiple conceptualizations that are "*patterns* of action and interaction between and among various types of social units (i.e., 'actors')" (Strauss & Corbin, 1998, p. 169). Grounded theory and other qualitative methods of knowledge development will be discussed in more detail in Chapter 11. Unlike the physical sciences, which determine unchangeable natural laws, the social sciences are continuously outdated and replaced with new findings, new interpretations of existing data, and new terminology.

Human sciences that apply to understanding adolescent development and behavior rely on types of theories that are mainly *descriptive, explanatory,* or *prescriptive.* Descriptive theories address processes such as the interaction between an adolescent and the people and circumstances in his or her environment. This type of theory is familiar to developmental psychologists, and examples of these theories will be discussed in Chapter 3. The explanatory type of theory addresses associations among concepts, such as the inverse relationship between the concepts of perceived self-efficacy and perceived barriers found in Pender's Health Promotion Model (described in Chapter 9). Prescriptive theories address specific propositions that can predict behavior change, such as those in the Transtheoretical Model (described in Chapter 10).

Four levels of theory found in behavior research are purported to improve interventions or practice related to human behavior. *Metatheory* is the level that is most abstract and establishes the philosophical base for a discrete discipline or body of knowledge (Meleis, 1997). Metatheory is concerned with identifying and analyzing the purpose of theory needed for a particular discipline. It also determines sources and methods of theory construction and development for the discipline. Metatheory allows scholars to establish criteria by which theories for that discipline are evaluated (Walker & Avant, 2005).

At the next level, *grand theory* is less abstract and establishes a worldview for understanding the phenomena of concern to a particular discipline. Grand or unified theories provide a conceptual map or paradigm for a discipline. The purpose of such theories is to help define a domain of knowledge for a specific area of study. Such theories are critical to the development and legitimization of a new discipline. They serve as heuristics for identifying the particular phenomena that are of central concern to a developing body of knowledge or discipline. Often, grand theories are problematic, because they are not sufficiently specific and thus have weak linkages among concepts and few operational definitions. This makes it difficult, if not impossible, to test them (Walker & Avant, 2005).

Middle-range theories are more limited in scope and contain limited numbers of variables (Walker & Avant, 2003). They "are abstract enough to extend beyond a given place, time, or population but specific enough and sufficiently close to empirical data to permit testing and to generate distinctive questions for study or specific interventions for practice" (Lenz, Suppe, Gift, Pugh, & Milligan, 1995, p. 2). Middle-range theories direct practice theory and help to refine grand theory (Walker & Avant, 2005). The Health-Belief Model and Pender's Health Promotion Model (discussed in Chapter 9) are examples of middle-range theories.

At the level of intervention, *practice theory* is constructed to control for the desired outcomes in a population. This type of theory has also been identified as prescriptive theory because such theories lead to prescribed actions that are associated with specified goals or objectives. When interventions are guided by practice-level theory and tested through research, they may also contribute to middle-range theories (Walker & Avant, 2005). Some theories at the level of intervention are also called situation-specific theories and are delimited in scope. They are developed within a social and historical context and focus on specific populations and phenomena (Meleis, 1997).

Middle-range and practice theories are also known as explanatory theories (*theories of the problem*) and change theories (*theories of action*). Explanatory theories or models are, as their name suggests, attempts to explain why a problem behavior exists. In contrast, change theories are created with the aim of controlling behavior, as through an intervention. These two types of theories are commonplace in the social sciences because they are concerned with phenomena that can be modified (Glanz et al., 1997). For example, if adolescent males have a high rate of STDs because they do not know how to use condoms effectively and are not confident about their skill in using them, we can intervene to modify their knowledge (e.g., give them information about why

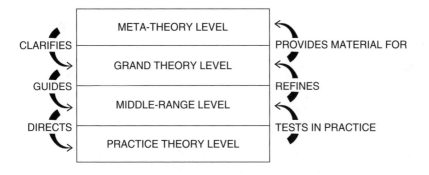

Figure 2.2   Linkages Among Levels of Theory Development

SOURCE: From Walker and Avant (2005, p. 13). Reprinted by permission of Pearson
Education, Inc., Upper Saddle River, NJ.

condoms protect them from contracting STDs and why it matters how they
are applied and removed) and their self-efficacy (e.g., confidence that they can
apply and remove a condom correctly and consistently).

Figure 2.2 depicts the relationships among the various levels of theory.
Metatheory clarifies the functions and methods of each level of theory development. Grand theory provides material for metatheory and guides middle-
range theory development. Middle-range theory refines grand theory
and directs practice or prescriptive theory. Tests of this latter level of theory
then contribute to middle-range theory and so on up the hierarchy to the
metatheory level within a discipline (Walker & Avant, 2005).

Theory Construction

There are numerous ways to construct and develop theories. Walker and
Avant (2005) have identified nine basic methods that result in theory construction and development. These methods are based on the three elements
that comprise theory: concepts, statements, and the theories themselves.
Approaches for theory construction are synthesis, derivation, and analysis.
The nine methods, shown in Figure 2.3, are thus concept synthesis, concept
derivation, and concept analysis; statement synthesis, statement derivation,
and statement analysis; and theory synthesis, theory derivation and theory
analysis. Although a thorough explanation of each of these methods is beyond
the scope of this text, each of the nine methods is described briefly.

Concepts

Concepts are the basic components out of which theories are constructed.
A concept is a basic abstraction of reality and is expressed through language.

Method	Synthesis	Derivation	Analysis
Concept	Concept synthesis	Concept derivation	Concept analysis
Statement	Statement synthesis	Statement derivation	Statement analysis
Theory	Theory synthesis	Theory derivation	Theory analysis

Figure 2.3   Methods Used in Theory Construction

NOTE: As conceptualized by Walker and Avant (2005).

For example, both *adolescence* and *health* are concepts. They are terms we use to express our ideas about real objects (e.g., the concept of *adolescent* refers to a human being during the second decade of life) and characteristics or situations (e.g., health, health-risk behavior). Such terms are not the concept itself (i.e., adolescence is not all the human beings who are between the ages of 10 and 20 years, nor is health the characteristic state of these human beings). However, these concepts allow us to communicate about them, to organize our observations of them, and to create an understanding of them. Concepts are also known as *variables* for which we can produce operational definitions essential to conduct research. Concepts or variables can be observed or measured. Similarly, relationships among concepts or changes in concepts over time can be observed and measured.

Statements

Statements are another abstraction of reality that express the existence of a phenomenon, define a concept, or declare the relationship between concepts. Statements give meaning to theories and may be statements of existence, definition, or relations (Walker & Avant, 2005). For example, a theory of health-risk behavior in adolescents might contain a statement about the existence of a phenomenon, such as "adolescents exhibit behaviors that place them at risk for adverse health outcomes." Such a statement simply states that something *is* (adolescents display health-risk behaviors). A definitional statement identifies the attributes of a concept (e.g., an adolescent is a human being who is older than 10 years of age and younger than 21 years of age). A relational statement declares or hypothesizes the association between two concepts (e.g., when an adolescent's self-efficacy to engage in daily physical activity is low, that adolescent's self-esteem will also be low). Such a statement identifies a relationship between the concept of self-efficacy to engage in physical activity and the concept of self-esteem.

Theories

Theories are composed of a set of interrelated concepts and statements that serve a purpose. They may be derived inductively from real-life cases, borrowed from another discipline and adapted to a new setting, or derived deductively from an existing set of statements. Concepts are the names given to specific phenomena such as objects, mechanisms, or processes. Statements clarify the meaning of the concepts and how they fit together for the purpose of description, explanation, prediction, or control. When a theory is logically constructed, one can then identify hypothetical relationships between or among the concepts that give validity to the theory.

Understanding the elements and methods of theory construction can enable the researcher and practitioner alike to appreciate the value of theory in organizing our understanding of adolescents, their health, and their behaviors. Consequently, we can apply this understanding to the development of policies, programs, interventions, and other services that will promote and enhance the health and well-being of our developing youth.

Synthesis in theory construction is a creative process and involves connecting ideas or data that have not previously been connected. Derivation is a matter of using theoretical material existing in one arena and, through the use of analogy or metaphor, transposing it into a new arena. Analysis is the process whereby theorists sharpen their focus by clarifying or refining concepts, statements, or theories. Much as the medical student dissects a cadaver to understand the structure and function of the human body, the theorist or researcher may dissect a concept, statement, or theory to clarify meaning and reduce ambiguity in communication about phenomena of concern within an area of science (Walker & Avant, 2005).

Concept Synthesis

The strategy of concept synthesis begins with empirical evidence. Primarily, this involves direct observation of data. Clinical or in vivo experience with a particular population is often the starting point for theorizing and leads to conceptualizing phenomena in new ways. The purpose of this strategy is to provoke new ways of thinking about familiar experiences. The qualitative research method of grounded theory is an example of concept synthesis. Observations about human behavior are collected, the data are compared, and patterns and categories are organized into descriptive or explanatory models that can then be further developed through other methods of research. Quantitative research also may be an example of concept synthesis. Patterns of behaviors may be demonstrated and classified through statistical analyses such as factor analysis and Q-sorts. A final approach to concept synthesis is examination of the literature, in which the literature itself comprises the extant database.

There are several sequential steps involved in concept synthesis, but the process is generally iterative in reality. The process of concept synthesis begins with familiarizing and immersing yourself in the literature or other data that provide examples of the concept of interest. As you become familiar with the data, you begin to code the data or label them in some way, looking for patterns or clusters of attributes of the phenomenon. Following this coding or classification, the next step is to examine the codes for hierarchical structure. This involves examining each code for overlap with other codes. If one coded category can be subsumed under another one, it should be reduced to the more abstract or higher order concept. When as much reduction as possible has occurred, the new concept can be labeled.

After the new concept has been labeled, it must be verified by finding empirical support for the phenomenon in extant literature. The concept may also be verified through discussion with professional colleagues or through the participants of studies that provided data about the concept. This process of verification must be pursued until no new information about the concept is identified. This stage of the process is referred to as saturation. At this point, a theoretical definition that contains all the defining attributes of the concept is written. The final step is to determine whether or not the concept fits into any existing theory about the general phenomenon of concern (Walker & Avant, 2005).

This process is familiar to those who have conducted grounded theory studies in which qualitative data are analyzed and new phenomena are named and defined. For example, the concept of drug abuse as "slow suicide" was identified in a qualitative study of street youth living in Canada (see details in Chapter 11). However, the authors completed only the first few steps of this strategy in theory construction (Kidd & Kral, 2002). They labeled the concept but did not provide a solid definition or support from extant literature. Nevertheless, the concept is intriguing and worthy of further exploration as we search for ways to understand the health and associated behaviors of homeless as well as household adolescents. In contrast, in a grounded theory study of low-income African American female adolescents (19 to 26 years old), Martyn and Hutchinson (2001) clearly identified and defined concepts that they used to develop a theory of how these young women avoided unintended pregnancy. For example, the concept of "rewriting negative scripts" was described as "recognizing negative scripts, being disenchanted with negative scripts, determining to be different, and creating a different life" (p. 242).

Concept Derivation

Concept derivation is a way of examining a new area of interest by determining how closely it resembles or is analogous to an existing area. New concepts may be created by redefining old concepts that have already been defined within an established context. The strategy involves moving a particular concept from one established field into another one. It is much like transposing the key of a musical composition. The technique of concept derivation requires creativity and imagination and often happens by serendipitous circumstance (Walker & Avant, 2005).

The purpose of concept derivation is to provoke new ideas about a phenomenon of interest. Unlike concept synthesis, concept derivation is faster because it begins with an existing field where theoretical constructs already exist and are well defined. Four basic steps are followed and do not have to occur in a linear sequence. The first two steps are (a) to become very familiar with the limits of existing literature about the phenomenon of interest to you and then (b) to look to literature in other disciplines. These steps are often born out of frustration because the existing literature does not fully capture the phenomenon you have encountered in working with or observing adolescents. It may also be that certain concepts exist in the area of adolescent health and health behavior but have not stimulated further development. The last two steps are to identify concepts from another field and redefine them for the new field.

The story of Kekulé, a German chemist, who searched for a long time to find the chemical structure of the carbon compound benzene, illustrates the process of concept derivation. Kekulé was said to have had an "aha" experience while relaxing in front of the fireplace one evening in 1865. He was mesmerized as he watched the flames twisting around like snakes. Then suddenly Kekulé saw a snake chasing and seizing its own tail, forming the exact shape that he recognized was analogous to the relationship of the elements in the benzene ring (Goldberg, 1983). The conceptual structure of this chemical compound, thus, can be said to have been derived from the concept of a snake seizing its own tail.

In his book *The Stress of Life,* Hans Selye (1978) illustrated the many steps he took in developing his classic theory, better known as the General Adaptation Syndrome (GAS) or stress syndrome. Along the way, Selye described his search for a name for the particular phenomenon he had studied for so long. The English word *stress,* which he knew had a particular meaning in engineering as "the effects of a force acting against a resistance" (p. 45), came to mind. Selye went on to show how his use of the term stress (i.e., a specific syndrome in the human body that "consists of all the nonspecifically induced changes within a biological system," p. 64) led to some confusion. The term was used to refer to both the cause and the effect of the general adaptation syndrome. Selye claimed that because English was not his first language, he had been unable to distinguish between the terms *stress* and *strain.* Thus, he created a neologism, *stressor,* which came to be defined as the causative agent of stress. At that point, Selye stated that these terms are generally accepted in the biological sciences, and he added "I would like to state here clearly that the concepts of stress and strain in physics correspond, respectively, to those of stressor and stress in biology and medicine" (p. 51).

Although Selye did not set out to develop a theory of stress by using the strategy of concept derivation, his work was obviously influenced to some extent by his understanding of the science of physics. His attention to the naming of the concepts that comprise the central focus of the theory shows the importance of naming phenomena in terms that many people can grasp and accept easily. This example also illustrates the necessity to define each term in a theory clearly, differentiating it from related terms.

Concept Analysis

Concept analysis is the process of critically examining the characteristics of concepts that comprise a theory. The purpose of this strategy is to differentiate one concept from another. It is useful in clarifying terms that may have been used frequently in the literature on a particular subject but that have ambiguous or even conflicting meanings. Moreover, it is an essential step in developing research instruments to operationalize variables (concepts) in a study.

Concept analysis begins with the selection of a concept (e.g., health-risk behavior) that is of focal interest to the theory to be constructed or critically evaluated. The example used here is central to the theme of this book, *health-risk behavior* in adolescents. After selection of the concept, the next step is to identify the purpose of the analysis. Examples of why you might perform a concept analysis, aside from the sheer academic enjoyment of doing so, are (a) to clarify the meaning of a concept, (b) to differentiate the common meaning of the concept in ordinary language from the scientific use of the term, or (c) to develop an operational definition of the concept. After determining the purpose of the analysis, identify all the uses of the concept that you can find in the literature, through dialogue with colleagues, in dictionaries or thesauruses, or through interviews with adolescents themselves. During this step of the process, you may find terms that are similar but not exactly the same as the concept of interest. It is important to make note of these as well because they will be used later in constructing borderline and contrary cases. For example, a concept in adolescent literature that is related to the concept of health-risk behavior is risky behavior. To clarify the meaning of *health-risk behavior* for theoretical purposes, one must differentiate the meaning of these two terms.

After all the uses of the concept have been identified, the next step is to determine the defining attributes of the concept. First, develop a list of provisional criteria for the concept. These criteria are the characteristics that occur repeatedly in the literature and help the reader to distinguish the concept of interest from related concepts. Second, specify the defining attributes of the concept as you intend to use it. Third, compose an exemplar of the concept that clearly demonstrates all the defining attributes of the concept. Such a model case cannot include any characteristics of another concept, and all attributes must be essential to the meaning of the concept of interest. Next, create two more cases: the borderline case, which will contain some but not all of the defining attributes of the concept, and a contrary case, which will contain few or none of the defining attributes. After the model cases are created, identify the antecedents and consequences of the concept. These steps help to sharpen your focus on the defining or critical attributes of the concept. Antecedents, by definition, are situations or events that take place prior to the occurrence of the concept of interest. When these are identified, you may have a clearer understanding of some of the assumptions about the concept that might otherwise have been implicit. Consequences, by definition, are situations or events that take place after the occurrence of the concept. For example, adverse health outcomes are consequences of health-risk behaviors.

The final step in concept analysis is to locate and list the empirical referents (operational definitions or indicators of the concept that can be observed or measured) of the concept. It may be that the defining attributes constitute the empirical referents. In other cases, measurement instruments may have been constructed to reflect the occurrence of the concept in the real world. At this point, it is good to remember that a concept, like a theory, is an abstraction of reality. It may not be possible to observe the occurrence of the phenomenon directly, but it may be inferred from situations. In studying the health-risk behavior of adolescent sexual activity, for example, it is not feasible to observe directly the use or nonuse of condoms during sexual intercourse, but one may infer the occurrence of the behavior through self-report from the adolescent or the absence of the behavior in the presence of an unplanned pregnancy or sexually transmitted infection (STI).

Summary

Concepts are the basic elements that comprise theories. Concepts may be synthesized directly from observation of a phenomenon of interest in real life or through factor analysis of quantitative data. Concepts may also be derived through analogy to an existing idea or term in another area of experience. Finally, concepts can then be analyzed to clarify their meaning for a particular theory. The process of concept analysis is imperative when developing operational definitions or in determining empirical indicators of a phenomenon so that theory can be tested.

Statement Synthesis

Statement synthesis is the process of examining empirical evidence and specifying relationships between two or more concepts. Procedures followed in statement synthesis involve a logical, dynamic process of proceeding from observation to inference and generalizing from a specific inference to one that is more abstract. This process may occur by using either qualitative or quantitative data or both. This strategy for theory construction is really synonymous with the research process (Walker & Avant, 2005). It is beyond the scope of this book to discuss the research process in depth, but a few comments here will serve to illustrate this point. Qualitative methods of research, such as phenomenology, ethnography, or grounded theory, are based on the assumption that a scientist will be able to amass thick descriptions of phenomena directly from research participants, who will ultimately benefit from what is learned in the process. Statements about the phenomena of interest can, therefore, be considered valid for application in the real world because the findings are grounded in the experience of the participants. The analysis of quantitative data through statistical tests assumes that tools for measuring theoretical constructs are valid and reliable. That is to say, such tools actually measure the concept of interest, and they do so in a consistent manner. The use of statistical tests, such as the Pearson product-moment correlation, provides evidence of relationships among variables that can then be translated into relational statements used to formulate a theory.

In addition to qualitative and quantitative research designs, a third method that may be used to conduct a statement synthesis is that of examining extant literature. This involves extracting only those statements of relationship that have empirical support. Two possible outcomes of this strategy are that (a) the meaning of a concept within a statement is made more general or (b) the scope of the phenomena addressed by the statement is expanded. In the first case, several concepts may be merged into one that is more abstract. In the second case, the boundaries are extended so that additional populations or circumstances may be addressed by the relationship specified in the statement (Walker & Avant, 2005).

Statement Derivation

Just as concept derivation is a way of examining a new area of interest as analogous to an existing area, so statement derivation is a continuation of this process. Rather than moving just one concept from one specific field of study to another, the theorist moves a whole set of statements from one domain to another. The statements retain their structure, but the meanings now reflect the context of the new field of study. Both structure and content may be transposed from one domain to another, and both must be considered when using this strategy. The strategy is designed for use when there are no extant data or literature on a particular phenomenon or where current thought is considered to be old-fashioned or not very useful (Walker & Avant, 2005).

There are five basic steps in statement derivation: (a) becoming immersed in the existing literature about the phenomenon of interest; (b) examining theoretical and research literature in other disciplines and noting statements of relationship that may be applicable to your phenomenon of interest; (c) selecting the parent domain from which statements will be derived, carefully considering both structure and content; (d) restating the statements from the original or parent domain in terms of the new area of interest; and (e) redefining new concepts in the new field of study as needed. Statement derivation has the advantage of being economical in terms of time and financial resources, but it is limited to discovery only. That is to say, just because the statements are valid in the parent field, does not mean they will be credible in the new field. Evidence for their credibility in the new field must be established.

Statement Analysis

The strategy of statement analysis is the process of inspecting statements to determine their form and to determine how concepts within them are related to one another. Statement analysis involves three essential processes: (a) the critical examination of each concept contained within the statement, (b) the critical examination of each concept in the light of each other concept contained within the statement, and (c) the role of the entire statement within the theory. Some statements within a theory are not relational. That is, they do not express a relationship between concepts. Such nonrelational statements are referred to as *existence* statements and merely make the claim that a phenomenon or object exists. This type of statement is used in a theory to provide a backdrop or context for the relational statements that form hypotheses of the theory. Another kind of nonrelational statement is a *definitional* statement. As this term implies, such a statement delineates the attributes of a concept. A definitional statement may be theoretical, meaning that it is abstract with no empirical referents identified, or it may be operational, meaning that it does have identified empirical referents.

Relational statements constitute the core of theories. Relational statements may be classified as one of several forms: causal, probabilistic, conditional, or time ordered. A causal statement expresses the relationship in which one concept (concept 1) causes another concept (concept 2). Causal statements are common in basic sciences such as physics, where these statements are deductively derived from laws. Such statements are found infrequently in behavioral and social sciences because the caused outcome (concept 2) must always occur if the causal event (concept 1) occurs. A more common type of statement in the behavioral and social sciences is the probabilistic statement, often derived from quantitative data. A probabilistic statement illustrates that if one concept occurs (concept 1), the second concept (concept 2) is also very likely to occur (Walker & Avant, 2005). An example of a probabilistic statement is that driving a motor vehicle after drinking alcohol is very likely to lead to an accident in which the driver or someone else will sustain considerable injuries. Fortunately, not everyone who drinks and drives ends up having an accident with considerable injuries.

A conditional statement shows that there is a relationship between two concepts (concept A and concept B), but only in the presence of a third concept (concept C). For example, the previous probabilistic statement about the relationship between driving while drinking and having an accident with injuries could be made conditional by adding that the relationship between driving while drinking and sustaining a life-threatening injury happens only if the driver is not wearing a seat belt. A time-ordered statement displays an intervening amount of time between the occurrence of concept A and concept B. An example of this type of statement is found in Pender's Health Promotion Model (Pender, Murdaugh, & Parsons, 2002; see Chapter 9 for details). Two major concepts in this theory are (a) commitment to a plan of action and (b) performing a health-promoting behavior. A theoretical proposition depicting the relationship between these two concepts is stated as "Commitment to a plan of action is less likely to result in the desired behavior when competing demands over which persons have little control require immediate attention" (p. 64). The latter portion of the statement about competing demands requiring immediate attention implies that there is a space of time between concept 1 (commitment to a plan of action) and concept 2 (performing a health-promoting behavior). This statement is also conditional because a third phenomenon (competing demands) is introduced to further explain the relationship between the two concepts (commitment to plan of action and desired behavior).

The purpose of statement analysis is to determine if statements that comprise a theory are informative, useful, and logically correct. The analysis begins with selection of a statement and may be prompted by the analyst's doubt or excitement. Some theories may sound exciting, but when one begins to analyze the statements within them, one finds that they are not useful or logical. It is probably not feasible to examine all the statements within a particular theory, so begin with one that has a broad rather than a narrow scope. It is more fruitful to select a relational statement rather than an existence statement because the relational statement is the basis for hypothesizing from the theory. After selecting the statement, simplify it if needed. A statement that is very long and complex may need to be reduced to more than one statement before the analysis can proceed. This is especially true if the statement contains more than two theoretical concepts.

After the statement has been simplified and its concepts clearly identified, examine the concepts for definitions and for theoretical validity. Although the statement being analyzed does not contain definitions of the concepts within it, these concepts should be clearly defined elsewhere in the theoretical formulation, and they should contain all the defining attributes that characterize the concept. The theoretical validity of the concepts as they are defined in the theoretical formulation should be congruent with other uses of the concept in the extant literature on the topic, or the concept may be considered valid if it has been exposed to a critical concept analysis (Walker & Avant, 2005).

The next step in statement analysis is to assess the relationships among concepts for type, sign, and symmetry. Remember that there are several types of relational statements, such as those that are causal, probabilistic, or time ordered. The signs of relationships are positive (+), negative (−), or unknown (?). Symmetry refers to the directionality of relationships among concepts. That is, if concept 2 is affected by concept 1 but concept 1 is not affected by concept 2, the relationship goes in one direction only; it is asymmetrical. If, on the other hand, each concept has an effect on the other, the relationship is considered to be symmetrical (Walker & Avant, 2005). To illustrate a symmetrical relationship, another proposition from Pender's Health Promotion Model will be used. The proposition is "Positive affect toward a behavior results in greater perceived self-efficacy, which can, in turn, result in increased positive affect" (Pender, Murdaugh, & Parsons, 2002, p. 63). This symmetrical relationship is depicted as follows: concept A ← → concept B; positive affect ← → self-efficacy.

The last two steps in statement analysis are to examine the logic and determine the testability of the statement. The logic is determined by examining its origin. If the statement is developed deductively from a more general law, it should be a true conclusion if the premises were true. If the statement is developed inductively from qualitative data, the logic can be judged by the amount of empirical support or comparison to existing knowledge (Hempel, 1966). Logic is further analyzed by comparing the statement to extant knowledge and determining if it is reasonable and makes sense within the context of what is known. Finally, to determine if the statement is testable, you must decide if there are operations that can be performed to measure the relationships specified by the statement (Walker & Avant, 2005).

Summary

Statement synthesis involves examining evidence to support the relationships specified between two or more concepts. Statement derivation involves moving one or more statements from a theory in one field into a new context but retaining the structure of the original statement(s). Statement analysis involves determining if the statements contained within a theory are useful and logically correct.

Theory Synthesis

Theory synthesis is the process of constructing a theory based on empirical evidence. The purpose of this strategy is to represent a real phenomenon through an interrelated set of concepts and statements that are systematically developed. The process of theory synthesis consists of three general steps:

(a) isolating a single phenomenon or a framework of phenomena of interest, (b) reviewing the literature for concepts and statements about the phenomena, and (c) organizing the statements into a coherent whole. Theory synthesis is a way to integrate myriad research evidence from extant publications, field observations, analysis of qualitative data, and statistical analysis of quantitative data. This strategy is useful in presenting many relationships economically. It is a method for summarizing similar findings into a coherent whole, which can then be used to guide further development of theory, policy, and intervention (Walker & Avant, 2005).

Theory Derivation

Theory derivation uses analogy from one field to provide explanations or predictions about a phenomenon in another field. Theory derivation differs from theory borrowing in that in the former, the entire set of concepts and their structure are moved, whereas in the latter, the theory is not changed when applied to the new field of inquiry. The process begins with a thorough literature review that leads you to the conclusion that none of the available theories in the area of interest is suitable for your purpose. The second step, then, is to conduct a literature review in other fields. This reading will allow you to see how other disciplines construct their theories. After reading widely, select a parent theory for its ability to provide a more thorough explanation or make better predictions about an analogous phenomenon or situation. Then carefully identify the content or structure from this parent theory that you wish to transpose into the new area of inquiry. Finally, you may have to redefine concepts for the new field and reconstruct sentences so they are meaningful for use within the new context (Walker & Avant, 2005).

Theory Analysis

Theory analysis is done to determine both the strengths and weaknesses of an extant theory. This analysis takes place through systematic examination of the theory for its structure, meaning, and completeness. Theory analysis is not the same as evaluation. Analysis is done to enhance our understanding of the theory; evaluation is done to determine its worth or value for some use. There are six steps in theory analysis, many of which may also be used in theory evaluation.

The origins of the theory can be traced to the first development of the theoretical formulation of interest. The particulars of how the theory was developed, either deductively from a general law or from another theory or inductively from data, must be determined. It may be important at the time of this first step to examine the explicit and implicit assumptions on which the theory was based. The second step is to analyze the meaning of the theory. Doing this involves identifying the concepts, how they are defined and used, how the statements delineate relationships among concepts, and how much empirical evidence there is to support these relationships. The third step is to determine the *logical adequacy* of the theory by assessing whether or not (a) the content makes sense, (b) there are logical fallacies in the statements, (c) predictions can be made independent of the content, and (d) scientists agree about the predictions. The *usefulness* of the theory is determined by asking whether (a) it helps explain things better than other theories, (b) it offers new insights, or (c) it allows us to make more accurate predictions. *Generalizability* refers to how widely a theory can be applied; *parsimony* refers to how simple (but elegant) a theory may be. The last step of *testability* refers to whether or not the theory can be tested, at least in principle (Walker & Avant, 2005). The major limitations of theory analysis are that it does not generate new information, and it is time consuming. However, it can lead to new insights and shed light on gaps in the knowledge about a particular phenomenon (Walker & Avant, 2005).

Theory Analysis and Evaluation

Before selecting a theory to guide research or practice, it is important to analyze and critically evaluate the theory. In an area where many professional disciplines contribute to the knowledge base about a subject, as is the case with adolescent health and health-risk behavior, it is essential that the user of the theory carefully evaluate the content and the structure of the theory. Several criteria have been proposed to guide the selection of a theory that is appropriate for research as well as policy or program development. The criteria offered here may not be the only ones applicable to your need for theory evaluation, but they have been suggested by various scholars and are similar, in many respects, to the strategy of theory analysis just described (Barnum, 1990; Ellis, 1968; Harter, 1999; Mithaug, 2003).

Usefulness

Foremost in evaluating theory is the criterion of usefulness. How useful a particular theory is will depend on whether it is going to be used to build knowledge (i.e., research process) or to apply knowledge (i.e., practice setting). In applying this criterion, the evaluator must keep in mind what the purpose of the theory is (e.g., to describe, explain, predict, or control). As long as a theory is deemed useful for one of these purposes, it will continue to be developed and applied. However, if a theory is no longer useful for one of these purposes, it will be modified or replaced.

If a clinician is evaluating the usefulness of a theory for practice, he may want to ask whether the theoretical formulation helps him to solve problems encountered in the practice setting. He should also ask whether there are conceptual problems generated by the theory and whether there are anomalies characteristic to the practice that interfere with the application of the body of knowledge represented by the theory (Fry, 1995).

A theory may also be considered useful if it contributes to our understanding of a phenomenon. A new theory will be adopted if it provides not just a new view of an old phenomenon but a clearer view that enhances understanding among scholars and practitioners. Theory helps us generate new information in the form of testable hypotheses. A related criterion is that of agreement of scientists. Theories survive and are used as frameworks for policy and interventions when scientists and practitioners agree on the contribution that such theories make to their understanding of the phenomena of concern.

Meaning and Logical Adequacy

The meaning and logical adequacy of a theory depend on the assumptions on which the theoretical formulation is based. In some theories, these assumptions are made explicit, whereas in other theories they are implicit. In either case, the evaluator must determine the validity of the assumptions. That is, are they true? To evaluate the meaning and logical adequacy of the theory, one must examine the concepts and the relationships among them. Again, the evaluator must determine the validity of the meaning of the concepts and look for a logical system of relationships. One must examine the argument presented to determine whether there are contradictions among terms, discrepancies in statements of relationships, or actual omissions. A helpful strategy for evaluating this component of theory is to construct a matrix of concepts and diagram the relationships among them. For example, in Figure 2.4, a theory is shown to consist of three major concepts: A, B, and C. On reading the theory, the evaluator determined that the statements that comprised the theory showed clearly positive relationships among these concepts. That is, A was positively related to B and A was positively related to C; therefore, B is positively related to C. Regardless of the content of the theory, all of the relevant concepts and statements are accounted for and are logically related to one another. If the meaning of the concepts and the statements in which they are related makes sense, the theory may be evaluated as having met the criterion of logical adequacy.

Scope

The usefulness of a theory also depends on the number of situations to which it can apply. A theory is more useful when it can apply to more than one situation. A theory that is abstract is more likely to be applicable to a larger number of situations than one that is very concrete and specific to a single situation. For example, social cognitive theory (see Chapter 8), which

	Concept A	Concept B	Concept C
Concept A	=	+	+
Concept B		=	+
Concept C			=

Legend: + means the concepts are positively related to each other; = means it is the same concept.

Figure 2.4   Matrix to Examine Relationships Between Concepts Within a
Theory to Determine Logical Adequacy

postulates that learning takes place within the context of social relationships, is useful because it has a broad scope. It applies not only to how young people learn about drinking and driving but to how they learn to engage in safer sex practices. In contrast, Marcia's theory of identity status (see Chapter 4) is limited because it applies to only a few categories of adolescent identity.

Elegance and Parsimony

The elegance and parsimony of a theory are determined by its scope relative to the number of concepts it includes. A classic example of an elegant yet parsimonious theory is Einstein's theory of relativity or $E = mc^2$. Such a theory explains many things with very few concepts (Ellis, 1968). When it comes to human behavior, however, things are less consistent and predictable. It generally takes many abstract concepts to explain complex relationships among development, behavior, and health. However, a theory that contains few concepts and statements, yet is applicable to many situations, is, by definition, more elegant and parsimonious than one with many concepts, statements, and redundancies.

Predictability

Theories that permit the scientist to make predictions about phenomena are more useful than those that merely describe or explain. Again, the natural sciences may have an easier time developing theories that meet this criterion than those of us dealing with sciences of human behavior. When evaluating a theory for its ability to predict phenomena related to adolescent health behavior, it is probably best to think in relative terms. That is, it is important to realize that human behavior is generally not very predictable, but if we can increase the probability that our predictions about behavior will be true, then our theories will have met this criterion.

Testability

A theory should have operational and empirical adequacy. Simply put, a theory must be testable. That is, concepts that comprise the theory should be measurable. For a theory to provide an adequate framework for research, the theoretical definition of a specific concept such as health-risk behavior should be congruent with the operational definition of the same term. For example, when the theoretical definition for the term *distress* is given as "a general, unpleasant response of the body to a stimulus," then measuring distress as one's self-report of symptoms of depression may not be the appropriate operation to perform to reflect the theoretical construct. Because theory is an abstraction of reality, it is sometimes very difficult to determine its operational and empirical adequacy. This is particularly true in the early stages of the development of a theory. Theories grounded in qualitative data from a target population are often conveyed in the words of the participants, having not yet been formalized into abstract concepts (see Chapter 11 for details). However, if it is possible to imagine that an instrument might be developed to measure an abstract concept, and if such instruments or operations might be possible for obtaining empirical evidence for all the concepts within the theory, then this criterion is met.

Pragmatic Adequacy

Similarly, theories that permit the scientist to control the phenomenon of concern or to control the outcomes of processes are more useful than those that do not permit such control. A theory that addresses a phenomenon in a practical way is more applicable than one that is very abstract or ideal. This is where the scientists and scholars may differ with clinicians in their evaluation of a particular theory. To meet the criterion of pragmatic adequacy, a theory must be suitable for human beings and the social orders within which they live (Meleis, 1997). This criterion has special importance when addressing the health behaviors of adolescents from various cultural backgrounds. A theory that has practical value for one culture (e.g., students attending an affluent private school) may have little practical value for another culture (e.g., adolescents who are homeless and living on the streets). This criterion is also known as generalizability.

Conceptual Models

Another way to represent the real world is through the use of conceptual models. In fact, a theory may begin as a conceptual model and, through repeated testing and refinement, become a testable theory. A model is simply a schematic representation of phenomena in the real world. It is a way to

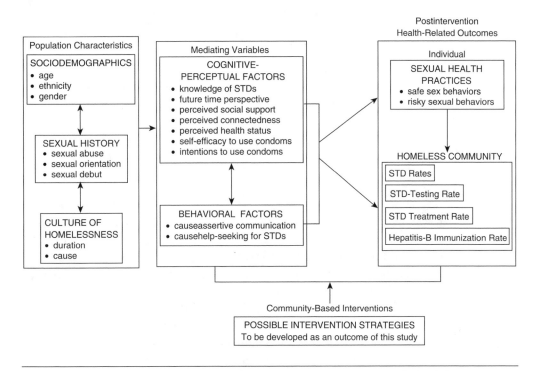

Figure 2.5   Conceptual Model of Sexual Health Practices Among Homeless Adolescents

SOURCE: Rew (2001). © 2001 Taylor & Francis, Inc. Reproduced by permission.

NOTE: STD indicates sexually transmitted disease. "This study" refers to Rew (2001).

organize what is known and unknown about a subject, facilitates communication about that topic, and guides research or practice related to the topic. A model can be useful for generating hypotheses (Lum, 2002). An example from my early work with homeless adolescents is depicted in Figure 2.5 (Rew, 2001). The model is based on the assumption that no single extant theory is adequate to explain or predict the complexity of factors that influence the sexual health practices of homeless adolescents. Thus, concepts based on a review of the literature, as well as health promotion, social cognitive theory, and the theory of reasoned action, resulted in a conceptual model that could be verified empirically and that could serve as a framework for interventions for this population.

Relationship of Theory to Research

The relationship between theory and research is dynamic. Theory serves as a framework for planning and conducting research. Theory contains the concepts or variables to be measured and the statements or hypotheses to be

Table 2.1   Relationship Between Theory and Research

	Theory	Research
Components	Concepts	Variables
	Statements	Hypotheses, questions
Purpose	Organize ideas	Support or refute ideas
Outcomes	Theory construction	Theory verification
	Framework for practice	Scientific body of knowledge

tested. Without a framework, research would be like a visitor going into a new country without a map or guide. Research that is conducted without a guiding framework has been referred to as "going on a fishing expedition" for good reason. The investigator has no idea what she or he is looking for and simply casts around, hoping to catch something useful and meaningful.

Research that is based on a framework of theory yields evidence to support or refute the theory. Theory is thus verified, refined, and enhanced by the research process. Each new study contributes to the body of knowledge about the particular phenomena of concern to a discipline or to a team of interrelated disciplines with a common goal. Table 2.1 depicts this relationship.

Relationship of Theory to Practice

The relationship between theory and practice is also dynamic. Most scientists who are interested in adolescent health and behavior have this interest because they are in a discipline that purports to aid in the healthy growth and development of human beings in the second decade of life. Rarely will we find a scientist in adolescent health who is merely interested in testing theoretical propositions for the sheer joy of doing so. Therefore, the sociologist, psychologist, nurse, social worker, or teacher who is a member of a helping discipline and whose focus is on adolescents will, of necessity, consult theory to guide his or her practice. Literature now abounds with articles on theory-based or evidence-based practice in several disciplines. There is also some tension between the purist, who wishes to test the efficacy of a specific theory in practice, and the practitioner, whose main focus is solving problems.

Practitioners often use a multiple-theory approach to solve a problem in practice. This perspective argues that "all theories are 'right,' within the parameters that the theory describes, and the challenge is to find the best theory or combination of theoretical constructs to understand or solve the problem at hand" (Bartholomew, Parcel, Kok, & Gottlieb, 2001, pp. 48-49). These practitioners argue that limiting oneself to a single theory may result in an inadequate solution to the problem or to conclusions that are not applicable within the context of a given problem.

Table 2.2 Relationship Between Theory and Practice

	Theory	Practice
Components	Concepts Statements	Phenomena of concern Problems to be solved
Purpose	Organize ideas	Delimit ideas
Outcomes	Theory construction Framework for practice and policies	Evidence-based practice Generalizable programs and interventions

Evidence-based practice is often atheoretical in nature. That is, practitioners may extract relevant concepts from various theories and put them together as a framework for programs or interventions. However, this approach is not theoretical and begs the question, What is the basis of the evidence? Scholars argue that theory "is the reason for and the value of the evidence" (Fawcett, Watson, Neuman, Walker, & Fitzpatrick, 2001). Without theory, how can one frame the evidence or determine what really counts as evidence? Without theory to identify concepts of importance and relationships among these concepts, we end up with nothing more than a glorified procedural manual, with its usefulness limited to a single setting. This makes it difficult to generalize to other problems in other settings. The healthy growth and development of complex human beings interacting with a complex environment requires the development of a systematic body of knowledge. In other words, it requires theory.

Table 2.2 depicts the ideal relationship between theory and practice. The concepts of which theory is constructed reflect the phenomena of concern in a practice discipline. The definitions and propositions of theory are abstractions of the practical problems to be solved in the practice arena. Whereas the purpose of theory is to organize ideas for some purpose, its application to practice is to delimit the ideas that abound in a practice setting. Outcomes of theory construction are reflected in frameworks that can guide practice and policy development. When theory is used to guide practice, evidence-based practices become generalizable programs and interventions that can be transposed to a variety of settings.

Atheoretical Perspectives of Adolescent Health and Health-Risk Behavior

Much of what we currently know and understand about adolescents, their health, and their health-risk behaviors is atheoretical. That is to say, it is not based on or framed by a specified scientific theory. Much of our research is organized using concepts that are in vogue at a particular time or that are of interest to a particular political movement at a given time. As Jessor and

Jessor (1977) noted more than a quarter of a century ago, such an approach to knowledge development "does not leave a legacy of understanding" (p. 10). The Jessors noted that facts do not speak for themselves; facts have to be located in a set of concepts that are linked together for some purpose. "Theory, thus, is the instrument of explanation or understanding, a source of meaning for facts or observations that endows them with a wider significance" (Jessor & Jessor, 1977, p. 10).

Although some of the variables or concepts identified in studies may be connected to theories of adolescent health or behavior, it is often not clear or explicit that a specific theory or framework guided the study. It is possible that the research was actually conducted using a theoretical framework, or at least a conceptual framework, but when the findings are published, the finished work does not identify a specific theory, model, or framework. Thus it is difficult for the student, scholar, or practitioner to see the progress of science. An example of this type of atheoretical perspective is a longitudinal study of protective and vulnerability factors in maltreated youth placed in foster care (Taussig, 2002). In a footnote to the title, the author acknowledges that the study was "a portion of the author's doctoral dissertation" (p. 1179). In the introduction to the study, Taussig notes that little is known about the long-term consequences of foster care in children who have been maltreated. She notes that what is known is that they have problems that are developmental, emotional, social, and behavioral in nature. These claims could be addressed through theories of development, social learning theory, problem behavior theory, and ecology. Taussig goes on to note that children who have been mistreated and who are then placed in foster care suffer from various stressors and because of their turbulent backgrounds may lack positive coping strategies. This suggests that a stress and coping theory might frame her analysis. She then suggests that previous research conducted on foster children who became adults points to the phenomenon of risk, and she proceeds to identify some research that specifically identifies self-destructive behaviors as an outcome of maltreatment. However, she does not present a coherent conceptual model to guide the study, and thus it is limited in its ability to contribute to a particular body of knowledge.

Although information obtained from studies done without a theoretical framework may be useful, it often remains isolated from an organized body of knowledge that practitioners and researchers can bring to bear on solving the problems of adolescent health-risk behavior. An example will illustrate this. A secondary analysis of data from the Teen Assessment Project at Cornell University was done to determine if there were differences in specific health-risk behaviors (i.e., use of alcohol and other drugs, use of tobacco, carrying weapons to school, and engaging in sexual activity) among adolescents attending schools in urban, suburban, and rural areas in New York. Results of the study were that a greater percentage of adolescents who lived in rural areas than in the other two areas exhibited these health-risk behaviors. The authors concluded that the location of an adolescent's residence had a strong influence on engaging in health-risk behaviors. In fact, for some of the behaviors (e.g., carrying weapons) the percentage of adolescents living in rural areas exhibited the behavior at twice the frequency of those living in urban and suburban areas (Atav & Spencer, 2002). Although this fact is important when planning interventions, it tells us nothing about why place of residence makes so much difference in these health-risk behaviors. There is nothing here that can be modified (i.e., manipulated in a scientific experiment). The investigators cited no theory in the introduction to the study but implied that stress may be a theoretical consideration: "Rural environment was previously thought to be an idyllic setting equated with the absence of stressors for rural adolescents" (p. 55). Studying health-risk behaviors of adolescents in a rural setting using a stress and coping model might have been more useful.

Theories Applicable to Adolescent Health and Health-Risk Behavior

Theories from a number of disciplines contribute to the knowledge base of adolescent health and health-risk behavior. Many of the theories presented in this text may be used to frame interventions to improve the health of adolescents. Health educators (Bartholomew et al., 2001) have developed a series of steps to follow in using theory, literature, and data to construct a plan for intervention (see Table 2.3).

Table 2.3   Steps in Using Theory to Plan a Health Promotion Intervention

1. Ask a question about the behavior of interest.
2. Seek answers to the question from literature, including theoretical, empirical, and clinical or practice sources.
3. Brainstorm provisional answers to the question.
4. Search the literature again to seek theoretical support and explanations.
5. Revisit the brainstormed list of provisional answers by using theory.
6. Add new concepts, if relevant.
7. Clarify definition of terms and relational statements.
8. Review theories from other disciplines to identify possible additional concepts.
9. Determine what additional data are needed from target population.

SOURCE: Based on Bartholomew et al. (2001).

Chapter Summary

Theory is the hallmark of any science. It exists for the purposes of helping us describe, explain, predict, and control phenomena in the real world despite our inability to manipulate those phenomena directly. Unlike our colleagues in the basic or natural sciences, those of us who are concerned about the health behaviors of and health outcomes for adolescents are often unable to observe these phenomena directly. As social scientists, we have been criticized for our lack of clarity in our theoretical writing and for our ignorance in how our science should look (Reynolds, 1971). In this chapter, the purpose of theory was delineated and several strategies for developing and evaluating theory have been presented. Developing a comprehensive and scientific understanding of adolescent health and health-risk behavior requires a commitment among scientists and practitioners to move from atheoretical to theoretical approaches that will help us to understand, explain, and make predictions.

Suggestions for Further Study

One of the purposes of this book is to raise awareness among students and professionals in a variety of disciplines that serve adolescents. Much of the current literature on adolescent health and health-risk behavior is not clearly linked to theory. Many theories about health and health behavior that were developed to explain and predict the behavior of adults have been borrowed and applied to adolescents. It is important to examine these more closely to determine if the assumptions on which they are based apply equally to adolescents. For example, the Health Belief Model (see Chapter 9) was originally proposed as a way to explain why adults did or did not engage in preventive screening for tuberculosis (Rosenstock, 1974c). Are the assumptions of the model and the theoretical constructs applicable to adolescents today? It is possible that assumptions and constructs based on developmental theories (see Chapter 3) should be incorporated to extend such theories for appropriate applicability to adolescents.

Inductive approaches to developing theories are also germane to the developmental levels and experiences of adolescents. Based on qualitative designs and data, such theories are cumbersome in their early stages but are worthy of fuller development because they emerge directly from the population we want to understand and help (see Chapter 11).

Suggestions for Further Reading

Im, E. O., & Meleis, A. I. (1999). Situation-specific theories: Philosophical roots, properties, and approach. *Advances in Nursing Science, 22*(2), 11-24.

Kulbok, P. A., & Cox, C. L. (2002). Dimensions of adolescent health behavior. *Journal of Adolescent Health, 31*, 394-400.

Meeker, M. (2002). *Epidemic: How teen sex is killing our kids.* Washington, DC: LifeLine Press.

3

Adolescent Development

U nderstanding health and health-risk behavior in adolescence begins here with a review of basic human development. Figure 3.1 is an abstraction of a holistic model of human development. It is not meant to depict a single unifying theory; rather, it is to illustrate the interrelatedness of families of theories that pertain to health and health-risk behaviors of adolescents. As Bronfenbrenner (1989) asserts, human development is a process of interaction between the developing person and the environment. Thus the behaviors that characterize the major morbidities and mortalities of adolescence are grounded, to some extent, in developmental changes that occur across multiple domains.

The purpose of Figure 3.1 is to be a heuristic—a guide to motivate the reader to seek a deeper and fuller understanding of how development in multiple domains shapes an individual's pattern of behavior. At the core of this schematic is the biogenetic domain. Human life begins with a single-cell organism, the fertilized ovum containing the unique genetic blueprint for the developing embryo and later for the maturing adolescent and young adult. From this physiological center emanates the social development of the individual. Even unborn children have not only a biological and genetic (biogenetic) connection to the mother but a social connection as well. As the mother-child relationship grows, in utero and beyond, the individual develops within the context of other people and their purposeful behaviors. The human infant cannot survive without help and social interaction with other people. Healthy growth and development depend on social interactions.

Simultaneously, the individual develops a uniqueness that is categorized as psychological. This dimension of human development is vast and incorporates myriad aspects, including changes in cognition or thinking and in personality construction, the differentiation of one's self as unique and separate from others. In many ways, this domain of development is closely connected to the social domain, because most of the cognitive and personality changes occur within the context of social relationships and institutions such as family, schools, and community organizations.

The final aspect of growth and development is the spiritual domain. Unfortunately, this is an aspect of development that has been seriously overlooked

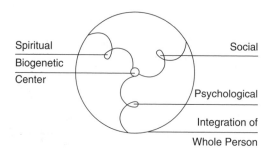

Figure 3.1   A Holistic Model of Human Development

and understudied. This spiritual domain of development also springs from the biogenetic center and unfolds along with the social and psychological domains. In adolescence, the awakening of a person's sexuality may also coincide with an increased awareness of one's spiritual nature. The parallels between sexual and spiritual development or maturation are remarkable and worthy of further study. The genetic blueprint, which dictates how and when the human body reaches sexual maturity, with its accompanying ability to reproduce, coincides to some extent with society's expectations about spiritual and religious maturity and commitment. During puberty, many adolescents seek intimacy with peers in ways that are prompted by new physical awareness and sanctioned by social mores. This time of increased awareness of self and others raises important questions about the purpose and meaning of life, as well as allowing the development of a broader and deeper understanding of what it means to love and to be loved.

Through the process of identity development (see Chapter 4), individuals gradually incorporate their social, psychological, and spiritual development around their central biogenetic core. Like the whole butterfly that emerges from the chrysalis, the young adult emerges from the adolescent phase of human development as an integrated whole person. The behavior in which the person then engages predicts the state of health or wholeness she or he experiences in this process.

Theories of Human Development

The discussion of the health-risk behaviors that are manifested in adolescence begins with acknowledging that adolescence is a unique phase in human development. Defined here as the second decade of life, adolescence is the time when the developing individual undergoes dramatic changes in the physical, psychological (emotional and cognitive), social, and spiritual domains of life. This chapter contains a brief overview of physical development in adolescence as the biological basis for understanding adolescent development that occurs also within the psychological, social, and spiritual domains.

Development in each dimension contributes to variations in health-risk behaviors exhibited by adolescents.

Numerous theories explain the sequential changes that occur over time in the human mind and body. Human growth and development are of interest to natural scientists, who seek to explain how and why the human organism changes in many predictable ways. Human growth and development are also of interest to psychologists and social scientists, who seek to explain how the human psyche and cognitive abilities change over time and in response to social and cultural influences. These theories are too numerous to explore in depth in this chapter, but a few have been selected to demonstrate the utility of developmental theories in understanding adolescent health in general and health-risk behaviors in particular. The author's bias throughout this text is to focus on the adolescent in a holistic manner; that is, not to separate adolescents' physical growth and development from their cognitive, social, emotional, or spiritual aspects. However, to paint the clearest picture, these dimensions will be explored in the light of existing theories and models, some of which are domain specific (e.g., physical and pubertal development). Other theories and models, such as Bronfenbrenner's ecological theory of human development, developmental contextualism, and the developmental assets and youth development models, provide a more holistic lens through which to observe adolescent growth and development. These models were selected because they focus on adolescence as a phase within the lifespan of development and emphasize the notion that behavior develops within the context of social relationships. The chosen theoretical approaches are also holistic in the sense that they address the integration of the biological, psychological, social, and, to a lesser extent, spiritual dimensions of human beings. All of these approaches are systems oriented, meaning that the unit of analysis is the person-within-environment.

Jessor and Jessor (1977) noted that the growth and changes that take place in this period of time provide a foundation for future action. They added,

> It is the time of acquisition of skills and interests, occupational, educational, and interpersonal, that will be relied on into old age; and it is, finally, the time of more lasting self-definition, the working out of a sense of identity that will serve to organize experience and guide behavior through much of adulthood. [This] period is something of a crucible for the shaping of later life. (p. 5)

Adolescence is a time of rapid change with far-reaching consequences.

Physical Development

The process of change within the human organism is known as development. The child develops from the infant, the adolescent from the child, and the adult from the adolescent. Development from an immature state to a mature state occurs in multiple dimensions simultaneously. For example, the organism develops physically in response to a genetic blueprint but also in response to sociocultural factors, such as family relationships and life events (Lerner & Castellino, 2002). The human being develops emotionally, cognitively, socially, and spiritually concurrently with physical development, but growth and development in one dimension does not guarantee a similar amount or quality of growth and development in another dimension (Susman, Reiter, Ford, & Dorn, 2002). Although theories of human physiology are beyond the scope of this book, it is important to consider basic information about physical development in general and sexual maturation in particular because they are directly related to the health-risk behaviors of adolescents. The physiological changes of adolescence are referred to as puberty, a term derived from the Latin *pubertas,* meaning *adult* (Pickett, 2000). During puberty, dramatic changes occur in several areas (Neinstein & Kaufman, 2002):

- Changes in the brain and endocrine system stimulate rapid acceleration in weight and height, often referred to as the *adolescent growth spurt.*
- Primary sexual characteristics develop, including the ovaries in females and testes in males.
- Secondary sexual characteristics develop, including growth of pubic, body, and facial hair, as well as changes in the breasts and genitalia.
- Body composition changes, including distribution of muscle and fat.
- The circulatory and respiratory systems change, resulting in increased strength and physical tolerance.

Physical development and sexual maturation depend on physical changes that occur among the various systems of the human body. Following the orthogenetic principle, development proceeds from lesser to greater differentiation within the organism (Wapner & Demick, 1998). However, these changes also take place within social and environmental contexts. The social setting in which a child develops not only affects the social behaviors, values, and habits of the individual, it has a powerful impact on the development of the child's body as well. Bowlby (1969) suggests in his attachment theory that the interactions between infants and their caregivers provide the foundation for healthy self-development. The environment also plays an important part in pubertal growth and development. Specifically, nutrition and general health status make critical contributions to this process. There is ample empirical support that puberty occurs earlier in children who receive good nutrition and is delayed in those who are deficient in protein and calories. Chronic illness has also been associated with delayed puberty (Neinstein & Schack, 2002).

Puberty marks a phase in human development that is characterized by the individual's ability to reproduce sexually. Pubertal changes are controlled by pituitary hormones that lead to rapid changes in body composition, size, and shape. These changes result in development of mature secondary sexual characteristics (e.g., beard in males, breast enlargement in females) and maturation of the genitalia, with concurrent processes of ovulation and spermatogenesis (Plant, 2002). The transformation from child to adult takes place in a generally predictable sequence, but this phase of development is neither sudden nor completed overnight.

Distinct differences between males and females are apparent long before puberty. Human life begins with the single cell, an egg or ovum from the mother that is fertilized by a sperm from the father. The single cell, or fertilized egg, carries two chromosomes that define the sex of the embryo: two X chromosomes (XX) for a female and a single X plus a Y chromosome (XY) for a male. There are, of course, variations in this plan, and once in a while there are abnormal chromosomal arrangements. For example, Turner's syndrome (45, X) in females occurs approximately once in 2500 births and generally refers to a missing X chromosome, hence the 45, X designation (Ploof, 1999). Similarly, Klinefelter's syndrome in males occurs in approximately once in 500 to 1000 births and is associated with one or two extra X chromosomes, hence the designation 47, XXY or 48, XXXY ("Sex chromosome variations," n.d.).

For the first 28 days after conception, male and female embryos are identical except for their chromosomal makeup. During the 5th or 6th week of development, however, the gonads begin to form, each with an outer cortex and an inner medulla, two sets of ducts (Wolffian and Müllerian), and external structures that include a tubercle, folds, and swelling (Masters, Johnson, & Kolodny, 1995). Within 2 weeks, the male phenotype (XY) develops testes. The female phenotype (XX) develops ovaries about the 11th or 12th week of gestation. The human fetus produces sex hormones, including both estrogen and testosterone, which can be detected in both males and females by the 10th week of gestation. The hypothalamus in the brain, responding to hormonal stimulation, is imprinted to become either female or male (Neinstein & Kaufman, 2002).

During the first decade of human life, the central nervous system directs the relationship among the hypothalamus, pituitary gland, and gonads, suppressing their interaction to prevent puberty. The levels of testosterone in the blood of male infants and estradiol in the blood of female infants rise shortly after birth and remain elevated for the first year of life. These gonadal steroids then fall to prepubertal levels until the onset of puberty, which occurs in response to changes in the axis between the hypothalamus and pituitary gland. The level of growth hormone, produced by the pituitary gland, rises and affects the growth spurt generally seen during adolescence. This growth spurt lasts 24 to 36 months and results in increases in height and weight that occur earlier in females than in males. In females, lean body mass decreases and body fat increases, whereas in males, lean body mass increases and body fat decreases. During this growth spurt, skeletal bone mass and internal organs also mature (Neinstein & Kaufman, 2002).

Sexual Maturation

The onset of puberty for males and females generally occurs between 9 and 13 years. The average age of puberty is 11.2 years for females and 11.6 years for males. The onset of menstruation, or menarche, in females ranges from 9 to 17 years, with the average age 12.3 years. The onset of sperm emission, or spermarche, in males ranges from 11.7 to 15.3 years, with the average age 13.4 years (Neinstein & Kaufman, 2002). Sexual maturation is the hallmark of adolescent physical development. This maturation process occurs in predictable stages. Tanner (1962) and his colleagues (Marshall & Tanner, 1969) identified and described five distinct stages that have become the gold standard for identifying sexual maturation in adolescence. The two aspects of physical development that are considered in determining the sexual maturity rating or Tanner stage for females are degree of breast development and pubic hair development. Three aspects are considered in determining the sexual maturity rating or Tanner stage for males. These are the size of the testes, the length of the penis, and pubic hair development.

The changes that accompany puberty are known to affect the psychological adjustment of both male and female adolescents. Pubertal status and pubertal timing have been studied for their effects on the psychological perception of distress among adolescents. Pubertal status refers to one's level of physical development or maturation, and pubertal timing refers to the person's perception that she or he is on time relative to peers (i.e., early, on time, or late). Ge, Conger, and Elder (2001) conducted a longitudinal study in which they examined relationships among pubertal status, pubertal timing, externalized hostile feelings, and internalized feelings of distress among adolescent males between 12 and 14 years old. They found that boys who were more physically mature in 7th grade had more externalized hostile feelings and internalized feelings of distress when they were in 8th through 10th grades. They also found that pubertal timing was significantly related to externalized hostile feelings and internalized feelings of distress in this sample.

Timing of puberty is related to an individual's lifetime exposure to estrogens. Bone accretion in adolescence depends on endocrine changes, diet, and exercise and may result in osteopenia in later life. Neuroendocrine changes may affect an adolescent's sleep, which, in turn, affects mood and emotional regulation. High-risk behaviors are more likely in youth with sleep problems (Susman et al., 2002). During maturation, sleep regulation changes in the following ways: duration of non-REM and REM sleep decreases, a mature pattern of REM develops, daytime sleepiness increases, and circadian rhythms change so that the individual is more likely to stay up later and arise later than in childhood. Research on sleep patterns and problems in adolescents has shown that many youth do not obtain sufficient sleep. Sleep deprivation is related to emotion, attention, and behaviors that affect the adolescent's academic and social development and competence (Dahl & Lewin, 2002).

The timing of puberty in girls has been shown to vary widely, and menarche is the most critical indicator of this transition. Researchers have suggested that early maturation in girls is related to race and ethnicity and to the presence of significant stressors (Muscari, Faherty, & Catalino, 1998). Obeidallah, Brennan, Brooks-Gunn, Kindlon, and Earls (2000) investigated pubertal maturation in a total of 866 African American (n = 314), White (n = 148), and Latina (n = 404) girls from environments of low, medium, and high socioeconomic status (SES). This sample of girls ranged in ages from 8.1 to 16.4 years (M = 12.08 + 2.38 years). Not adjusting for differences in SES, Latinas experienced menarche earlier (M = 11.68 + 1.3 years) than did African American (M = 11.93 + 1.1 years) or White (M = 12.04 + 1.3 years) participants. There were no significant differences in age of menarche between African American and White participants. After controlling for SES, the difference between Latinas' age at menarche and that of Whites disappeared, but the difference between Latinas and African Americans remained. There were no significant differences among racial and ethnic groups in perception of pubertal timing. The researchers suggested that the racial and ethnic differences in menarche might be related to environmental stress and are worthy of further exploration. They also concluded that pubertal timing might have differential effects on the vulnerability to engage in health-risk behaviors among girls of different ethnic, racial, and SES backgrounds. Other researchers have found that girls who mature early are at risk for engaging in health-risk behaviors, such as unprotected sexual intercourse and drug use (Wiesner & Ittel, 2002), and in experiencing psychological distress and symptoms of depression (Brooks-Gunn, Graber, & Paikoff, 1994; Graber, Lewinsohn, Seeley, & Brooks-Gunn, 1997).

Pubertal Development and Gender Roles

The physical changes associated with puberty are also sociocultural events (Porter, 2002). Noticeable changes in the human body associated with sexual maturity are signals to the larger society that the developing individual is now capable of filling more complex, socially constructed roles and engaging in more complex interactions or behaviors. For females, the shift from identification as a little girl to a young woman is often accompanied by an unwelcome identification as a "sexual object" (Pipher, 1994; Porter, 2002). As illustrated in the poignant account of this phenomenon in Pipher's (1994) *Reviving Ophelia,* at puberty, females in our society receive conflicting messages about what it means to identify oneself as a young woman. Pipher adds that coming of age for young women often involves sex, alcohol, and drugs in "a culture preoccupied with money, sex and violence" (p. 291). In Shandler's (1999) *Ophelia Speaks,* hundreds of adolescent girls spoke out to describe their struggles to develop a strong and authentic self in the light of society's disparate expectations.

For males, the shift from little boy to young man is also accompanied by new expectations and demands for gendered behaviors. Gurian (1998) outlined three stages in the male's journey to manhood: the age of transformation (9-13 years), the age of determination (14-17 years), and the age of consolidation (18-21 years). The focus of Gurian's observations is on the emotional neglect of American adolescent males. He argued that in addition to the social, emotional, and vocational goals of adolescence, males in American society need to learn personal independence, a spirit of adventure and exploration, moral character, toughness and tenacity, and adaptability and flexibility. He added that they also need to learn a spiritual role.

Physical Maturation and Health-Risk Behavior

Every stage of human development is characterized by specific behaviors. In adolescence, the physiological maturity of puberty within a social context influences behavior and health in a variety of ways. Harrell, Bangdiwala, Deng, Webb, and Bradley (1998) included developmental theory as one aspect of a framework for a longitudinal study, the purpose of which was to describe the initiation of smoking behavior in school-aged children. They found that the mean age for initiation of smoking was 12.3 years. Experimental smoking was significantly related to pubertal development. Specifically, children who were at a more mature level of pubertal development than their peers were more likely to experiment with smoking. In a study of 4686 junior high school students in Norway, the relationship between pubertal timing and health-risk behaviors (i.e., alcohol use and intoxication, sexual behavior, and substance use) was investigated (Wichstrøm, 2001). Early timing of puberty was associated with alcohol use, especially among males.

Developmental and Behavioral Genetics

Behavioral scientists are increasingly willing to entertain the possible genetic basis for behavior change throughout the lifespan. Major topics related to the development of health-risk behaviors in adolescence are those of personality, psychopathology, and cognitive ability. Future studies may answer questions concerning how genetic factors influence behavior, how these factors interact with environment to influence health-risk behaviors, and how the intersection of genetic and environmental factors change and influence behavior over time (Plomin, 2000).

Investigators have shown that specific health-risk behaviors increase with biological maturation and age. Using longitudinal data from the Cardiovascular Health in Children and Youth Studies (phases I and II), Harrell and colleagues (1998) found that experimental smoking increased from 4% among third and fourth graders to 42% among eighth and ninth graders. These investigators also found that those children who were at a later stage of pubertal development were more likely to experiment with smoking than peers who were at an earlier stage of pubertal development. The investigators concluded that prevention of smoking needed to be addressed through interventions for children in elementary and middle schools, and interventions to assist young adolescents in cessation of smoking needed to be provided in both middle and high schools.

In a study of middle school children with a mean age of 13.1 years, Aten, Siegel, Enaharo, and Auinger (2002) found that the onset of sexual intercourse increased with age. This study was a nonrandomized control trial of a school-based intervention designed to delay the onset of sexual intercourse and to continue abstinence for a period of 1 year following the intervention. The research team found that maintaining abstinence was possible only among those participants who were abstinent when the study began. Students who were younger than 13 years old and abstinent when the intervention began were more able to remain abstinent than older students or than those who had already initiated sexual intercourse. The researchers concluded that primary prevention interventions were needed before children become adolescents.

Cognitive Development

Much of human behavior is volitional and goal directed. Thus it is essential to consider the cognitive or intellectual development that occurs in adolescence. This development is a critical aspect of moral reasoning and decision making. Space does not permit a thorough presentation of theories of cognitive development. However, the major contributions of Jean Piaget (genetic epistemology), Lawrence Kohlberg (moral reasoning), and Carol Gilligan (women's moral development) are presented briefly.

Genetic Epistemology

Jean Piaget, born in Switzerland in 1896, sought to discover a biological basis for knowledge development. Using naturalistic methods of inquiry, he termed his framework *genetic epistemology*, or the study of how knowledge develops. Piaget described cognitive structure as the mental and physical actions that undergird intelligence. This cognitive structure is manifested in skills or schemas that correspond to predictable stages of development. Cognitive development occurs as the child acts on the environment and as the environment acts on the child. Independent of this organism-environment interaction was the contribution of heredity.

The major concepts in Piaget's theory are the four cognitive structures or developmental stages (i.e., sensorimotor, preoperational, concrete operational, and formal operational) and the processes through which these structures change (i.e., assimilation, accommodation, and equilibration). The stage of *formal operations* occurs at around age 12, when the person begins to think less like a child and more like an adult. The use of logical operations in the abstract means that the person is able to engage in hypothetical thinking. This ability to engage in formal operations contributes to the reasoning that allows the person to investigate and solve problems systematically (Piaget & Inhelder, 1958, 1969, 1973). Piaget's theory has spawned countless other studies and theories to explain cognitive development. The theory has also been criticized for its somewhat rigid approaches to stages. Rather, the types of cognitive structures and processes described by Piaget and his disciples reflect a gradual process of transition from more concrete to more abstract ways of thinking (Lerner, 2002).

Information Processing

More recent theories of cognitive development focus on information processing and the development of competence in such processing. Human beings are viewed as actively receiving, storing, and retrieving information that is then used to inform behavior. Early work on this theoretical approach was done by George Miller (1956), who introduced the terms *bit* and *chunk*. These terms refer to the amount of information that can be held in immediate memory and made available for making judgments. Miller asserted that short-term memory was limited to holding five to nine (i.e., seven plus or minus two, hence the title of his classic paper) chunks of information.

Concepts of attention and memory are salient to theories of information processing. For example, adolescents are characterized by the ability to pay closer attention to stimuli than younger children. This may be seen as increases in both selective attention (e.g., focusing on one stimulus and tuning out another) and in divided attention (e.g., focusing on two stimuli simultaneously). Other changes that occur in adolescence are improvements in both short-term memory (i.e., the ability to remember for brief periods of time) and long-term memory (i.e., the ability to remember something that occurred long ago). The ability to retrieve information stored over time is crucial to the adolescent in solving problems and making decisions. Adolescents are also able to process information more rapidly and to organize that information into a plan better than younger children. During adolescence, there are also increases in *metacognition,* the ability of the person to think about his or her own thinking (Lerner, 2002; Steinberg, 1996).

Moral Development

Just as physical development occurs in the context of social structures, cognitive development occurs within this same context. The increasingly

Table 3.1   Stages in Kohlberg's Theory of Moral Reasoning

Level	Conceptual Stage	Characteristics of Stage
First	Preconventional morality	Naïve egoistic reasoning, focus on obedience and punishment
Second	Conventional morality	Concerned with being a good person and with adhering to social and institutional norms
Third	Postconventional morality	Concerned with what is legal; able to consider principles and one's conscience

complex social setting in which the adolescent matures calls for an increasing ability to think morally about his or her own behavior. Again, the work of Piaget (1932), which was further developed by Lawrence Kohlberg, invited a perspective that included both the person and the environment in reciprocal interaction. According to Kohlberg (1963a, 1963b, 1978), moral reasoning involved a progression through stages, as depicted in Table 3.1.

Kohlberg's theory has been criticized for its primary focus on the person and its secondary consideration of the environment (Lerner, 2002). Moreover, it has also been criticized because of its construction primarily considering research conducted with males rather than both males and females. The work of Carol Gilligan (1993) grew out of her experiences teaching at Harvard with Erik Erikson and her work as a research assistant with Lawrence Kohlberg. In her book *In a Different Voice*, Gilligan asserts that her description of moral development does not concern generalizations about gender differences as much as it does her empirical observations that there is more than one way in which cognitive and moral development occur. Moreover, her work clearly provides more information about this development in females than previous studies that focused almost exclusively on moral reasoning and development in males. In fact, Gilligan was puzzled about why females consistently rated lower than males on moral reasoning when using Kohlberg's conceptualization. What she found, then, was that males and females approach this cognitive task in very different ways.

Gilligan (1993) discovered that boys and girls resolve disputes using fundamentally different principles: Boys resolve the dispute directly, whereas girls stop playing to preserve the relationship. From her research, Gilligan asserted that males' moral reasoning was based on the ethical principle of justice (e.g., persons have rights that must be respected), whereas females' moral reasoning was based on the ethical principle of responsibility (e.g., persons have a moral imperative to care for other people). She stated:

Women's construction of the moral problem as a problem of care and responsibility in relationships rather than as one of rights and rules ties the development of their moral thinking to changes in their understanding of responsibility and relationships, just as the conception of morality as justice ties development to the logic of equality and reciprocity. (p. 73)

In adolescence, girls recognize a disparity between care and power and choose to abandon the concern for attaining and maintaining power and adopt the concern for caring.

Critical Thinking

The development of critical thinking skills is another dimension of cognition that is highly important in understanding adolescent decision making and subsequent behavior. Theories of critical thinking have their origin with the work of Bloom (1956), who classified learning objectives that paralleled learning behaviors. The six levels in Bloom's taxonomy are found in Table 3.2. These six levels of learning range from lower to higher levels of cognitive abilities. Critical thinking is said to occur in the levels of analysis, synthesis, and evaluation. Gagné (1965) also contributed to the early development of critical thinking theory. He outlined eight phases called *events of learning,* depicted in Table 3.3.

Critical thinking skills are learned primarily through a process of discovery rather than through mere memorization of facts. These skills are honed through both deductive and inductive reasoning, as well as during opportunities to debate and interact with peers and mentors alike.

Table 3.2   Bloom's Taxonomy of Learning

Level of Learning	Characteristic Features
Knowledge	Focus is on memorizing and reciting facts.
Comprehension	Focus is on relating and organizing new information with information previously learned.
Application	Focus is on using rules or principles to interpret the information to fit a particular set of circumstances. The learner puts information into practice.
Analysis	Focus is on how parts are functionally related to the whole. May include comparing and contrasting things to and with each other.
Synthesis	Focus is on putting things together to make a new whole. May include planning, creativity, and imagination.
Evaluation	Focus is on making judgments based on information. May include making decisions about value and effectiveness.

SOURCE: Bloom (1956).

Table 3.3   Gagné's Eight Events of Learning Critical Thinking

Phase	Characteristic Features
Motivation	Learner expects that the need to learn or have curiosity satisfied will be met.
Apprehension	Learner attends to or focuses on the task at hand.
Acquisition	Learner assimilates new information into cognitive associations.
Retention	Learner places new information in long-term memory through processes of practice and recitation.
Recall	Learner connects new information to previously stored information to facilitate memory.
Generalization	Learner applies information in real-life situation.
Performance	Learner exhibits mastery of information through behavior displayed.
Feedback	Learner receives information about the performance to correct or modify future performance of the learned behavior.

SOURCE: Gagné (1965).

Psychosocial Development in Puberty

Physical development and sexual maturation in the young adolescent are accompanied by profound changes in the social and psychological domains as well. Adolescents experience drastic changes in their bodies and in their emotions. Social support, or lack thereof, provided by parents, teachers, peers, and others can facilitate or inhibit healthy development. Hormonal changes within the body may be responsible for excessive mood swings. Adolescents are also beginning to separate from parents and move toward stronger relationships with peers.

Erik Erikson (1963, 1968) proposed a theory of human development that emphasized the psychosocial crises of developmental stages. Erikson viewed these crises as a continuum of development with both negative and positive poles. Although most individuals do not resolve a crisis entirely positively or negatively, they need to come through the stage more in the positive direction than the negative one to continue on to the next stage. In adolescence, the psychosocial crisis that must be resolved is one of identity versus identity diffusion. James Marcia (1966, 1980, 1989, 1993, 1994) extended our understanding of the crisis of adolescence and developed a theory of identity statuses. Both Erikson's and Marcia's conceptualizations will be addressed in greater detail in Chapter 4.

Spiritual Development

The development of the spiritual dimension of adolescents is not well documented. This dimension of the person is often conceptualized as religious beliefs and practices. Spirituality, however, is defined as a universal phenomenon characteristic of human wholeness (Cavendish et al., 2001). A holistic discussion of human development, including the search for a sense of identity and purpose in life during adolescence, must include this dimension. The terms *spiritual* and *spirituality* have not been clearly defined in the adolescent or health behavior literature. Spirituality and religiosity are often used interchangeably, although they are, arguably, different but related concepts. Religiousness and participation in religious activities have been shown to be protective factors against specific health-risk behaviors in adolescents, including substance use and sexual activity (Fehring, Brennan, & Keller, 1987; Hodge, Cardenas, & Montoya, 2001; Resnick et al., 1997). Limited research has been done linking religious and spiritual development with attachment (Lovinger, Miller, & Lovinger, 1999) and psychosocial development in adolescents (Markstrom, 1999).

In identifying spirituality as an important component of human development, Crawford and Rossiter (1996) caution against defining the spiritual (a) in religious terms, (b) excluding any reference to religion, or (c) as something so broad that it includes every possible aspect of life. Rather, they define spirituality as "the ways in which people look for and perceive meaning, purpose and values as well as other personal aspects like beauty, appreciation of nature, fulfillment, happiness and community" (p. 306).

Crawford and Rossiter (1996) identified 10 aspects of spirituality in the lives of children and adolescents:

1. Ideals: The need for guidance about how to manage life

2. Varied sources: Ideals and values come from family, friends, teachers, television, music, film, and screen stars

3. Personalized religion: If interested in religion, they prefer heuristics to prescriptives

4. No perceived separation between secular and religious aspects of life

5. Inspiration from secular sources, such as Amnesty International

6. Consciousness of social morality

7. Question economic rationalism and how it might damage persons

8. Question economic values in times of social stress

9. Challenge authority

10. Conscious and anxious about violence in society (pp. 310-311)

Kibble (1996) defined spiritual development as "A lifelong process of encountering, reflecting on, responding to and developing insight from what, through experience, one perceives to be the trans-personal, transcendent, mystical or numinous. It does not necessarily involve the concept of God"

(p. 71). Kibble added that spiritual development may be enhanced by asking students to share and reflect on the following:

- Feelings of awe and wonder
- Experiences of the transcendent
- Personal concerns
- Religious experiences
- Uses of imagination
- Experiences of things that are aesthetically pleasing or challenging
- Working to help others, particularly the disadvantaged (p. 71)

Three theorists who have contributed to our knowledge of the spiritual dimension of youth are Robert Coles (1986, 1990), who described the spiritual thoughts of and moral life of children, James Fowler (1991), who identified eight stages of faith development, and Ralph L. Piedmont (1999), who developed a scale to measure spiritual transcendence as a personality factor.

Coles's Model of Spiritual Development

Origins

Coles's work addressing the moral life (1986) and spiritual development of children (1990) was born out of his training as a pediatrician and psychoanalytic psychiatrist. Coles was influenced by both Sigmund and Anna Freud, as well as Erik Erikson. In addition, he acknowledged the influence of mathematician and physicist Blaise Pascal on his work, as well as the contributions of Piaget, Kohlberg, and Gilligan in differentiating the moral development of males and females. But most of all, his observations and theoretical formulations were influenced by his day-to-day listening to and prolonged engagement with children and adolescents.

Purpose

The purpose of Coles's contributions was to understand and describe what children think and believe about what is right and wrong and how they want to live when grown up.

Meaning of the Model

Through qualitative study, Coles identified themes about the spiritual development of the person. Rather than analyze the many narratives he collected from children over a 25-year period to develop conceptual categories that could comprise a theory, Coles provided rich and thick descriptions of individual children whose insights and transitions in thinking about moral dilemmas and spiritual beliefs provided an intimate view of these understudied phenomena of development.

In describing the spiritual life of children, Coles (1990) identified the following themes that reflected the spiritual content of their narratives or life stories:

- Ambitions
- Desires
- Hopes
- Fears
- Worries
- Deep despair
- Emotions of guilt and shame
- Meaning in life and death

The children he interviewed connected their experiences to Bible stories, religious rules of right and wrong, and learned rituals of prayer and meditation. Coles (1990) illustrated his belief that children "try to understand not only what is happening to them, but why; and in doing that, they call upon the religious life they have experienced, the spiritual values they have received, as well as other sources of potential explanation" (p. 100).

Coles (1990) asserted that his work was "*contextual*, that it aims to learn from children as they go about their lives: in the home, the playground, the classroom, the Hebrew school or Sunday school" (p. 342). He meant to represent both the secular and religious viewpoints of the developing child. What he found was that many children who had never been exposed to formal religious teachings nevertheless struggled with the same concerns about their futures and the meaning of their lives. Without religious rituals to practice, these children were asking the same questions as their peers about the meaning and purpose of life.

Scope and Parsimony

The model is not abstract enough to meet the criterion of parsimony, and the scope is rather large and vague, having to do with children's concepts of morality and hopes for the future.

Logical Adequacy

The model lacks specific concepts and statements; thus its logical adequacy cannot be determined.

Usefulness

The qualitative data presented by Coles is useful in grasping a fundamental appreciation for the validity of a spiritual dimension of human beings. Religious and spiritual educators have based their understanding of children's faith and spiritual development on the work of Coles (Caldwell, 2000, 2002; Nelson, 2002).

Testability

Coles's work has not been abstracted to the level of formal theory; thus, at this time, it is not testable.

Fowler's Stages of Faith Consciousness Theory

Origins

James Fowler's (1991) stages of faith theory has its roots in the philosophies of Immanual Kant and G. Hegel, the developmental theories of J. Mark Baldwin, Jean Piaget, John Dewey, and Lawrence Kohlberg, and the Judeo-Christian theological positions of Paul Tillich, H. R. Niebuhr, and Wilfred Cantwell Smith. Fowler also notes that this theory is grounded in the ego psychology of Erik Erikson. Fowler and several colleagues interviewed more than 500 people across a span of 18 years, and from the analysis of these interviews, he constructed the stages of faith consciousness theory.

Purpose

The purpose of Fowler's theory was to describe a series of stages through which people developed a conscious awareness of their faith.

Meaning of the Theory

Faith, according to Fowler (1991), is a universal and dynamic human experience and may or may not be synonymous with religious faith. He differentiates faith from belief by saying that although beliefs express faith, faith is deeper than beliefs. Moreover, he asserts that beliefs are conscious, whereas faith may include both conscious and unconscious motivations. Fowler makes the assumption that human beings evolved with not only a capacity but also a need for faith. He defines faith as "a dynamic pattern of personal trust in and loyalty to a center or centers of value" (p. 32). A center of value can be anything that ignites the person to invest time and energy in it (e.g., career, family, sexuality), and it guides behavior. Faith is also described as "trust in and loyalty to images and realities of power" (p. 32). It is a way to sustain one in the face of life and death issues. Another dimension of faith is "trust in and loyalty to a shared master story or core story" (p. 32) of some ultimate and powerful reality. And faith reflects a commitment among persons within a group who share a trust and loyalty to some powerful other or set of values. Finally, Fowler synthesizes the dimensions into a definition of a dynamic process or "an existential orientation formed in our relations with others that links us, in shared trusts and loyalties, to each other, to shared values, and to a transcendent framework of meaning and power" (p. 33).

There are seven stages of faith consciousness, according to Fowler (1991). The structural aspects and stages of faith development are depicted in Table 3.4. Primal or undifferentiated faith begins in infancy and enables the person to differentiate the self from the caregiver and to endure separation from this other without unnecessary anxiety about losing the self. It occurs in the interaction between infant and caregiver before the infant develops language. This early experience provides the framework on which further faith is constructed. Intuitive-projective faith develops in early childhood (ages 2 to 7 years), when language is learned and when the child's imagination and emotions are ripe for developing the enduring images of faith (Straughn, 2003). This stage is congruent with Erikson's (1980) hypothesis about the tension between autonomy and shame as the person begins to form a sense of identity. Mythic-literal faith occurs in elementary school, where the concrete operational thinking of the child is paramount. At this stage, the developing person is able to differentiate fact from fantasy, and the individual may experience a crisis when there is a perception of dissonance between prior belief and new understandings of what is real. Children at this stage of faith development are generally literal in their interpretation of stories and symbols of faith and religion (Straughn, 2003).

Synthetic-conventional faith occurs in early adolescence (beginning at about 12 to 13 years), when the developing person is becoming proficient at formal operations and abstract thinking. The young adolescent is capable of self-reflection and can analyze both past and future circumstances to look for meaning and purpose. The formal operational stage of thinking (Piaget & Inhelder, 1969) also enables the young adolescent to take the perspective of another person, making a kind of mutuality possible. Fowler (1991) argues that the adolescent's "personal relations with significant others correlate with a hunger for a personal relationship to God in which we feel ourselves to be known and loved in deep and comprehensive ways" (p. 38). Again, he draws the parallel with Erikson's (1968) view of the adolescent forming a sense of identity and incorporating "a set of beliefs, values, and commitments that provides orientation and courage for living" (Fowler, 1991, p. 38). The term *synthetic* denotes the adolescent's beginning to synthesize experiences and images and forming an identity or sense of self at the same time (Straughn, 2003).

Individuative-reflective faith occurs after the individual develops a coherent sense of self-identity. This stage may begin by age 17 but may not be completed until the person is in her or his third decade of life (Straughn, 2003). Fowler (1991) states that to attain this level of faith development, the person must be willing and able to reevaluate the values and beliefs adopted up to this time and make explicit, rather than tacit, commitments to these values and beliefs. In the synthetic-conventional stage, the person's identity is shaped to a large extent by his or her relationships with others and the roles that he or she fills within the family and community.

Table 3.4 Fowler's Stages of Faith Development

Structural Aspects	Primal	Intuitive-Projective	Mythic-Literal	Synthetic-Conventional	Individuative-Reflective	Conjunctive	Universalizing
Form of logic	Sensory-motor	Pre-operational	Concrete operational	Formal operational early	Formal operational full	Formal dialectic	Unitive
Symbolic function	Cross-modal	Archetype imagination	Narrative imagination	Associational	Conceptual	Mystic-critical	Participative
Moral reason	Intuition of standards	Punishment-reward	Fairness, reciprocity	Interpersonal expectations	Societal rules, roles, laws	Procedural justice	Universal care and justice
Perspective taking	Affect attunement	Rudimentary empathy	Construct other's interests	Mutual interpersonal	Third-person, systemic	Intersystemic multiple	Transcendental
Locus of authority	Bonding	Attachment, power	Authority roles, relations	Group consensus, charisma tradition	Self-judgment, selective norms	Balance self-judge and reconstituted tradition	Transcends ego-striving, principle of being
Bounds of social awareness	Primal others	Family, nurturing environment	"Those like us"	Composite of face-to-face groups	Beyond tribe, ideological construal	Extended identification in time and culture	Genuine cosmic solidarity
Form of world coherence	Presymbolic, proto-rituals	Episodic	Narrative dramatic	Tacit system, symbolic	Explicit system, conceptual	Multisystemic, symbolic, and conceptual	Unitive actuality cosmological integration

SOURCE: Fowler (1991). © 1991 Jossey-Bass, Inc. Reprinted with permission.

Conjunctive faith occurs in middle age (mid-30s to 40s), when individuals integrate the various polarities experienced in their lives. They recognize that they are both young and old, feminine and masculine, and so forth.

Universalizing faith is the final stage of faith development, and Fowler does not put an age limit on it, but he notes that few persons move into this stage (Straughn, 2003).

Scope and Parsimony

Fowler's conceptualization of the stages of faith consciousness is broad and applicable to various faiths across the lifespan. Moreover, it addresses these phenomena with just the labels of the eight stages.

Logical Adequacy

Fowler's formulation of the stages of faith consciousness development is primarily descriptive. The major concepts describe degrees of spiritual development. Although it is implied, there is no explicit statement that people pass through these stages in the order given in the description. The descriptions make sense and are supported by empirical evidence derived from interviews (Fowler, 1991).

Usefulness

Fowler (1991) acknowledged that his faith development theory has been used by counselors, religious educators, and religious pastors to shape curricula and educational methods. It has been applied in the United States, as well as in several other countries.

Testability

Fowler (1991) notes that there is a sizable body of research literature testing the application of this theory. However, the lack of relational statements in this descriptive theory makes it difficult, if not impossible, to test. Through the statistical analyses of interviews with 60 members of a kibbutz, Fowler (1991) claims that there is construct validity for the descriptive stages. Wallace and Williams (1998) remarked,

> Although not yet tested fully and verified empirically, Fowler's theory of the stages of faith development effectively integrates past theoretical work on identity development, moral development, and cognitive development into a useful framework within which to begin to investigate the family's role in religious development across the lifespan. (p. 462)

Empirical Referents

The Spiritual Well-Being Scale was developed from several sources, including Fowler's theory of faith development and interviews of children and adolescents (Paloutzian & Ellison, 1982, 1991).

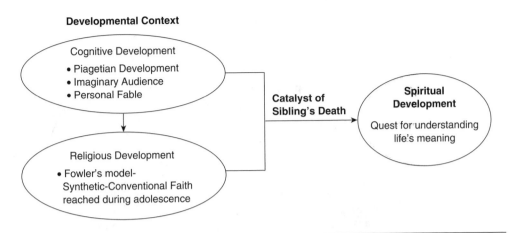

Figure 3.2   Sibling Bereavement as a Catalyst for Spiritual Development in Children and Adolescents

SOURCE: Batten and Oltjenbruns (1999, p. 531). © 1999 Taylor & Francis, Inc. Reproduced by permission.

Related Research

Batten and Oltjenbruns (1999) formulated a model of adolescent spiritual development, which they defined as a person's quest to understand the meaning of life. This model, shown in Figure 3.2, depicts how the loss of a sibling served as an impetus for spiritual development. To test the model, the researchers interviewed four adolescents, two females and two males, 15 to 18 years old, who had experienced the death of a sibling in the previous 2 years. Six themes that reflected spiritual development emerged from the data: (a) a new perspective of the self, (b) a new perspective of others, (c) a new perspective of a higher power, (d) a new perspective of death, (e) a new perspective of life, and (f) a new perspective of sibling relationship (see Figure 3.3).

Spiritual Development and Health-Risk Behaviors

Several recent studies indicate an inverse relationship between spiritual development and health-risk behaviors (Christian & Barbarin, 2001; Donahue & Benson, 1995; Pullen, Modrcin-Talbott, West, & Muenchen, 1999; Stewart, 2001). For example, Resnick, Harris, and Blum (1993) found that spiritual connectedness protected adolescent females from disordered eating and suicidal behaviors. Similarly, these researchers found such connectedness protected adolescent males from reckless driving, drinking, and drug use. More recently, analyzing data from more than 12,000 adolescents in a nationally representative sample, Resnick and colleagues (1997) found that 88% of the participants reported that religion and prayer were important to them. This aspect of their development acted as a protective factor; these youth were less likely than others to use any type of substance, and they began sexual activity at later ages.

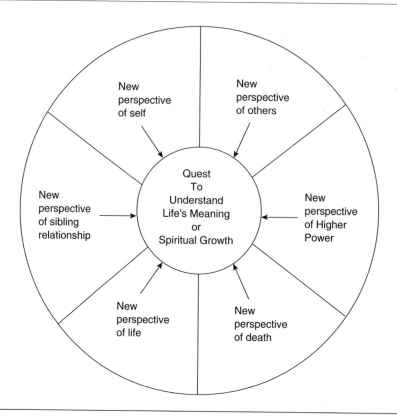

Figure 3.3   The Quest to Understand Life's Meaning and Spiritual Growth After a Sibling Dies

SOURCE: Batten and Oltjenbruns (1999, p. 539). © 1999 Taylor & Francis, Inc. Reproduced by permission.

A study of substance use in a multicultural sample of rural adolescents ($N = 414$) was conducted in the southwestern United States (Hodge et al., 2001). Two hypotheses concerning the associations among spirituality, religious participation, and substance use (alcohol, marijuana, and hard drugs) were tested. Results were that the higher the levels of participation in religious activities, the more likely it was that the participant had never used alcohol [$X^2(4, 414) = 46.65$, $p < .001$]; the higher the levels of spirituality, the more likely it was that a participant had not used marijuana [$X^2(4, 414) = 18.48$, $p < .001$] or hard drugs [$X^2(4, 414) = 20.14$, $p < .001$]. In the discussion of their findings, the researchers speculated that finding different relationships for different substances (i.e., spirituality was associated with never using hard drugs or marijuana, and religious participation was associated only with never using alcohol) might have something to do with the differences between spirituality and religious activity. Specifically, they suggested that because religion is a social activity and spirituality is an internal process, their results might help to explain these relationships. They argued that participation in religious activities and experimentation with alcohol both tend to occur at earlier ages than the more internal, introspective spiritual maturation. Moreover, they noted that use of illicit drugs and marijuana may be more substantial departures from scriptural messages, whereas alcohol use may not (Hodge et al., 2001).

Related Empirical Referents

The study of spiritual development has been limited to some extent by the paucity of empirical referents. However, a few scales exist.

Index of Core Spiritual Experiences

The Index of Core Spiritual Experiences contains seven items that use a 4-point Likert-type scale. The scale was designed as a measure of internal subjective spirituality (Kass, Friedman, Leserman, Zuttermeister, & Benson, 1991). It has a Cronbach alpha coefficient of .90 in adults but only .64 in a sample of adolescents (Hodge et al., 2001).

Spiritual Transcendence Scale

The Spiritual Transcendence Scale was developed to measure spirituality as a source of intrinsic motivation and a way of constructing purpose and meaning in life. The scale consists of 24 items representing three domains: (a) universality, or a belief in purpose and unity in life; (b) prayer fulfillment, or a feeling of contentment related to prayer or meditation; and (c) connectedness, or a feeling of connection with and responsibility toward others. The scale has a five-point Likert-type response format and can be used as a self-report or rater-report instrument. Reliabilities for the subscales on the self-report version range from .64 to .87 and from .72 to .91 on the rater-report version. Construct validity is supported through relationships with other concepts (Piedmont, 1999, 2001).

Purpose-in-Life Test

The Purpose-in-Life Test is a 20-item scale that measures Victor Frankl's (1978) construct of "will to meaning" (p. 29). The scale has a 7-point Likert-type response format. The scale has evidence of internal consistency (Cronbach alpha of .84) and validity (Crumbaugh, 1968; Piedmont, 2001).

Faith Maturity Scale

The Faith Maturity Scale contains 38 items, is criterion based, and measures eight dimensions of the maturity of one's faith. The core of the measure reflects two primary dimensions of faith that are consistent with both Christian and non-Christian faiths. The first of these dimensions, the vertical, is in reference to the personal self, the participant's relationship to a God, and the way that this relationship alters the participant. The second dimension, the horizontal, reflects a belief in interpersonal obligations of social justice and service to mankind. Coefficients of reliability (Cronbach alpha) for the overall scale is .87 for adolescents and .88 for adults. Coefficients of internal consistency were reported as 0.79 for the horizontal dimension and 0.81 for the vertical dimension in a study of 322 adolescents (Piedmont, 2001). There is evidence of validity supplied by three expert panels and development of items from literature and specific denominations. Mean scores for the overall scale show progressive increases from age 13 years to age 80 years and older ($M = 4.03$ and $M = 5.01$, respectively), adding to the construct validity of the scale. A short form of the scale also exists; this form consists of 12 items that balance both horizontal and vertical dimensions of the original scale (Benson, Donahue, & Erickson, 1993).

Bioecological Theories of Human Development

One of the theories that has particular relevance to understanding how adolescent behavior, particularly health-risk behavior, occurs in relation to development is the ecological theory of human development initially formulated by Urie Bronfenbrenner. This original theory is presented in some detail here to demonstrate both its scope and utility. Bronfenbrenner's (1979) work spawned a new domain for studying human change, known as the ecology of human development. The study of human development within the larger context of social entities such as family, school, neighborhood, community, and society was a shift from earlier models that were characterized as mechanistic or organismic. Newer models extend Bronfenbrenner's work and include the bioecological model and developmental contextualism (Lerner, 1998; Lerner & Castellino, 2002; Lerner & Miller, 1993).

Origins

In the preface to his classic work *The Ecology of Human Development: Experiments by Nature and Design,* Bronfenbrenner (1979) describes a snapshot of the experiences that formed the origins of his theory. He tells about growing up in the landscape of a state institution for "feebleminded" persons. His father was a neuropathologist and had both a medical degree and a doctorate in zoology, which prompted him to encourage his son to see the interdependence between all living things. The grounds of the institution consisted of 3000 acres of woods, farmland, and swamp, which gave the young Bronfenbrenner opportunities to interact with all sorts of living organisms, both plant and animal. He could observe and play with farm animals, such as cows, sheep, pigs, horses, and chickens, and he could interact with the residents of the institution, who worked within a protected community where they performed menial labor, accomplishing the business of farming, running a bakery and a general store, and doing carpentry.

Bronfenbrenner also described a faculty seminar in which he and several colleagues set out to design new theoretical models of human development. Through this seminar and subsequent work with some of its members, he developed an appreciation of culture and its effect on field research. He added that his work on the ecological theory of human development was strongly influenced by his realization that human beings were extremely resilient and versatile in their ability to adapt to a variety of ecological conditions and thus to grow in them. He also noted that public policy had a powerful influence on the healthy growth and development of human beings. He continued by saying that researchers who focus on human development must pay attention to public policy.

Bronfenbrenner (1979) asserted that human development was a product of the interaction between human beings and their environments (p. 16). He referred to Kurt Lewin's classic theorem $B = f(PE)$, which means that behavior is a function of the person and the environment, but argued that although most psychologists focused more on the person than the environment, both should have equal weight.

> The ecology of human development involves the scientific study of the progressive, mutual accommodation between an active, growing human being and the changing properties of the immediate settings in which the developing person lives, as this process is affected by relations between these settings, and by the larger contexts in which the settings are embedded. (Bronfenbrenner, 1979, p. 21)

Bronfenbrenner's ecological model has evolved into a bioecological model that allows for the study of the synergy between genetics and environment in the development of human beings (Bronfenbrenner & Ceci, 1994). Moreover, Bronfenbrenner's evolving model has contributed to the emergence of a new discipline known as *developmental science* (Bronfenbrenner & Evans, 2000). Urie Bronfenbrenner is currently the Jacob Gould Schurman Professor Emeritus of Human Development and of Psychology at Cornell University. He is internationally recognized as an expert in developmental psychology and the father of the interdisciplinary domain known as the *ecology of human development*. In the 1960s, the United States initiated the Head Start program to improve the learning opportunities for children from families with low incomes. This program incorporated Bronfenbrenner's model and research findings to date. At present, the Bronfenbrenner Life Course Center at Cornell University exists to "foster collaborative research, outreach, and educational efforts dedicated to understanding the forces and experiences that shape human development throughout all stages of the life course" ("About the Bronfenbrenner," 2003).

Purpose

Bronfenbrenner (1979) stated that the purpose of his theoretical formulation was to offer a new, "somewhat unorthodox concept of the environment" and the interaction between it and the developing person (p. 3). He argued that his new perspective provided a model whereby one could observe the development of an individual within the context of several levels of environment, which he visualized "as a set of nested structures, each inside the next, like a set of Russian dolls" (p. 3). Critical to his conceptualization of environment is the individual's perception of the environment.

Since his early conceptualizations, Bronfenbrenner's ecological theory of human development has expanded to include a behavioral genetic paradigm. The purpose of this expansion was to address the nature-versus-nurture controversy and incorporate genetic potential with environment to understand better the psychological functioning of the developing human being (Bronfenbrenner & Ceci, 1994).

Meaning of the Theory

Bronfenbrenner's (1979) theory of human ecology is highly structured. He presents the basic concepts of the theory, which lean heavily toward definitions of the environment. He provides clear definitions of major concepts (see Table 3.5). Each definition is clearly illustrated with examples from existing research or with implications that can be tested through propositions and hypotheses. Bronfenbrenner also provides eight propositions, which are basic tenets or principles held as true and which can be tested through the various experiments he describes.

Bronfenbrenner (1979) defined the human being's developmental process as one in which the individual becomes increasingly aware of the environment and his or her relationship to it. Hence, the person is motivated to engage in behaviors that maintain or restructure that environment in increasingly complex ways. Behavior, or activity, is not only an outcome of development but is seen as simultaneously the source and process of development. Developmental trajectory is evidenced by the individual's behavior or activity in a series of new settings. Bronfenbrenner (1986b) further asserts that behavior change alone is not evidence of development; rather, observable patterns of behavior that continue across time and space represent such development.

Scope, Parsimony, and Generalizability

The theory is complex, as seen in the number of concepts, propositions, and hypotheses it encompasses. This complexity, however, also suggests that the theory is applicable to a large number of diverse environments. The explicit articulation of hypotheses provides concrete direction for testing the

Table 3.5 Definitions in Bronfenbrenner's Theory of the Ecology of Human Development

Concept	Definition
Microsystem	A component of the ecological environment in which the developing individual engages in a pattern of relationships and roles. The setting has unique physical characteristics and is proximal to the individual.
Mesosystem	This component of the ecological environment represents relationships among two or more settings in which the developing individual engages in activities with others, such as home, school, and work. The microsystem is nested within this mesosystem.
Exosystem	The most distal component of the ecological environment in which both the micro- and mesosystems are embedded, it consists of settings in which the developing person does not actively participate but which affect or are affected by that person.
Macrosystem	This refers to a generalized pattern of organization within a particular social group or culture that is based on shared beliefs of the society or cultural group.
Ecological transition	When the developing person's role changes or the setting in which he or she interacts changes, an ecological transition occurs.
Human development	The process through which the developing individual becomes more differentiated from others and has a fuller understanding of her or his relationship to the ecological environment.
Molar activity	A form of behavior exhibited by the developing individual that is meaningful and that indicates psychological growth.
Relation	The activity of a person within a given setting who pays attention to the activities of another person.
Primary dyad	Two individuals who continue to think of their reciprocal relation to one another in spite of being separated.
Observational dyad	One person in relation to another in which one attends closely to the behavior of the other person.
Joint activity dyad	Two individuals perceive that they are engaging in an activity together.
Reciprocity	The activity of one member of a dyad affects and is affected by the activity of the other member.
Balance of power	One person in a dyadic relation may have more influence than the other.
Affective relation	Participants who engage in dyadic interactions may develop strong feelings about the other person.
Role	An individual who occupies a specific position within a social setting is expected to engage in a pattern of behaviors and relationships with others in that setting.

theory. Although developed in the United States, Bronfebrenner's conceptualization of human development taking place within a social ecological system can be generalized to any cultural group.

Logical Adequacy

Although this theory is not easily reduced to a mathematical model, a few of the major concepts have been useful in predicting much that we currently understand about adolescent behavior. Bronfenbrenner's ecological theory makes sense because there is evidence that human behavior is learned and has meaning because of the relationships among human beings in a social setting. There is agreement among scientists that the ecological theory of human development makes sense.

Usefulness

The usefulness of Bronfenbrenner's ecological model is apparent in the plethora of papers and studies that have been framed by major concepts and tenets of the theory. Many studies of children and adults in ecological settings have been done (Bronfenbrenner, 1986a, 1986b). The theory has been applied to such diverse studies as parental monitoring and its relationship to adolescent health behavior (Jacobson & Crockett, 2000) and adolescent fathers' involvement in the care of their infant children (Gavin et al., 2002).

Testability

A considerable body of research exists to affirm components of this bioecological theory (Bronfenbrenner, 1986a, 1986b; Bronfenbrenner & Crouter, 1983). In 1989, Bronfenbrenner updated his theory with corollaries to the original theory and reminded us that the aim of the original theory (Bronfenbrenner, 1979) was to generate hypotheses, not to test them. In his reformulation, however, he included a testable formula for expressing development (D) as a joint function of the person (P) and environment (E) over time (t = time developmental outcome is observed; t-p = period when outcome was produced):

$$D_t = f_{(t-p)}(PE)_{(t-p)}$$

Research Applications

Parental Monitoring and Adolescent Health Behavior

Basing their study on Bronfenbrenner's model, Jacobson and Crockett (2000) examined the relationship between parental monitoring and various health behaviors indicating adolescent adjustment. A total of 424 students (197 males and 227 females) in the 7th through 12th grades in a rural school district was surveyed. Bivariate correlations showed modest but significant inverse correlations between parental monitoring and delinquent behavior ($r = -.27$, $p < .001$) and sexual activity ($r = -.25$, $p < .001$); there was also a weak but significant positive correlation between parental monitoring and grade point average ($r = .22$, $p < .001$). Both grade level and gender moderated the correlation between parental monitoring and delinquent behavior;

parental monitoring increased across grade levels for males but decreased across grade levels for females. Mothers' employment moderated the relationship between parental monitoring and delinquent behavior and sexual behavior; among adolescents whose mothers worked full-time, monitoring was related to lower levels of delinquent behavior and sexual behavior in both males and females.

Adolescent Fathers Involved in Infant Care

Researchers at the School of Public Health, Johns Hopkins University, used an ecological framework to investigate the involvement of adolescent fathers in the care of their infants (Gavin et al., 2002). Gavin and her associates tested an adaptation of Bronfenbrenner's model that included a new concept of *developmental niche*. A developmental niche consists of ethnotheories of parenting, the social and physical setting, and the psychology of the child's caregivers. The researchers extended this conceptualization by adding the paternal niche and included both father and child in the framework (Figure 3.4).

All data were gathered through structured questionnaires in interviews. Fathers, mothers, and grandmothers were each interviewed in person. In addition, mothers provided some data by responding to questions on a laptop computer. The sample consisted of 181 first-time African American mothers

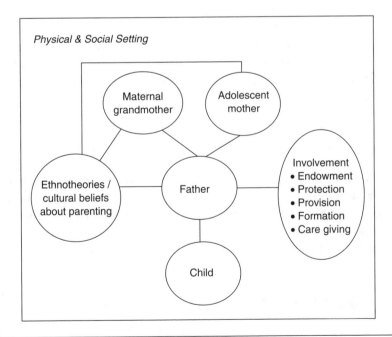

Figure 3.4   Conceptual Framework for the Paternal Niche: An Application of an Ecological Model of Human Development

SOURCE: Gavin et al. (2002, p. 267). © 2002 Society for Adolescent Medicine. Reprinted by permission.

younger than 18 years old who lived in a three-generation household (i.e., mother, grandmother, infant), their mothers, and 109 (60%) of the fathers.

Findings from the study were that the best predictor of paternal involvement with the child was the quality of the relationship between the child's parents. Other factors that influenced this involvement were the father's employment status, maternal grandmother's education, and father's relationship with the baby's maternal grandmother. In the discussion of their findings, Gavin and colleagues (2002) noted that because they used an ecological model to guide this study, the results extended understanding of paternal involvement beyond financial contributions. The use of an ecological model allowed the researchers to explore a concept of "paternal niche" that included fathers in the cultural, environmental, and social systems influencing their behavior. Paternal niche meant that the quality of the romantic relationship between a child's mother and father would affect how the father related to the child. Because all of the children in this study were living in a three-generation household (i.e., baby, mother, maternal grandmother), the father's relationship with the maternal grandmother of the child was also thought to influence the father's behavior.

Developmental Contextualism

Origins

Developmental contextualism is an outgrowth of Bronfenbrenner's (1979) ecological perspective on human development and the view of land-grant colleges that combines the knowledge function of higher education with specific needs of the community (Lerner & Miller, 1993).

Purpose

The purpose of this approach is to explain human development within the context of multiple levels of organization. It purports to provide an integrated and dynamic approach to understanding how human life changes in biological, psychological, and social domains. It serves to advance research that can promote the positive development of adolescents (Lerner, 1996).

Meaning of the Theory

Developmental contextualism is a way of studying the development of human beings throughout the lifespan within the context of various social entities, including family, school, and the community at large. This framework emphasizes the dynamic interaction or *relations* among the various levels of organization extending from the biological to the cultural. Such interactions provide the system or structure for human behavior (Lerner & Miller, 1993). Human development represents a fusion of changes in the internal (e.g., genetic and biological) structural organization and functioning of the individual with the external (e.g., family, friends, social institutions such as school) structure comprising the individual's ecology (Lerner, 1996, p. 781). Moreover, the system of *fused* levels of organization is temporal, reflecting the interaction of the various systems at a particular time in history. Human life and development are based on changes among the relationships of the various levels of organization (Lerner & Miller, 1993). No single factor influences adolescent development; rather, it is the relations among biological, cognitive, psychological, social, and cultural contexts that exert a fused influence on the developmental status of the individual (Lerner & Galambos, 1998).

Figure 3.5 depicts the developmental contextualism view of human development. Children and their parents both develop and change in relation to one another and within social institutions such as marriage, work, and school. Interactions among children, parents, and peer groups of each take place in a particular time in history and are embedded within a community that is embedded within a society and within a larger culture (Lerner, 1995a).

The concept of *plasticity* is critical to this perspective on human development and refers to the "relative flexibility, or capacity to modify behavior to fit contextual demands, shown by a species (or individual) at its most advanced level of development" (Lerner & Hood, 1986, p. 139). As it pertains to human development, plasticity, put simply, refers to the human potential or ability to adapt to change. The process of human development is probabilistic rather than deterministic. That is, individual development is guided, not determined, by genetics but is shaped by the individual's interactions with the environment. Consequently, the adolescent is at greater risk (i.e., higher probability) for problems when multiple changes occur simultaneously. For example, the female who experiences menarche at an earlier age than her peers and, at the same time, changes schools and experiences her parents' divorce is more likely to engage in health-risk behaviors than girls for whom there was not such a confluence of changes. Such an example reflects the concept of *diversity*, which means that there are many different pathways through adolescence. Both intraindividual and interindividual changes are characteristic of normal adolescent development (Lerner & Galambos, 1998). "*Diversity* is the exemplary illustration of the presence of relative plasticity in human development . . . and is the best evidence that exists of the potential for change in the states and conditions of human life" (Lerner, 1996, p. 783).

According to this view, human beings are viewed as both active producers and products of their own development. This happens through the reciprocal relationships of the individual with other significant people in the various contexts in which they live. "The concept of development is a relational one: Development is a concept denoting systemic changes—that is, organized, successive, multilevel, and integrated changes—across the course of life of an individual (or other unit of analysis)" (Lerner, 1996, p. 781).

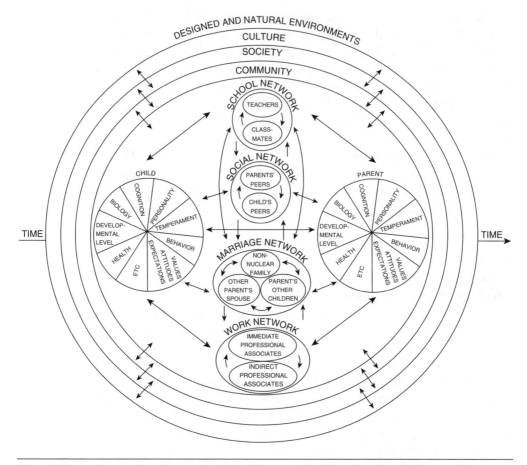

Figure 3.5   Human Development From the Perspective of Developmental Contextualism
SOURCE: Lerner (1995a, p. 31). © 1995 Sage Publications. Reprinted with permission.

The individual becomes *unique* over time because of these interactions and displays unique physical, psychological, and behavioral characteristics. The basic process of development is that of "changing person-context *relations*" (italics in original) with an emphasis on "relations between an individual's development and the changing familial, community, societal, and cultural contexts within which the person is embedded" (Lerner & Miller, 1993, p. 354). Reciprocal change refers to changes in cognition that are, in turn, related to changes in caregiving patterns. Change is interdependent, "changes within one level of organization . . . are reciprocally related to developmental changes within other levels" (Lerner, 1996, p. 781).

Scope, Parsimony, and Generalizability

The scope of developmental contextualism is very broad, yet there are only a few defined concepts. Because of its broad scope, developmental contextualism is generalizable and can be adapted to diverse cultures and target populations.

Usefulness

Developmental contextualism is useful in helping us to understand that it is the dynamic interplay of intraindividual factors, such as genetics and cognitions, with external factors, such as family and community context, that represent risk for or protection from harmful behaviors in adolescence. Lerner and Galambos (1998) reviewed trends in youth health-risk behaviors, including substance use and abuse, sexual activity, school underachievement and dropout, delinquency, crime, and violence and concluded that each of these behaviors represents interactions among intraindividual factors, such as biology and cognition, with interindividual factors, such as family functioning and social controls. They concluded that the model is useful to translate knowledge about human development into programs, emphasizing that risk behavior is more serious when (a) it begins early, (b) it is engaged in frequently, (c) friends are also involved in the behavior, (d) parents are either permissive or authoritarian, and (e) the neighborhood is characterized by poverty and dense population.

The developmental contextualism approach suggests that one can influence or alter change processes "by entering the system at any one of several levels, or at several levels simultaneously, depending on the precise circumstances within which one is working and on the availability of multidisciplinary and multiprofessional resources" (Lerner, 1996, p. 784). This perspective is useful in planning community-based interventions to address health-risk behaviors of youth. Lerner (1995b) summarizes features of successful programs based on this approach:

- Individualized attention to diversity of participants
- Responsive to needs of those individuals most at risk
- Focus on changing the developmental system, not the individual
- Integration of social context of family, peers, school, and workplace
- Collaboration among multiple agencies within a community

Testability

Because of the lack of formal propositions, developmental contextualism is supported by research done in real-world or naturalistic settings. The research approach includes policy development, program design and implementation, and evaluation. This calls for collaboration among professionals from multiple disciplines, community planners, policymakers, and community members (Lerner & Miller, 1993). Also, because the model emphasizes relational changes over time, research questions should focus on interactions among multiple sources of influence and use longitudinal designs. Research should also involve the youth themselves.

Empirical Referents

There are no known empirical referents for the major concepts of developmental contextualism. Objective measures of naturalistic environments and interactional relations are difficult to develop.

Developmental Assets Framework

Origins

The Developmental Assets Framework (DAF) was conceptualized by Benson, Leffert, Scales, and Blyth (1998) at the Search Institute in Minneapolis. Drawing on the concept of community as defined by Bronfenbrenner (1979), the work of Jessor and Jessor (1977) on the social and cultural influences on problem behavior (see also Chapter 4), and on Lerner's model of developmental contextualism, Benson's team applied these ideas to the study of "the human developmental infrastructure" (Benson et al., 1998, p. 142). Citing also the classic work of Werner and Smith (1992) on the resilience of the Hawaiian children of Kauai, Benson and colleagues identified a taxonomy of human attributes that, if present and encouraged, would contribute to healthy developmental outcomes.

Purpose

The purpose of the DAF is to identify the strengths or positive building blocks that all children and adolescents need to be successful, thrive, and move toward achieving their full human potential (Scales, 2000).

Meaning

The construct, *developmental assets,* refers to 40 attributes identified from data collected from more than 250,000 middle and high school students in the United States. These 40 attributes include 20 internal assets and 20 external or environmental assets. The internal assets are categorized as "(a) commitment to learning, (b) positive values, (c) social competencies, and (d) positive identity" (Benson et al., 1998, p. 143). Internal assets evolve slowly over time as the individual gains a variety of experiences. The internal assets categorized as *commitment to learning* include the motivation to do well in school, being engaged in learning, and caring about school. The internal assets categorized as *positive values* include accepting responsibility; valuing equality, justice, and honesty; and acting with integrity. The internal assets categorized as *social competencies* include having skills for making friends, knowing how to make choices and decisions, and being able to resist negative peer pressure. The internal assets categorized as *positive identity* include feeling a sense of control over what happens, having high self-esteem, having a sense of purpose, and feeling optimistic about the future. Table 3.6 contains the full list of internal and external assets.

The external assets are categorized as "(a) support, (b) empowerment, (c) boundaries and expectations, and (d) constructive use of time" (Benson et al., 1998, p. 143). External assets derive from continuous interaction of the individual with prosocial, caring adults and peers within the community and include assets of *support*, which include an array of opportunities in which the adolescent feels accepted, affirmed, and appreciated; *empowerment*, which include feeling safe, feeling valued by adults, and feeling that one fills a significant role within the community; *boundaries and expectations*, which include having adults who model responsible behavior, knowing what the rules are (at home, school, and within the community), and having parents and teachers who have high expectations for school participation and performance; and *constructive use of time*, which includes participation in creative activities such as music groups and youth programs at school or church or in community organizations (Benson et al., 1998).

The construct of *asset-building community* is not clearly defined (Benson et al., 1998), but it is central to the framework. The term *community* is defined as a geographic location with influence on the developing person. It is implied that an asset-building community is a geographic location "that effectively organizes social life (i.e., its residents and its systems) to consistently promote developmental assets among young people, from birth through age 20" (Benson et al., 1998, p. 151). When a community is healthy or is the type that builds assets, the youth of the community should enjoy greater health and well-being. In such communities, residents and organizations such as schools and churches have caring relationships with adolescents. Moreover, businesses that hire adolescents reflect the categories of external assets, such as providing support and boundaries, and contribute to internal assets, such as commitment to learning and development of social competencies (Benson et al., 1998).

Benson et al. describe *developmental outcomes* as follows:

The prevention of high-risk behaviors (e.g., substance use, violence, sexual intercourse, school dropout); (b) the enhancement of thriving outcomes (e.g., school success, affirmation of diversity, the proactive approach to nutrition and exercise); and (c) resiliency, or the capacity to rebound in the face of adversity. (p. 143)

Recent work using the DAF includes the concept of *thriving*, defined as "a state of well-being that encompasses more than avoidance of risk taking" (Scales, Leffert, & Vraa, 2003, p. S23). In addition to a focus on the absence of problem behaviors, the concept of thriving suggests positive development

Table 3.6 The Search Institute's List of 40 Developmental Assets

Asset Type	Asset and Description
External Support	1. Family support: Family life provides high levels of love and support. 2. Positive family communication: Young person and her or his parent(s) communicate positively, a young person is willing to seek parent(s) advice and counsel. 3. Other adult relationships: Young person receives support from three or more non-parent adults. 4. Caring neighborhood: Young person experiences caring neighbors. 5. Caring school climate: School provides a caring, encouraging environment. 6. Parent involvement in schooling: Parent(s) are actively involved in helping young person succeed school.
Empowerment	7. Community values youth: Young person perceives that adults in the community value youth. 8. Youth as resources: Young people are given useful roles in the community. 9. Service to others: Young person serves in the community 1 hr or more per week. 10. Safety: Young person feels safe in home, school, and the neighborhood.
Boundaries and Expectations	11. Family boundaries: Family has clear rules and consequences and monitors the young person's whereabouts. 12. School boundaries: School provides clear rules and consequences. 13. Neighborhood boundaries: Neighbors take responsibility for monitoring young people's behavior. 14. Adult role models: Parent(s) and other adults model positive, responsible behavior. 15. Positive peer influence: Young person's best friends model positive, responsible behavior. 16. High expectations: Both parents and teachers encourage the young person to do well.
Constructive Use of Time	17. Creative activities: Young person spends 3 or more hr per week in lessons or practice in music, theater, or other arts. 18. Youth programs: Young person spends 3 or more hr per week in sports, clubs, or organizations at school and/or in community organizations. 19. Religious community: Young person spends 1 or more hr per week in activities in a religious institution. 20. Time at home: Young person is out with friends "with nothing special to do" 2 or fewer nights per week.
Internal Commitment to Learning	21. Achievement motivation: Young person is motivated to do well in school. 22. School engagement: Young person is actively engaged in learning. 23. Homework: Young person reports 1 or more hr of homework every school day. 24. Bonding to school: Young person cares about his or her school. 25. Reading for pleasure: Young person reads for pleasure 3 or more hr per week.
Positive Values	26. Caring: Young person places high value on helping other people. 27. Equality and social justice: Young person places high value on promoting equality and reducing hunger and poverty. 28. Integrity: Young person acts on convictions and stands up for her or his beliefs.

Asset Type	Asset and Description
	29. Honesty: Young person "tells the truth even when it is not easy."
	30. Responsibility: Young person accepts and takes personal responsibility.
	31. Restraint: Young person believes it is important not to be sexually active or to use alcohol or other drugs.
Social Competencies	32. Planning and decision making: Young person knows how to plan ahead and make choices.
	33. Interpersonal competence: Young person has empathy, sensitivity, and friendship skills.
	34. Cultural competence: Young person has knowledge of and comfort with people of different cultural, racial [and] ethnic backgrounds.
	35. Resistance skills: Young person can resist negative peer pressure and dangerous situations.
	36. Peaceful conflict resolution: Young person seeks to resolve conflict nonviolently.
Positive Identity	37. Personal power: Young person feels he or she has control over "things that happen to me."
	38. Self-esteem: Young person reports having high self-esteem.
	39. Sense of purpose: Young person reports "my life has a purpose."
	40. Positive view of personal future: Young person is optimistic about her or his personal future.

SOURCE: Reprinted with permission from *The Asset Approach* (Minneapolis, MN: Search Institute). © Search Institute, 2002. http://www.search-institute.org.

in areas of "school-work, helping others, valuing diversity, feeling healthy, exhibiting leadership, delaying gratification, overcoming adversity, and active coping" (p. S25). Adolescents who experience an environment with multiple assets have higher levels of thriving than those with fewer assets. A logic model, Figure 3.6, depicts these relationships.

Scope, Parsimony, and Generalizability

The Developmental Assets Framework is broad in scope and generalizable to various cultures with the United States. The large number of assets, however, is not consistent with the criterion of parsimony.

Usefulness

The DAF has been the foundation for work of the Search Institute since 1990. The Search Institute, a not-for-profit organization, was organized by Merton P. Strommen in 1958 to advance the well-being of children and adolescents through the processes of generating and applying new knowledge about development. Currently based on the conceptualization of the 40 developmental assets, the Search Institute, now headed by Peter L. Benson,

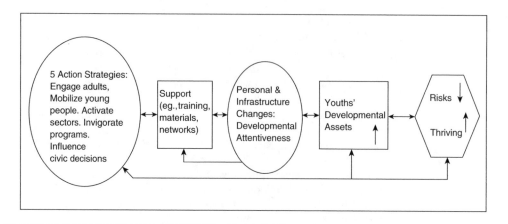

Figure 3.6   Logic Model for Increasing Developmental Assets

SOURCE: Scales et al. (2003, p. S23). © 2003 PNG Publications. Reprinted with permission.

originally focused on research related to adolescents in religious contexts and settings. Findings from the applied research of this institute have been translated into a variety of publications to assist community organizations with improving their developmental infrastructure. The Search Institute also provides networking opportunities for communities through a national conference and on-line bulletin boards, training for community leaders, and consultation ("About Search Institute," 2004). The DAF has been criticized as presenting "only abstract concepts, not tangible products and services" (Lafferty, Mahoney, & Thombs, 2003), thus making it difficult to apply in a community setting. However, the focus on developing strengths rather than correcting deficits in adolescents has been acknowledged as an important shift in thinking about adolescent development and health.

Testability

Blyth and Leffert (1995) conducted a cross-sectional study to compare the experiences of youth in grades 9 through 12 in 112 different communities. Findings demonstrated that vulnerable youth, defined as those with few personal assets, had better outcomes (i.e., exhibited fewer problem behaviors, such as smoking marijuana or drinking) when living in communities with greater resources to support their healthy development. Similarly, those youth with the greatest number of assets did more poorly (i.e., exhibited more problem behaviors) if they were living in the least healthy communities (Scales, 1999).

From a sample of 6000 adolescents in grades 6 through 12, Scales, Benson, Leffert, and Blyth (2000) examined the ability of developmental assets to predict *thriving behaviors,* which were defined as school success, leadership, valuing diversity, physical health, helping others, delaying gratification, and overcoming adversity. The sample was composed of youth from 213 public or alternative schools who completed the Search Institute Profiles of Student Life: Attitudes and Behaviors survey. There were 1000 research participants in each of the following racial or ethnic groups: African American, Native Indian, Asian American, Hispanic, multiracial, and White. Multivariate analysis of covariance of grade by sex by asset level (levels were 1-4, where 1 = 10 assets and 4 = 40 assets) was performed on the seven thriving behaviors. Adolescents with higher levels of developmental assets were more likely than those with lower levels to report more thriving behaviors [$F(8, 5022) = 2.37$, $p < .02$], and there was a significant interaction between grade and sex [$F(24, 14566) = 121.7$, $p < .0001$]. Developmental assets explained 47% to 54% of variance in a composite index of thriving behaviors. There is evidence from this study that the conceptualization of developmental assets has a fair amount of explanatory power for at least six of the indicators of thriving behaviors (i.e., school success, leadership, helping others, physical health, delaying gratification, and valuing diversity).

In a study designed to investigate the effects of service learning in 6th through 8th graders in 29 schools across the United States, Scales, Blyth, Berkas, and Kielsmeier (2000) found that students who had such experiences maintained a concern for the social welfare of others, but students in a control situation did not. The purpose of service learning was to strengthen the developmental asset of empowerment by providing students with opportunities to volunteer and provide community service. Participants who had more than 30 hours of service had higher scores on post-tests of perceived efficacy in helping others [$F(4, 936) = 6.22$, $p < .0001$] than those with fewer hours or with no hours of service learning. Participants who were more highly motivated to do well in school, which they attributed to their service learning experiences, were also higher than all other participants in their commitment to classroom work [$F(4, 931) = 10.47$, $p < .0001$]. Girls scored significantly higher than boys on perceptions of opportunities for personal development within their schools [$F(1, 538) = 4.15$, $p < .04$], sense of duty to help others [$F(1, 541) = 15.77$, $p < .0001$], and concern for the welfare of others [$F(1, 540) = 8.26$, $p < .004$] (Scales et al., 2000, p. 348). The study was limited by a lack of standardization in the intervention (i.e., the service learning program), and parents of participants had higher levels of education than the average. In spite of these limitations, the findings lend support to the developmental assets framework.

Other research conducted by the Search Institute provides support for the cumulative effect of developmental assets. Using aggregated data from 99,462 youth enrolled in grades 6 through 12 (of either public or alternative schools) from 213 cities and towns in the United States, Leffert and colleagues (1998) found significant two-way interactions between grade and asset level. While risk behaviors of gambling, use of alcohol, school problems, and antisocial behavior increased from the 6th to the 12th grade, adolescents with more assets displayed fewer risk behaviors across all grade levels. A statistically significant interaction of grade, sex, and asset level on violence was also demonstrated [$F(3, 88363) = 2.78$, $p < .04$]. Males reported higher levels of violence than females in all grades; youth in higher grades (9-12) reported less violence than those in the 6th through 8th grades; and for both males and females in both age groups, those with higher assets displayed fewer violent behaviors.

Empirical Referents

The Search Institute's *Profiles of Student Life: Attitudes and Behaviors* (PSL-AB) is a self-report instrument designed for adolescents in grades 6 through 12. Developed by researchers at the Search Institute, the PSL-AB was developed specifically to test the developmental assets model. The instrument was initiated in 1989 and revised in 1996 based on data from 254,000 youth. The survey consists of 156 items that measure each of the 40 developmental assets (92 items), as well as indicators of thriving (e.g., school success, 8 items) and high-risk behaviors such as substance abuse, violence, gambling, and sexual intercourse (31 items). The survey also contains five items that measure deficits and 20 items that are demographics plus lifetime prevalence of risk behaviors. Subscales for the 40 developmental assets have Cronbach alpha coefficients of reliability that range from .31 to .82. There is evidence to support the content validity of the scale, and factor analysis supports construct validity (Leffert et al., 1998).

The *Youth Supplemental Survey* was developed to provide a more reliable measure of the major concepts that comprise the Developmental Assets Framework than the PSL-AB, which contains single-item measures of assets. The Youth Supplemental Survey consists of 150 forced-choice items that reflect domains of asset exposure and thriving. The response format is a five-point scale ranging from *strongly agree* to *strongly disagree*. For the thriving factors measured, Cronbach alphas of internal consistency ranged from .63 to .81 for a combined sample of males and females (there were no significant differences in these alphas by gender). For the exposure to assets measured, Cronbach alphas ranged from .70 to .92 for a combined sample with no significant differences noted by gender (Scales et al., 2003).

Research Applications

Using Benson's conceptualization of developmental assets, French and colleagues (2001) sought to examine relationships between binge-purge eating and weight loss behaviors and developmental assets among adolescents. The developmental assets that most strongly discriminated between youth who engaged in these health-risk behaviors and those who did not were those of positive identity. Specifically, those adolescents who engaged in weight loss and binge-purge eating behaviors were less likely than their peers to report high self-esteem, feeling a sense of purpose in life, and having values concerning abstinence from alcohol, other drugs, and sex.

Youth Development Model

Origins

Two commissions are credited with focusing the nation's attention on the need for youth development programs in this country. In 1988, the Grant Foundation Commission on Work, Family and Citizenship noted that our society should provide an integrated approach to the experiences of young people in their homes, schools, at work, and in the communities where they live. The Grant commission targeted adolescents who were not planning to go to college. In 1989, the Carnegie Council on Adolescent Development commissioned its Task Force on Education of Young Adolescents to identify the characteristics of young adolescents (i.e., 10- to 15-year-olds) that would reflect competence and preparation for a fulfilling and healthy future. These two groups produced lists of community resources and associated youth outcomes that emphasized positive preparation for adulthood rather than problem prevention (Pittman, Irby, & Ferber, 2001).

Purpose

The youth development model (YDM) is not a formal theory. It is, rather, a "public idea" whose purpose is to create policy and programs that support the competent and healthy development of all adolescents (Pittman et al., 2001). This model, in contrast to risk-reduction models, purports to promote positive developmental processes, such as competence, connection, and caring, that are assumed to contribute to health and well-being (Benson & Saito, 2001).

Meaning of the Model

The youth development model contains three essential principles or tenets. The first is that youth are not to be defined in terms of their problems but in terms of their potential to become socially responsible adults. The phrase "problem-free is not fully prepared"(Pittman et al., 2001, p. 6) illustrates the philosophy that our nation wants more for its young people than simply the reduction or amelioration of problems. The second principle is that in spite of the critical importance of academic competence, it is not sufficient preparation for the challenges of being an adult. Other competencies that are essential for healthy adults include skills in emotional, civic, physical, vocational, and cultural domains. The third principle in the youth development model acknowledges that in addition to competence, youth need to develop character, confidence, and connections. This principle reflects the notion that although youth may develop useful skills in each of the domains identified as essential for healthy adults, they may misuse or abuse these skills unless they also develop a sense of social responsibility (Pittman et al., 2001).

Additional principles that are evident in the youth development model include the following:

- Youth need a full range of community support and opportunities.
- Youth require full-time access to resources and attention to development (i.e., 24 hours, 7 days a week).
- All community members, not just professionals, are included.
- Adolescents contribute to their own development and that of society.
- Youth with special problems should be free of labels and stigma.
- A comprehensive approach should be developed that includes as many youth as possible.

Internal Structure

The youth development model reflects the three essential principles outlined earlier. The desired outcomes of youth development are summarized by five "C"s: (a) competence, (b) character, (c) connection, (d) confidence, and (e) contributing. When youth develop these five characteristics, they are deemed fully prepared to participate actively and productively within society. The relationships among these outcomes are as follows. When youth develop competence and character, they learn to connect to others. When youth are competent, they feel confident about their ability to contribute to society and often do so through connections with others. When youth are able to contribute to society, they understand that they can make a difference in the world (Pittman et al., 2001).

Logical Adequacy

This model is not at the level of abstraction where predictions can be made independent of the content. However, there is agreement among scientists that the model makes sense.

Usefulness

The YDM is closely related to the Developmental Assets Framework, with its emphasis on developing the whole person within the context of an asset-building community (Benson et al., 1998). The model has been successful in shifting the focus of many community-based programs from deficit reduction models to improving the environment and increasing resources to ensure positive human development. Many organizations have responded to the need for such programs within communities and have developed programs such as the drug and alcohol prevention program of the Boys and Girls Clubs of America. Figure 3.7 depicts a conceptual framework for youth development theory and research.

In a comprehensive comparison of youth development programs with other youth programs, Roth and Brooks-Gunn (2003) found that a greater percentage of youth development programs addressed the five Cs that comprise the expected outcomes of the YDM than did other youth programs. Moreover, these researchers concluded that YDM programs

> seek to enhance not only adolescents' skills, but also their confidence in themselves and their future, their character, and their connections to other people and institutions by creating environments, both at and away from the program, where youth can feel supported and empowered. (p. 180)

The youth development model was used to explore the relationships among familial factors, such as parental monitoring and connectedness, and adolescent behavioral outcomes in a Latino population (Kerr, Beck, Shattuck, Kattar, & Uriburu, 2003). It has also been used to develop age-specific profiles (13- to 14-year-olds versus 15- to 17-year-olds) of sexual abstinence in inner-city neighborhoods in the Midwest (Oman, Vesely, Kegler, McLeroy, & Aspy, 2003).

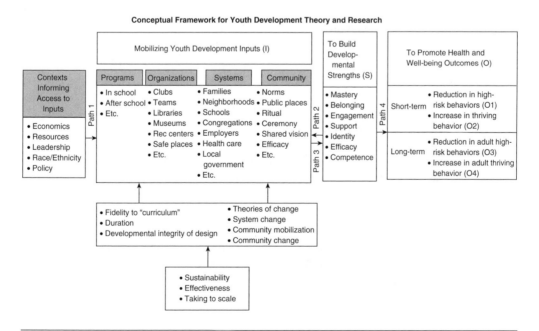

Figure 3.7   Conceptual Framework for Youth Development Theory and Research

SOURCE: Benson and Pittman (2001). © 2001 Kluwer Academic Publishers. Reprinted with permission.

Testability

Most of the testing of the YDM has been done through evaluation of programs within communities rather than through formal research. The Center for Youth Development and Policy Research, established in 1990 at the Academy for Educational Development in Washington, DC, is devoted to creating more optimistic futures for American youth. Their mission is to increase public support that would make it possible for communities to support the positive development of all adolescents, to increase opportunities for youth to develop to their maximum potential, to increase the availability of successful programs for youth development, and to establish comprehensive infrastructures for youth development programs. The work of the center is based on the three principles of the youth development model identified earlier (Center for Youth Development and Policy Research, n.d.).

A 5-year, community-based initiative to promote positive youth development in southeastern Indiana illustrates the challenges and successes inherent in the planning, implementation, and evaluation of a program based on this model (Barton, Powers, Morris, & Harrison, 2001). Key informants were interviewed (total number of interviews = 44) concerning their involvement in the initiative, their understanding of the mission, their view of accomplishments and shortcomings, and their perceptions of community improvements. Positive outcomes included (a) the development of neighborhood family centers that key informants credited with cultivating a sense of neighborhood identity, (b) a summer jobs program for students completing 10th grade, (c) after-school programs for elementary children, and (d) a healthy families action group that included home visitation for families with newborns. Although this initiative did not meet all its goals throughout the community, the community has increasingly acknowledged the importance of involving youth in making decisions about community programs and use of the community's economic resources.

Empirical Referents

The Youth Asset Survey was designed by Oman and colleagues (2002). It includes original items and valid and reliable items from published literature. Using factor analysis, these researchers developed eight youth assets subscales, comprising two to seven items each. In addition to the eight subscales, there are two single-item measures of cultural respect and good health practices (i.e., nutrition and physical activity). Cronbach alpha coefficients of reliability ranged from .61 to .81 for the eight subscales. These subscales and one sample item from each follow.

Non-parental adult role models: "Most of the adults you know are good role models for you."

Peer role models: "Do most of your friends do well in school?"

Use of time (religion): "How often do you participate in church/religious groups?"

Use of time (groups): "You participate in out-of-school sports teams or groups."

Community involvement: "You know where to volunteer in your community."

Future aspirations: "As you look to your future, how important is it to you to stay in school?"

Responsible choices: "You make decisions to help you achieve your goals."

Family communication: "How often do you talk to your mother or father about your problems?" (Oman et al., 2002, p. 251)

Atheoretical Research Applications

An atheoretical approach to examining the developmental relationship between substance use in adolescence and risky sexual behavior in young adulthood was taken by Guo and colleagues (2002). Participants (N = 808) from public schools in a high-crime neighborhood in Seattle were recruited to participate in a survey and were followed until they were 21 years old. This longitudinal design was employed to determine the trajectory of cigarette smoking, marijuana use, binge drinking, and illicit drug use. Trajectory groups were then used to predict risky sexual behavior, defined as a high number of sexual partners and inconsistent condom use at age 21. A method known as semiparametric group-based modeling was used to identify the patterns of sub-stance use during adolescence. Results showed that the distinct trajectories of cigarette smoking, marijuana use, binge drinking, and illicit drug use in ado-lescence were significantly and uniquely related to risky sexual behavior when participants became young adults. Specifically, adolescents who were cigarette smokers were inconsistent in their condom use. Adolescents who were engaged in marijuana use had high numbers of sexual partners and inconsistent con-dom use as young adults. Those who engaged in binge drinking had high numbers of sexual partners. The researchers concluded that interventions to prevent onset of marijuana use and binge drinking in high school may prevent risky sexual behavior when these adolescents become young adults.

Chapter Summary

Adolescence is a socially constructed phenomenon that includes multiple domains of change that occur in the second decade of life. The growth and development that take place during this period are directed by a biological genetic blueprint. This blueprint unfolds to reflect a pattern of change that takes place within the ecology of social interactions. These social interactions are increasingly intimate, extensive, and diverse during adolescence. The complexity of growth and development in multiple domains is reflected in behaviors that may add risk to the health and safety of the person in this developmental phase of life. Health-promoting behaviors that include what we eat, our level of physical activity, and how much we sleep become habits that are learned from observing the behavior of our caregivers. These behaviors are reinforced by the larger social culture that dictates what is normal and expected. The potential for healthy growth and development throughout adolescence does not lie entirely within the individual. Rather, it is affected by the social setting and activities of others with whom the developing person interacts on a daily basis. The theories presented here suggest numerous research questions and hypotheses that could be tested with complex multivariate, longitudinal, and triangulated studies.

Suggestions for Further Study

The theories of human development presented here are not limited to guiding only the study and science of how human beings change over the life span. They have implications for understanding human behavior as well. Bronfenbrenner's (1979) description of the ecological system in which development takes place can inform our study of adolescent health and health-risk behaviors. Many of the explicit propositions and hypotheses of his theory could be tested in longitudinal studies of the activities and social settings in which health behaviors are learned and reinforced from preadolescence through adolescence.

The concept of plasticity in developmental contextualism suggests that human beings are capable of great variability and uniqueness in their patterns of behavior. The idea that human beings are very complex and have great potential for change may call into question some of our tendencies to generalize about the factors within an individual that increase or decrease health-risk behaviors. The diversity of behavioral patterns that accompany development reflects the reciprocal interactions of the changing person and the changes that occur within the social settings in which the person lives. This theory suggests that health and health-risk behaviors should be studied by looking beyond the individual to the context in which that individual learns and exhibits those behaviors. This calls for complex research designs that go beyond collecting data from individuals to collecting data about various social institutions and settings.

The Developmental Assets Framework suggests that the more resources a person has, the less likely it is that he or she will engage in health-risk behaviors. However, this prediction is by no means 100% accurate. Again, if our tendency is to look only at the behaviors of the individual, we may miss important opportunities to understand the part that the environment plays in promoting healthy growth and development. The question of how our social institutions might ensure that all children receive the maximum number of developmental assets has implications for public policy. This framework could be developed further to construct a theory of assets and their relationship to specific health behaviors.

The youth development model expands on the DAF to address the need for social policies that support healthy growth and development. With its basic tenets that youth should be defined in terms of their potential rather than their problems; that academic competence is not sufficient preparation for adulthood; and that youth also need to develop character, confidence, and connections, programs and policies can be developed and tested for efficacy in contributing to adolescent health and reducing health-risk behaviors.

These theories suggest that research questions and hypotheses must be addressed by conducting complex multivariate, longitudinal, and triangulated studies. Simple correlations between individual characteristics and behaviors provide superficial answers to complex phenomena. Thus research models that include interaction of variables and that consider the pathways by which variables are related to each other will enhance our understanding of the complexity of behaviors that occur in this developmental phase. These theories also suggest that longitudinal studies must be done to capture changes over time, which would then clearly depict the process and not merely the outcomes of development. Moreover, triangulated studies that include multiple sources of data, such as the adolescent, the peer network, the family, and the institutions with which the adolescent interacts on a daily basis, are also needed to broaden our understanding of development within the context of social interactions. Finally, triangulated studies that include qualitative (see Chapter 11) as well as quantitative data have great potential for contributing to a more holistic and humanistic approach to understanding adolescent health and behaviors and to building the science of adolescent health.

Related Web Sites

Bronfenbrenner Life Course Center: http://www.blcc.cornell.edu/about.html

Center for Youth Development and Policy Research: http://cyd.aed.org/mission.html

Critical thinking theory:

(Cognitive Technologies, Inc.) http://www.cog-tech.com/projects/CriticalThinking/CriticalThinkingTheory.htm

(Institute for Critical Thinking) http://www.chss.montclair.edu/ict/homepage.html

James Fowler: http://www.lifespirals.com/TheMindSpiral/Fowler/fowler.html

Carol Gilligan:

(Notes on *In a Different Voice*) http://www.acypher.com/BookNotes/Gilligan.html

(Review of the first three chapters of *In a Different Voice*) http://www
.stolaf.edu/people/huff/classes/handbook/Gilligan.html

(Biography) http://www.webster.edu/~woolflm/gilligan.html

Information processing theory:

(Article by George A. Miller) http://www.well.com/user/smalin/miller.html

(Information process theory of learning) http://tiger.coe.missouri.edu/~
t377/IPTheorists.html

(Summary) http://www.educationau.edu.au/archives/cp/04h.htm

Lawrence Kohlberg:

(Summary of the stages of moral development) http://www.nd.edu/~
rbarger/kohlberg.html

(Tutorial on the theory of moral development) http://web.cortland.edu/~
andersmd/kohl/content.html

Jean Piaget:

(Jean Piaget Society) http://www.piaget.org

(Biography) http://www.piaget.org/biography/biog.html

(Genetic epistemology) http://tip.psychology.org/piaget.html

Search Institute:

(Home page) http://www.search-institute.org

(About the institute) http://www.search-institute.org/aboutsearch/

Spiritual development:

http://www.brainprod.com (Brings up nothing)

(Council on Spiritual Development) http://www.csp.org/development/
development.html

Youth development:

(Academy for Educational Development) http://www.aed.org

(Center for Youth Development and Policy Research mission statement)
http://cyd.aed.org/mission.html

(Center for Youth Development and Policy Research projects) http://www.
aed.org/aedgroups/socialchange/cydprinfo.html

(Center for Children at the University of Chicago: Chapin Hall
Publications) http://www.chapin.uchicago.edu

(Forum for Youth Investment) http://www.forumforyouthinvestment.org

(Juvenile Law Center) http://www.jlc.org

Suggestions for Further Reading

Benson, P. L., Donahue, M. J., & Erickson, J. A. (1989). Adolescence and religion: A review of literature from 1970 to 1986. *Research in the Social Scientific Study of Religion, 1,* 153-181.

Benson, P. L., Donahue, M. J., & Erickson, J. A. (1993). The Faith Maturing Scale: Conceptualization, measurement, and empirical validation. *Research in the Social Scientific Study of Religion, 5,* 1-26.

Bloomberg, L., Ganey, A., Alba, V., Quintero, G., & Alcantara, L. A. (2003). Chicano-Latino Youth Leadership Institute: An asset-based program for youth. *American Journal of Health Behavior, 27*(Suppl. 1), S45-S54.

Brown, J. D. (2001). Body and spirit: Religion, spirituality, and health among adolescents. *Adolescent Medicine, 12,* 509-523.

Caldwell, E. F. (2000). *Making a home for faith: Nurturing the spiritual life of your children.* Cleveland, OH: Pilgrim Press.

Caldwell, E. F. (2002). *Leaving home with faith: Nurturing the spiritual life of our youth.* Cleveland, OH: Pilgrim Press.

Dell'Orfano, S. (2002). The meaning of spiritual care in a pediatric setting. *Journal of Pediatric Nursing, 17,* 380-385.

Fowler, J. W. (1996). *Faithful change: The personal and public challenges of postmodern life.* Nashville, TN: Abingdon Press.

Goggin, S., Powers, J., & Spano, S. (2002). *Profiles of youth engagement and voice in New York state: Current strategies.* New York: Cornell University.

Lerner, R. M., & Benson, P. L. (Eds.). (2002). *Developmental assets and asset-building communities: Implications for research, policy, and practice.* New York: Kluwer Academic/Plenum.

Lerner, R. M., Jacobs, F., & Wertlieb, D. (Eds.). (2003). *Handbook of applied developmental science: Promoting positive child, adolescent, and family development through research, policies, and programs. Vol. 1. Applying developmental science for youth and families: Historical and theoretical foundations.* Thousand Oaks, CA: Sage.

Meyer, C. (1999). *Twelve smooth stones.* Kelowna, BC, Canada: Northstone.

Nelson, C. E. (2002). Reforming childish religion. *Insights: The Faculty Journal of Austin Seminary, 117*(2), 3-11.

Rogol, A. D., Roemmich, J. N., & Clark, P. A. (2002). Growth at puberty. *Journal of Adolescent Health, 31*(6S), 192-200.

Saito, R. N., Sullivan, T. K., & Hintz, N. R. (2000). *The possible dream: What families in distressed communities need to help youth thrive.* Minneapolis, MN: Search Institute.

Scales, P. C., & Gibbons, J. L. (1996). Extended family members and unrelated adults in the lives of young adolescents: A research agenda. *Journal of Early Adolescence, 16,* 365-389.

Stoltzfus, J. A., & Benson, P. L. (1994). The 3M alcohol and other drug prevention program: Description and evaluation. *Journal of Primary Prevention, 15*(2), 147-159.

4

Theories of Self

Identity and Self-Care

In the previous chapter, we examined theories of human development, with an emphasis on the person growing and maturing within a social and cultural environment. A holistic model of human development depicted the process of development, which begins with a biogenetic center from which the person develops into a whole through social, psychological, and spiritual dimensions that are then reflected in his or her behavior (see Figure 3.1, Chapter 3).

In this chapter, we will examine more closely the development of a personal sense of self and identity. In addition to the biological and social changes that characterize the developmental stage of adolescence, dramatic and important changes take place in cognitive and psychological domains as well. These changes occur in the way the person thinks and feels about him- or herself. To engage in behaviors that either promote or compromise one's health, an individual needs to have both an objective and a subjective sense of self. That is, adolescents must develop a way of realizing that what they decide to do and then do has an effect on their body, mind, spirit, and social relationships, not just now, but in the future, as well.

Conceptualization of a Sense of Self

William James, often referred to as America's first psychologist, was also a philosopher who struggled to understand the workings of his own mind. His legacy, found in numerous writings, includes a conceptualization of the difference between the objective (i.e., me) and subjective (i.e., I) sense of self (James, 1950). This description of the sense of self has influenced many social and developmental psychologists for the past 100 years (Bretherton, 1991; Harter, 1999).

In Volume 1 of *The Principles of Psychology* (first published in 1890), James (1950) begins with a description of the *empirical self* or objective sense of "me." *"The words ME, then, and SELF, so far as they arouse feeling and connote emotional worth, are OBJECTIVE designations, meaning ALL THE THINGS which have the power to produce in a stream of consciousness excitement of a certain peculiar sort"* (p. 319). He asserts that people find it difficult to differentiate between what is me and what is mine. Thus, he says, one's sense of "Self *is the sum total of all that he CAN call his,* not only his body and his psychic powers, but his clothes and his house, his wife and children, his ancestors and friends, his reputation and works, his lands and horses, and yacht and bank-account" (p. 291).

James (1950) goes on to identify the constituents of the Self as the material, the social, the spiritual, and the pure Ego. The material Self refers to the body, whereas the social Self refers to the recognition a person gets from other people with whom he or she interacts. James describes the spiritual Self as "the most enduring and intimate part of the self, that which we most verily seem to be" (p. 296). Further, James suggests a hierarchical order for the constituents of the Self, with the material Self at the bottom, the social Self (or selves; he suggests that we have as many different social selves as there are other persons who recognize us) in the middle, and the spiritual Self at the top. Without elaborating on the pure Ego, James describes the Self-feelings aroused by the various constituents of the Self. He refers to two primary feelings: Self-complacency and Self-dissatisfaction. These opposing feelings prompt Self-seeking and Self-preservation. James also differentiates between the actual or immediate sense of Self and the remote or potential.

According to James (1950), the subjective sense of Self, or "I," is not the same as the empirical aggregate identified as "me." Rather, it consists of thought and a conscious awareness of being the same person over time. The ability to perceive one's sameness is critical to development of a sense of personal identity.

> The sense of our own personal identity, then, is exactly like any one of our other perceptions of sameness among phenomena. It is a conclusion grounded either on the resemblance in a fundamental respect, or on the continuity before the mind, of the phenomena compared. (p. 334)

Figure 4.1 is a schematic interpretation of James's description of the self. Following his hierarchy, the material self, the multiple social selves, and the spiritual self are presented in ascending order. These dimensions of the self are integrated around the subjective sense of "I" and can be viewed from the objective sense of "me."

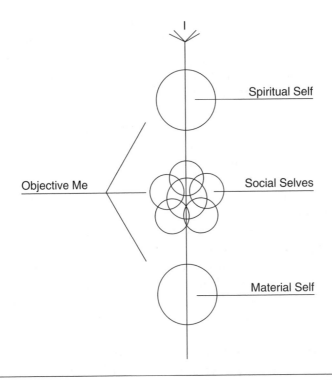

Figure 4.1   A Schematic Interpretation of William James's Conceptualization of the Self

Construction of the Self

Just what is the self, and how does it come into being? It is generally agreed that the self refers to the enduring nature of the individual that distinguishes that individual from others and gives her or him a sense of sameness or continuity over time and space (Markus & Wurf, 1987). Beginning with James's (1950) differentiation of the objective (I) and subjective (me) self, the symbolic interactionist George Herbert Mead (1934) expanded our view of the social self or selves. Mead suggested that to develop the objective sense of self, a person had to develop a representative model from the perspective of another person. Through social interaction, the developing child learns to fill particular roles in relation to significant others in the environment. Later on, children learn to see themselves as objects through playing games wherein, by following the rules, they come to see themselves as they are viewed by the group. This two-pronged process helps the person to internalize rules for social behavior and to integrate multiple views of self into a coherent sense of identity. Thus the individual develops a sense of self out of social interactions as well as assessment of and reflection on the self.

Harter's (1999) description of the construction of the self reflects the influences of William James, symbolic interactionists (including George Herbert Mead), Charles Horton Cooley, and James Mark Baldwin, as well as Jean Piaget and postmodern developmental theorists. Harter asserts that self-development proceeds through predictable stages that begin at birth. She focuses on the way that cognitive changes in development affect both an objective and subjective sense of self (congruent with those of James, 1950). Harter further asserts that the self is both a cognitive and a social construction. The sense of self develops over time, first as a cognitive process of self-representation. Using a developmental perspective, Harter describes how the self develops in a continuous fashion as the person is increasingly capable of cognitive self-representations. Language permits individuals to verbally express their self-representations. Over time, the structure of these self-representations changes. That is, individuals construct a self-theory in which they conceptualize themselves in "various domains of experience" (Harter, 1999, p. 9). Individuals become increasingly capable of comparing themselves to others, of differentiating between an ideal self and a real self, and, in adolescence, of creating many selves that reflect a variety of relational situations.

Psychoanalytic and attachment theorists have shown how the interaction between infant and mother provides a foundation for differentiating self from other. Bowlby's (1969, 1973) view of attachment is that in the course of early development, the infant and then the child develops internal working models that influence his or her perception and interpretation of the social environment. As children are socialized, they develop language, which allows them to change their cognitive self-representations. These changes occur in a predictable pattern throughout childhood and adolescence. Construction of the self proceeds as the person's ability to construct a narrative or life story develops. In early childhood, self-representation of the self is in very concrete terms and may include abilities, possessions, and emotions readily visible to the child and others. Some self-representations may also be "unrealistically positive" (Harter, 1999, p. 41).

In midchildhood, the person's cognitive development is accompanied by the ability to make comparisons between past and present performance. In other respects, the self-representations are much like those of earlier childhood: concrete and positive. In later childhood, both cognitive maturity and increased socialization result in individuals' describing themselves in terms of traits such as happy. Older children are capable of self-evaluation and begin to form a representation of their self-worth. These children are increasingly capable of abstract thinking and are beginning to develop the ability to recognize that they can possess both positive and negative attributes (e.g., happy and sad) at the same time. In adolescence, the person develops even greater capacity for abstract thinking. Thus the adolescent is capable of constructing a theory of self that is valid, organized, internally consistent, and organized in a coherent manner. As adolescents move from early to middle adolescence, they begin to recognize multiple selves who play different roles in different social contexts. They also begin to experience different levels of self-worth in the process of relating to different people. During the middle adolescent period, individuals also become markedly more concerned about how others see and evaluate them. Conflicting roles and self-representations often lead to instability in the sense of self during middle adolescence. As the adolescent phase of development draws to a close, the person begins to focus on a more coherent view of the self, incorporating opposing traits, owning a set of selected beliefs and values, and increasing his or her capacity to perceive future selves. The older adolescent comes "to the conclusion that it is desirable to be different across relational contexts" (Harter, 1999, p. 81). Harter's evidence and conclusion support James's conceptualization of the multiple selves that a person develops in the social context of relationships.

In addition to the cognitive and social aspects of development, the sense of self is also shaped by affective reactions, which Harter (1999) refers to as *self-conscious emotions*. These emotional representations of the self are primarily pride and shame, similar to Erikson's (1980) conceptualizations of the crisis of autonomy versus shame and doubt. Such dichotomous views of the self have an impact on the development of self-worth, the evaluation of oneself as competent across a variety of domains. From childhood through adolescence, each domain of competence becomes more or less salient. For example, in early childhood, cognitive and physical competence are more central to the child's self-concept than are physical appearance and peer acceptance, which dominate the thoughts of adolescents. Also, in adolescence, job competence and romantic appeal become important self-evaluative components in the development of the self (Harter, 1999).

How does a person's representation of self influence behavior? According to Markus and Wurf (1987), the dynamic self-concept contains a variety of self-representations that vary in structure and function. The consequences of self-development are both positive and negative. One positive aspect is that the development of a sense of self allows the person to organize beliefs about behavior and experiences. Such beliefs are reflected in expectations and predictions about the future. The structure of a self permits the person to interpret experiences and make meaning out of them. The self becomes a vehicle for social intercourse as well as self-regulation. The sense of self serves a motivational function that permits a person to identify goals and standards for performing selected behaviors. The process of self-development and self-representation also provides protection for the person. That is, this process allows individuals to value themselves and to pursue goals that maximize pleasurable life experiences (Harter, 1999).

In contrast to the positive outcomes associated with self-development, there are negative possibilities as well. Throughout the developmental stages of life, a person's self-representation may be threatened by either cognitive or social limitations. A person whose cognitive and social development are challenged and recognized as valuable assets will develop a very different sense of self from a person who experiences negative evaluations or abusive treatment from significant others. Particularly in adolescence, individuals may experience conflict among the various self-representations they have developed, or they may be unable to experience themselves as authentic because they have received approval from caregivers only when their behavior is congruent with powerful others' expectations (Harter, 1999). The model depicted in Figure 4.2 shows that self-worth is constructed out of competencies developed by a person in various aspects of her or his life, along with approval and support from significant others.

The concept of self-worth is closely connected to health-related behaviors that may be life enhancing or life threatening. The model shown in Figure 4.3 depicts the complex relationships among perceptions of oneself as competent in various domains, self-worth, and suicidal ideation. This model suggests that physical appearance, being liked by peers, and athletic competence bring greater peer approval and support than parent approval and support, whereas scholastic competence and prosocial behavior elicit just the opposite approval and support responses. In both domains, however, the affective outcomes of depression versus adjustment can lead to suicidal ideation, a precursor to suicide, the ultimate health-risk behavior (Harter, 1999).

Harter (1999) further points out that as adolescents develop multiple selves in response to a variety of socializing interactions, they begin to ask "Who am I?" or "Who is the real me?" Thus the concept of *authenticity of the self* becomes critical during adolescence. Harter notes that concern about authenticity may result in suppression of true feelings, particularly the voice of adolescent women. Gilligan (1993) also recognizes the sacrifice that many adolescent and young adult women have made in "rendering oneself selfless in order to have 'relationships'" (p. x). As noted in Chapter 3, Pipher (1984), in *Reviving Ophelia*, also reflects this identity crisis in young adolescent girls.

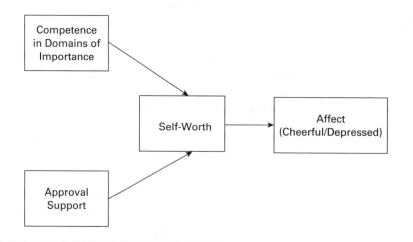

Figure 4.2   Original Model of the Determinants and Consequences of Self-Worth

SOURCE: Harter (1999, p. 198). © 1999 Guilford Press. Reprinted with permission.

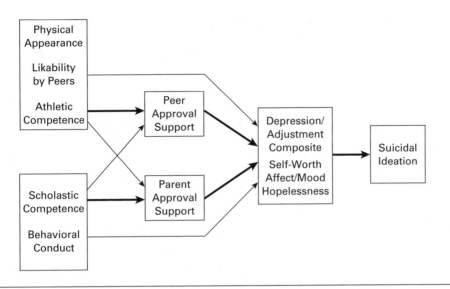

Figure 4.3   A General Model of the Predictors of Depression and Adjustment

SOURCE: Harter (1999, p. 199). © 1999 Guilford Press. Reprinted with permission.

An important aspect of socialization in adolescence is the arena of peer relationships, including romantic partnerships. Figure 4.4 shows findings from a path analysis of data (Harter, 1999) supporting relationships between validation by a partner and perception of one's authentic self in relationship and outcomes of self-worth and affect or mood. The model clearly shows that the perception of validation by a partner contributes directly to both self-worth and affect or mood, as well as to the perception of oneself as having an authentic identity within the relationship.

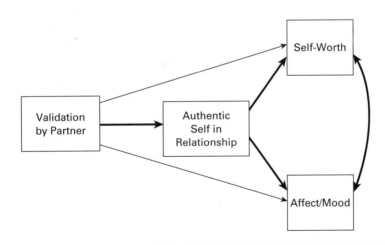

Figure 4.4   Process Model of the Effects of Validation and Authentic-Self Behavior on Self-Worth and Affect or Mood

SOURCE: Harter (1999, p. 307). © 1999 Guilford Press. Reprinted with permission.

Measurement of Self-Concept

The Self-Perception Profile of Adolescents was developed by Harter (1983, 1988) to measure the several dimensions of self-concept plus a global measure of self-worth. The instrument consists of nine subscales (scholastic competence, social competence, athletic competence, physical appearance, morality, friendship, romantic appeal, job competence, global self-worth), each having five items. Internal consistency reliabilities ranging from 0.70 to 0.83 have been reported when the scale was used in a longitudinal study of 248 same-sex twins (McGuire et al., 1999).

Self Theories

A major approach to self-identity as the task of adolescence was established by Erik Erikson (1963, 1968) in his classic works *Childhood and Society* and *Identity: Youth and Crisis*. Other theories that are applicable to the study of adolescent health and health-risk behavior include Marcia's theory of identity status, Grotevant's model of identity exploration process, Berzonsky's theory of identity style, Kerpelman's theory of identity control, and Orem's theory of self-care.

Erikson's Stages of Psychosocial Development

Origins

Erikson was born in Frankfurt, Germany, in 1902 and immigrated to the United States in 1933, where he taught at both Yale University and Harvard University. Before coming to the United States, he studied child psychoanalysis with Anna Freud. Erikson (1968) credited both William James and Sigmund Freud with the seeds of his conceptualization of the development of a sense of identity, referring to them as "conceptual ancestors" (p. 19). His work with veterans of war who suffered from various neuroses and with severely disturbed children influenced his thinking and writings. He was concerned that Freud's psychoanalytic approach did not include the environment and that the ego did not account for organizing one's life around social constructs of ethnicity and history. Erikson was also influenced by anthropological observations he made of the Sioux Indians after coming to the United States. In particular, he noted the identity challenges of their historical identity as hunters of buffalo and their new occupational identity as civil service employees.

Purpose

The purpose of Erikson's work is to describe human development or development of the ego as a series of psychosocial crises. Erikson describes stages of psychosocial development, beginning at birth and continuing through old age and death, as a series of inner and outer conflicts.

Meaning of the Theory

Erikson's work is based on the epigenetic principle, which states that "anything that grows has a ground plan, and that out of this ground plan the parts arise, each part having its time of special ascendancy, until all parts have arisen to form a functioning whole" (Erikson, 1968, p. 92). The eight stages of development are labeled as crises to "connote not a threat of catastrophe, but a turning point, a crucial period of increased vulnerability and heightened potential, and therefore, the ontogenetic source of generational strength and maladjustment" (p. 96). The "vital personality" survives each crisis, "re-emerging from each crisis with an increased sense of inner unity, with an increase of good judgment, and an increase in the capacity to 'do we' according to his own standards and to the standards of those who are significant to him" (p. 92). The eight stages of psychosocial development, as conceptualized by Erikson, are shown in Table 4.1.

Erikson (1968) asserted that only in adolescence does the individual have sufficient "physical growth, mental maturation, and social responsibility to experience and pass through the crisis of identity" (p. 91). He identified personal identity as the process residing within the core of a person and within the core of the person's "communal culture" (p. 22). The process of identity formation involves observation and reflection, which occur simultaneously. As individuals experience this process, they become increasingly more differentiated from others and, at the same time, are able to include more in their own sense of self. Personal identity is "the perception of the selfsameness and continuity of one's existence in time and space and the perception of the fact that others recognize one's sameness and continuity" (p. 50).

Erikson's conceptualization of identity was along a continuum between identity synthesis and identity confusion. Identity synthesis represents the culmination of beliefs and ideals about the self that form one's coherent and consistent

Table 4.1   Erikson's Stages of Psychosocial Development

Developmental Stage	Crisis or Basic Conflict
Infancy (birth to 18 months)	Trust vs. mistrust
Early childhood (18-36 months)	Autonomy vs. shame and doubt
Play age (3-6 years)	Initiative vs. guilt
School age (6-12 years)	Industry vs. inferiority
Adolescence (12-18 years)	Identity vs. identity diffusion
Young adult (19-40 years)	Intimacy vs. isolation
Middle adult (40-65 years)	Generativity vs. self-absorption
Maturity (65 years–death)	Ego integrity vs. despair

SOURCE: Erikson (1980).

view of that self. Identity confusion, however, represents a lack of coherence and consistency in one's view of self. This confusion may range from uncertainty in making decisions to a lack of purpose in life (Schwartz, 2001).

Scope, Parsimony, and Generalizability

Erikson's theory of identity is broad in scope. He applies the concept of identity to social, cultural, cognitive, and moral dimensions of life (Schwartz, 2001). The concepts are primarily descriptive of stages of development and are highly generalizable to persons of various cultures across the life span.

Logical Adequacy

Scientists from a variety of psychological and social disciplines agree that Erikson's work makes sense (Lerner, 2002; Schwartz, 2001). Other scientists have viewed Erikson's concepts as innovative and credible within the context of discovery (Berzonsky & Adams, 1999).

Usefulness

Erikson's contribution to the field of developmental psychology has been enormous. Lerner (2002) notes that his "richly evocative descriptions of the changes involved in adolescent ego development have fired the imaginations and empirical energies of many scientists studying adolescents, perhaps more so than any other theorist" (p. 137).

Testability

The lack of clearly defined concepts and straightforward relational statements make it difficult to test Erikson's theory (Schwartz, 2001). However, the work of James Marcia (see below) has extended Erikson's conceptualizations and created a way to operationalize many of the concepts inherent in Erikson's work.

Empirical Referents

Although Erikson's conceptualization of identity as a central task of adolescence opened the doors for further exploration into this phenomenon, it lacked empirical referents and hence was more heuristic than operational (Josselson, 1994; Schwartz, 2001).

Marcia's Theory of Identity Statuses

Origins

Marcia's theory of identity status originated with the concepts of ego identity and identity diffusion or confusion, which are possible outcomes of the psychosocial crisis or task Erikson hypothesized would occur in late adolescence (Erikson, 1963). Marcia (1980) asserted that Erikson had greatly influenced the field of identity development and that Erikson's delineation of stages of human development was very much rooted in Freud's psychoanalytic theory.

Purpose

The original purpose of Marcia's work was to operationalize the terms of ego identity and identity diffusion found in Erickson's formulation of the stages of human development (Marcia, 1966). Initial research on identity statuses was conducted to establish validity of the constructs and was not intended primarily as a study of adolescence (Marcia, 1993). Marcia's conceptualization of identity statuses has been integrated, over time, into a larger body of life cycle development.

Meaning of the Theory

Marcia built on the work of Erikson and viewed adolescent identity as a social phenomenon. He thought of adolescent identity as making a commitment to an identity (one's place in the world) following a period of exploring possibilities. Marcia (1980) clearly situated the task of identity achievement within the psychosocial theory of ego development as proposed by Erikson. According to Erikson's (1963) formulation, the period of development preceding adolescence is characterized by the crisis of industry versus inferiority. In this period, the individual develops a variety of skills that can later be applied to the vocational commitment that is an essential part of Marcia's identity statuses. Similarly, Marcia pointed out that the chief task of young adulthood, according to Erikson, is intimacy versus isolation, and the individual who has an internalized sense of self or identity is thus able to risk the vulnerability of having an intimate relationship with another individual.

In addition to the polar opposites of ego identity and identity diffusion set forth by Erikson, Marcia elaborated on two task variables: moratorium and foreclosure. The individual in moratorium was viewed as struggling with a commitment to an identity, whereas the individual in foreclosure was viewed as making a commitment to an identity without experiencing a crisis. Marcia identified two independent dimensions of *exploration* and *commitment* as central concepts in his description of adolescent identity formation. He further delineated four categories of identity resolution that he named *statuses,* which are related to the concepts of exploration and commitment. From the lowest to the highest form of identity achievement, the statuses are as follows:

- *Identity diffusion:* The individual has no identity commitment and is not exploring possibilities for a definitive identity.
- *Moratorium.* The individual is in a crisis or period of exploration, attempting to identify values and goals that suit him or her. Commitment, if present, is vague.

- *Foreclosure.* The individual makes a commitment to a particular identity but does so without a period of exploring possibilities, thus foreclosing on an identity that may have been strongly colored by childhood beliefs and desires of influential others.
- *Identity achievement.* The individual makes a commitment to a particular identity after a period of exploring possibilities.

The defining criteria of identity statuses (i.e., identity achievement, moratorium, foreclosure, and identity diffusion) are related to the concepts of exploration of alternatives and commitment as follows: (a) for those in identity achievement, both exploration of alternatives and commitment are present; (b) for those in moratorium, exploration is in process and commitment is present but vague; (c) for those in foreclosure, exploration of alternatives is absent but commitment is present; and (d) for those in identity diffusion, exploration of alternatives may be present or absent, but commitment is definitely absent (Marcia, Waterman, Matteson, Archer, & Orlofsky, 1993).

Marcia (1980) explained that his conceptualization of identity was that of an internal structure of the self, a "dynamic organization of drives, abilities, beliefs, and individual history" (p. 159). He outlined the process of developing this identity structure as beginning with the infant's awareness of self as differentiated from mother and ending with the elderly individual's awareness of self as integrated with all humankind. Thus, identity development neither began nor was finally achieved in adolescence. Rather, the intersection of physical, social, and cognitive development during adolescence meant that the individual had the potential to construct a flexible identity. With a well-developed structure, one would be aware of one's uniqueness and of one's preparation to deal with the world, whereas with a less developed structure, one would be confused and less prepared to face life's challenges without external reinforcements. Marcia confirmed that identity was a dynamic process rather than a static product, with various portions or details of identity continuously being incorporated or rejected.

Identity statuses are flexible and open to restructuring. From a lifespan context, Marcia (1980) envisioned successive periods of exploration and commitment called moratorium-achievement-moratorium-achievement (MAMA) cycles (Stephen, Fraser, & Marcia, 1992).

Identity also has a phenomenological aspect that allows individuals to experience themselves as having "a core or center that gives meaning and significance to one's world" (Marcia, 1993). This inner core of identity may be either conferred or constructed. As infants separate from the mother and recognize the difference between self and other, they also begin to develop a sense of identity that is conferred by others. They are their parents' child, their teacher's pupil, citizens of a country, and so on. When individuals make decisions about what to believe, how to spend their time, what values they want to defend, they begin to construct an identity. Individuals with only a conferred identity are said to hold the status of foreclosure, whereas individuals with a constructed identity are said to hold the status of identity achievement. Individuals with neither a conferred nor constructed identity that is firmly in place hold the status of identity diffusion, and those in transition from no identity, or from conferred to constructed identity, are said to hold the status of moratorium. These varied perceptions of oneself are related to differences in the way individuals with different identity statuses perceive the future. Individuals with constructed identities look forward to the future as something for them to shape, whereas individuals with conferred identities look to the future as having to live up to the plans made for them by influential others.

A third aspect of identity, according to Marcia (1993), is the behavioral. Two behavioral areas that express individual identity are ideology and occupation, and these are related to the process of commitment. Marcia (1989) further elaborated on the concept of identity diffusion in late adolescence (ages 18-22). Based on studies of college students, his research team identified five types of identity diffusion: self-fragmentation, disturbed, carefree, culturally adaptive, and developmental.

Self-fragmentation diffusion is pathological and describes borderline functioning. This type of identity is seen in persons diagnosed with borderline personality disorder who lack a consistent definition of self. *Disturbed* diffusion refers to the individual who is characterized as a loner with a possible diagnosis of schizoid personality disorder. *Carefree* diffusion refers to the individual who has developed many interpersonal skills but is not capable of making commitments to an occupation or ideology. This type of identity is associated with a person who appears competent on the outside but on the inside is shallow. *Culturally adaptive* diffusion refers to those individuals who have skills and are capable of making commitments but who are in an environment that offers few viable ideological or occupational choices. The healthiest of the types of identity diffusion is that referred to as *developmental*. Individuals with this type of identity diffusion have an identity structure and values that should move them into the status of identity achievement, but they prefer to remain in the current state of development rather than moving on.

Scope, Parsimony, and Generalizability

Marcia's model has been seen as both parsimonious and elegant in its simplicity (Lerner, 2002). Archer and Waterman (1990) expanded on Marcia's work and created subcategories of diffusion and foreclosure that allow for greater variability within the four statuses and for greater scope in and predictability of the theory. Other scholars have also extended Marcia's theory (Grotevant, 1987; Kerpelman, Pittman, & Lamke, 1997a, 1997b).

There is evidence from more than 20 years of research of geographically diverse populations that the model is highly generalizable (Marcia, 1993). However, more recent evidence shows significant variability related to ethnic groups (Phinney & Rosenthal, 1992). Schwartz and Montgomery (2002) found support for the stability of the theory in a study of culturally diverse university students.

Logical Adequacy

Developmental psychologists have agreed that Marcia's theoretical formulation has been useful in extending our understanding of how adolescents develop a sense of self (Lerner, 2002; Phinney & Kohatsu, 1997).

Usefulness

Marcia's work "has provided the basis for generating operational definitions of the construct of identity and it has inspired hundreds of scientific investigations" (Berzonsky, 1997; Berzonsky & Adams, 1999, p. 560).

Testability

Both qualitative and quantitative methods have been used to measure identity statuses in adolescents. Using formulae for calculating continuous measures of the identity statuses, Schwartz and Dunham (2000) conducted two studies of university undergraduate students who were between 18 and 27 years old. The results supported the testability of the theory.

Schwartz (2002) conducted a study of 758 undergraduate students (560 females, 174 males, 24 did not report gender) attending a public university in the southeastern part of the United States. Participants were primarily Hispanic ($n = 467$), non-Hispanic White ($n = 129$), and non-Hispanic Black ($n = 74$). Participants were 18 to 27 years old, with a mean age of 21.3 years. Two measures were used to determine identity status and to determine if identity status related to theoretical definitions of identity exploration and commitment. Results were equivocal. Statuses of achievement and diffusion (conceptualized as opposing poles in Marcia's model) were negatively related to one another ($r = -.42$, $p < .001$). Foreclosure and moratorium (also conceptualized by Marcia as opposites) were mildly, but positively, related to each other ($r = .18$, $p < .001$). Diffusion was negatively related to commitment ($r = -.33$, $p < .001$), foreclosure was negatively related to exploration ($r = -.34$, $p < .001$), and achievement was related both to commitment ($r = .29$, $p < .001$) and to exploration ($r = .24$, $p < .001$), findings that support the model. However, foreclosure was not related to commitment and moratorium was not related to exploration. Overall, however, this study does lend support to Marcia's theoretical formulations.

With a sample of 356 young adolescents (6th, 7th, and 8th graders between 10 and 14 years old), Allison and Schultz (2001) used Marcia's identity statuses to classify their identity development. More than half (55%) of the participants were clearly identified as being in one of the four status categories, and more than half of these (62%) were classified into statuses of diffusion (uncertain or lacking commitment) or foreclosure (committed to beliefs and values of significant others). Thirty-eight percent of those falling into the discrete status categories were classified as being in moratorium (actively exploring alternatives) or achievement (commitment subsequent to exploration). Diffusion was found in more seventh and eighth graders than in sixth graders ($X^2 = 12.791$, $p < .01$) and in more females than males ($X^2 = 9.733$, $p < .05$). Grade and gender also showed an interaction effect ($X^2 = 6.335$, $p < .05$).

Significant main effects for grade and gender were also found for the status of foreclosure. Eighth graders more than seventh and sixth graders ($X^2 = 23.892$, $p < .001$) and girls more than boys ($X^2 = 3.616$, $p < .05$) were classified by this status. No significant main or interaction effects for grade or gender were found for the statuses of moratorium or achievement. The researchers concluded that their findings supported the transitional character of identity development, which could be demonstrated even in young adolescents (Allison & Schultz, 2001).

Empirical Referents

Since 1964, a number of nonstandardized identity status interviews have been used to measure the concepts inherent in Marcia's formulation of identity statuses. One form of the interview, the Ego Identity Interview (Waterman, 1983), addresses these core domains: vocational choice, religious beliefs, political ideology, gender-role attitudes, beliefs about sexual expression, avocational interests, relationships with friends, and relationships with dates. Additional domains that are more applicable to older age groups include role of spouse, role of parent, priorities of family, and career goals.

To be used appropriately in research, interviewers and scorers must be trained to operationalize the concepts of exploration and commitment in determining the status that best describes the individual's identity status. The type of scoring used depends on the hypotheses being tested. Identity status interview guides and scoring criteria are available for early and middle adolescents (Archer, 1983), late adolescents (Marcia & Archer, 1993), and adults (Waterman & Archer, 1983).

Another instrument that has been used to determine identity status is the Ego Identity Process Questionnaire. The questionnaire consists of 32 items (16 for exploration and 16 for commitment). Scores are determined from a 6-point Likert-type scale (*strongly agree* to *strongly disagree*). The Cronbach alpha for exploration is .76 and .75 for commitment (Balistreri, Busch-Rossnagel, & Geisinger, 1995).

Identity Exploration Process Model

Origins

Grotevant (1987, 1992, 1997) extended Marcia's theory of identity status by adding the dimension of process. His work had its origins, therefore, in the approaches to identity formation of Erikson and Marcia.

Purpose

The purpose of the Identity Exploration Process Model was to identify the antecedents, components, and concurrent processes involved in the exploration of identity.

Meaning of the Model

The focus of this model is on exploration as the process underlying identity formation. Two major concepts in this model are ability and orientation, which are assumed to be independent components of the exploration process. Ability refers to a person's skills of critical thinking, problem solving, and perspective taking. Orientation refers to attitudes that influence a person's willingness to engage in a process of exploration (Grotevant, 1987).

Exploration is viewed as problem solving that involves using information about oneself and the environment to make choices. This process is critical in the adolescent's construction of an identity. A person's ability to explore options is influenced by personality traits, abilities, and self-concepts. Identity is developed through exploration over time and is not conceptualized as an achievement in any one stage of life. The process of constructing an identity is contextual and develops in response to the person's experiences with family, school, and work (Grotevant, 1992).

Identity is conceptualized as "a sense of coherence and wholeness about the self" (Grotevant, 1992, p. 82). A person's identity is seen as a narrative or life story. This holistic perspective includes those domains or components of identity that are assigned and those that are chosen by the individual. Assigned components include gender, ethnicity, certain physical attributes (e.g., eye color and size), and adoption status. These assigned aspects of identity, over which the individual has no control, are the context in which chosen aspects of identity are developed. Thus a person's assigned identity (e.g., as an adopted child or as a Black child) may constrain the person's development in other domains.

Scope, Parsimony, and Generalizability

The Identity Exploration Process Model is limited to a few major concepts, thus meeting the criterion of parsimony. It is broad in scope because it is intended to address the construction of identity over the life span. Because of the assumption that the construction of identity is contextual, the model is generalizable to adolescents in various cultures.

Usefulness

The Identity Exploration Process Model has been particularly useful in the study of children and adolescents who were adopted (Grotevant, 1992).

Testability

Grotevant's (1987, 1992) model has been used primarily to guide qualitative, narrative research to test hypotheses.

Identity Style Model

Origins

Based on the work of James, Erikson, and Marcia, Michael D. Berzonsky (1989) proposed a process model of human development. The four identity statuses proposed by Marcia were conceptualized in terms of styles of personal problem solving and decision making (Berzonsky, 1989).

Purpose

The purpose of the Identity Style Model was to describe the processes people use to solve problems and make decisions that affect identity. The theory refers to how people revise and maintain a sense of identity (Berzonsky, 1992). It was developed to reflect William James's conceptualization of the subjective and objective senses of self (Berzonsky, 1993a).

Meaning of the Model

Berzonsky (1992, 1993a, 1993b, 1997) conceptualized identity as a constructed theory of self rather than as a discovery model. That is, individuals construct a theory about themselves that is an integration of assumptions, constructs, and hypotheses about how they will adapt and cope with the world. An effective self theory means that a person can cope with information and situations in an adaptive manner. Berzonsky proposed three identity styles: (a) informational, (b) normative, and (c) diffuse-avoidant. Persons with an *informational* orientation actively seek new information, process that information thoroughly, and then evaluate what is relevant before making a decision. If the person receives conflicting information, he or she will revise the self theory accordingly. This process is likely to contribute to the formation of a coherent and integrated self theory. Persons with a *normative* orientation express greater concern for conforming to the standards and expectations of a reference group, such as parents. Individuals with a normative orientation are concerned primarily with conserving their current identity status and may distort or disallow information that is contrary to internalized messages. The result is a person with limited differentiation from others and a rigidity of response. Persons with a *diffuse* orientation tend to avoid dealing with their problems directly, procrastinate, and finally make decisions only when circumstances are such that rewards or other consequences are close at hand. The three orientations are not mutually exclusive or independent (Berzonsky, 1989, 1992).

These three styles of solving problems and making decisions are closely associated with Marcia's conceptualization of identity statuses. For example, persons with an identity status of foreclosure or diffusion have difficulty in processing and analyzing conflicting information that affects their self-representations. The three styles or orientations reflect different social, cognitive, and behavioral approaches for incorporating experiences and information that a person encounters in daily living. Such experiences and information are relevant to the construction of a sense of identity. The selection of style may be related to differences in motivations and in both demands and incentives provided by the environment (Berzonsky, 1989).

Berzonsky (1989, 1992) assumes that the identity orientations operate on different levels: (a) cognitive and behavioral, (b) social and cognitive, and (c) identity style. The primary level (a) refers to the cognitive and behavioral responses that a person makes to the activities and problems encountered in daily living. The intermediate level (b) refers to the way in which individuals organize their basic cognitive and behavior repertoire in daily living. The third, or most general, level (c) refers to the preferred style or strategy that a person employs in response to issues that may affect personal identity.

Identity style theory proposes that people prefer to use different styles to regulate their behavior. Whereas in early developmental periods a person is mostly externally controlled, in later developmental stages, a person has assimilated and integrated a large repertoire of cognitions and responses that reflect more self-regulation of behavior. When individuals incorporate standards and values based on a style of taking in new information and revising the self theory accordingly, they are likely to experience themselves and their behaviors as "being authentic and self-endorsed" (Berzonsky, 1997, p. 350).

Scope, Parsimony, and Generalizability

The identity style theory is parsimonious because it contains few concepts that do not overlap in meaning. The theory is applicable to various stages in human development and has similar applications to both males and females (Berzonsky, 1993b).

Logical Adequacy

The logical adequacy of identity style theory is questionable because, as Berzonsky (1989) states, "These process orientations are not conceptualized to be completely independent" (p. 270).

Usefulness

The theory has been useful in identifying coping strategies used by late-adolescent college students (Berzonsky, 1992).

Testability

The theory has been tested primarily in college students (Berzonsky, 1992, 1993a, 1993b).

Empirical Referents

Identity Style Inventory. The Identity Style Inventory consists of 30 self-report items with a 7-point, Likert-type response format (*like me* or *not like me*). The inventory includes four subscales: Information Orientation, Normative Orientation, Diffuse Orientation, and Commitment. Cronbach alphas for the four subscales ranged from .52 to .77. Test-retest reliability over five weeks ranged from .78 to .86 for the four subscales. Evidence of validity of the inventory was obtained from correlations with measures of personality traits (Berzonsky, 1989). The inventory was revised to contain 39 items (10 that measure information style, 9 that measure normative style, and 10 that measure diffuse style). The 10 items in the original commitment subscale were also retained. Cronbach alphas for the three revised subscales were .62, .66, and .73, respectively. Test-retest reliability for a two-month interval for these three subscales was .75, .74, and .71, respectively (Berzonsky, 1992).

Identity Control Theory

Origins

Identity control theory is an outgrowth of Erikson and Marcia's work on ego identity formation. It also extends the work of Grotevant on exploration as a process in identity formation.

Purpose

The purpose of the Identity Control Theory is to describe the microprocesses involved in identity development (Burke, 1991; Kerpelman et al., 1997a).

Meaning of the Theory

The identity control process consists of five basic components. Two of these are interpersonal (i.e., social behavior and interpersonal feedback) and three are intrapersonal (i.e., self-perception, identity standard, and the comparator). The process of identity control is cybernetic. That is, it is a nonlinear process that involves a negative feedback loop, analogous to a thermostat. When adolescents engage in social behavior (i.e., how they act around other people), they receive feedback from those with whom they interact. This interpersonal feedback is then converted into a self-perception. The self-perception is then compared (through the comparator component) to the person's identity standard. If the self-perception and the identity standard are not congruent, an error or dissonance occurs. This awareness of error or dissonance leads to new behavior with the aim of restoring the previous identity. Cognitive behavior may contribute directly to self-perception, or social behavior may result in new interpersonal feedback. Identity is maintained when behaviors lead to congruence between the self-perception and the identity standard of the individual. If repeated behaviors fail to yield congruence between self-perceptions and the identity standard, the person may alter the identity standard itself (Kerpelman et al., 1997a).

Relationships among the major concepts of the theory are illustrated in Figure 4.5.

Scope, Parsimony, and Generalizability

The identity control theory could be applied to multiple dimensions of the person or domains in which an identity is being formed over time. The theory contains only five major concepts, making it parsimonious.

Logical Adequacy

The logical adequacy of the theory is clear, as illustrated in the primary relationships depicted in Figure 4.5. A number of scientists agree that the theory makes sense (Grotevant, 1997; Kerpelman et al., 1997a, 1997b).

Usefulness

The theory has been useful in studying the career identities of college women (Kerpelman & Lamke, 1997) and in exploring identity among adjudicated adolescent girls (Kerpelman & Smith, 1999).

Testability

The identity control theory can be tested with hypotheses about the relationships among the concepts within it.

The Identity Control Process

Social behavior "→" Interpersonal Feedback

Social behavior "→" Self-perception

Self-perception "→" Comparator "↔" Identity Standard

Self-perception ≈ Identity Standard "→" Identity Maintained

Self-perception < Identity Standard "→" New Behavior

Figure 4.5   Relationships in the Identity Control Process

Empirical Referents

Ego Identity Process Questionnaire. The Ego Identity Process Questionnaire is a 32-item, self-report inventory that assesses dimensions of exploration and commitment in eight areas: sex roles, politics, occupation, religion, dating, friendships, family, and values. Content validity was established through review of literature and expert agreement on the dimensions. Further validity was supported through confirmatory factor analysis yielding a two-factor solution. Twenty items on the questionnaire are worded positively, and the remaining 12 items are worded negatively; the 12 negatively worded items are reverse-scored. Responses are given on a six-point, Likert-type scale (*strongly agree* to *strongly disagree*). A kappa coefficient of agreement among five experts was .76 ($p < .01$). Reliability coefficients ranged from .75 to .90 for the commitment subscale and .76 for exploration (Balistreri et al., 1995).

Sexual Identity

Gender Identity

Throughout childhood, males and females learn to assign gender to themselves and others. Gender assignment at birth is generally made by observation of external genitalia, but sometimes this assignment is not straightforward and genetic material must be considered. For the majority of persons, however, the gender assigned at birth is the one with which the child begins to associate the sense of self. Socialization also plays a big part in the cognitive and emotional components of gender identity. Gender identity disorder is a diagnosable condition in which the child has a strong and persistent desire to be the opposite sex (Perrin, 2002). Boys often prefer to wear girls' clothing and girls insist on wearing clothes that are typically designed for boys. These children also show persistent fantasies of being a person of the opposite sex and tend to play the stereotypical games of the opposite sex. Unlike their peers who prefer to play with children of their own sex, these children prefer playmates who are not of the same sex. In adolescence, this disorder may be manifested by frequent passing as a member of the other sex and continued conviction that the person is a member of the other sex. This disturbance is not concurrent with an inter-sex condition and causes significant distress and difficulty in social areas of functioning (American Psychiatric Association, 1994).

Sexual Orientation Identity

Sexual orientation identity formation is the developmental process of recognizing that one is attracted to the opposite or same gender (Patterson,

1995). Among gay, lesbian, and bisexual youth, this process, which is known as "coming out," reflects changes in development status. Although this process is not clearly explicated for heterosexual youth, several models have been offered to hypothesize developmental stages experienced by adolescents who are gay, lesbian, or bisexual. One model consists of four stages: (a) *sensitization,* which usually begins in childhood or early adolescence as the person initially becomes aware of an attraction to same-sex individuals; (b) *identity confusion,* which occurs following a period of identity exploration that reflects inner turmoil as the person recognizes the stigma attached to such an identity; (c) *identity assumption,* which occurs following initiation of sexual experiences with partners of the same gender and includes limited disclosure of the orientation; and (d) *commitment,* which occurs when the individual accepts his or her sexual identity and proceeds to live with it (Troiden, 1989).

Troiden (1989) identified six states in homosexual identity formation: identity confusion, identity comparison, identity tolerance, identity acceptance, identity pride, and identity synthesis. This model was supported by findings from a study of 118 women over the age of 18 years who self-identified as lesbian. Participants in the study were found to move through the stages in the predicted order (Levine, 1997).

Although proposed models of sexual orientation identity formation suggest a linear development of this identity, researchers have shown that a developmental sequence of coming-out events occurs with much variation in adolescence and early adulthood (Floyd & Stein, 2002). These findings suggest that social context, including independence from parents, plays an important role in delaying the trajectory of this developmental sequence. Similarly, social alienation may prevent many questioning youth from integrating their emerging sexual awareness into a solid self-identity (Ryan & Futterman, 2001; Sullivan & Wodarski, 2002). Feeling a need to hide their true identity, nonheterosexual youth may become isolated and fearful in social situations. Those youth at most risk for not disclosing this identity are those whose families are abusive or lack cohesion and youth who have low self-esteem and limited ability to cope with hostility (Harrison, 2003).

Graber, Brooks-Gunn, and Galen (1998) noted that sexuality is a critical and normal aspect of adolescent development. In their words, "development of a sexual sense of self occurs prior to first intercourse as well as after this event; furthermore, the potential for the redefinition of self and the role that sexuality plays in it exists throughout the life course" (p. 272). Graber and colleagues argued that scholars focus too much on sexual intercourse as a defining behavior, a problem behavior, or a risky behavior; that it is taken out of context. They urged researchers in multiple disciplines to examine adolescent sexuality within the multiple domains of adolescents' lives. They also emphasized that program planners should focus on health promotion interventions rather than on preventing intercourse. This approach will be discussed in detail in Chapter 9.

Self-Identity and Sexual Diversity

In a study of 72 gay, lesbian, and bisexual youth (36 males and 36 females, 16-27 years old), Floyd and Stein (2002) identified five patterns of emerging self-awareness. Participants were recruited through flyers, announcements, and newspaper and community bulletin board advertisements in two communities, one in the Midwest and the other in the southeastern United States. Participants were interviewed and provided additional survey data on milestone events related to coming out, current social immersion, sexual orientation, comfort with orientation, emotional distress, and self-esteem. Milestone events occurred in predictable stages. Awareness about same-gender attraction occurred much earlier, on average, than disclosure or engaging in a serious same-gender relationship. The findings showed wide diversity in timing of coming out. Those with early trajectories from awareness to disclosure were more likely to be comfortable with current social immersion in sexual diversity experiences and with their identity. Those with later trajectories and who were not well connected to gay, lesbian, or bisexual networks were least comfortable with their sexual orientation identity. Overall, most of the participants had low levels of emotional distress and high levels of self-esteem.

Sexual Orientation Identity and Behavior

The process of sexual identity, particularly among gay, lesbian, and bisexual persons, influences the adolescent's behavior. Rosario, Hunter, Maguen, Gwadz, and Smith (2001) interviewed 156 gay, lesbian, and bisexual youth who were between 14 and 21 years old ($M = 18.3 \pm 1.65$ years). They conceptualized the coming-out process as one of identity formation and integration, reflecting an acceptance of one's sexual orientation and a willingness to disclose this to other people. These researchers eschewed a stage model because of their belief that this process of identity is multidimensional (e.g., attitudinal, cognitive, and behavioral), and that as a developmental process, it occurs in slightly different ways among individuals. In their study, they found that those youth who had limited involvement in gay and lesbian group activities and who held negative attitudes toward homosexuality were more distressed than their peers and engaged in more risky sexual behaviors.

Empirical Referent

The Multidimensional Sexual Self-Concept Questionnaire (Snell, 1998) is a self-report measure of 20 psychological dimensions of human sexuality: sexual anxiety, sexual self-efficacy, sexual consciousness, motivation to avoid risky sex, chance or luck regarding sexual control, sexual preoccupation, sexual assertiveness, sexual optimism, self-blame concerning sexual problems, sexual monitoring, sexual motivation, sexual problem management, sexual esteem, sexual satisfaction, power-other sexual control, sexual self-schemata, fear of sex, sexual problem prevention, sexual depression, and internal sexual control. This questionnaire contains 100 items with a five-point Likert-type response format. Each dimension forms a subscale with Cronbach alphas ranging from .72 to .94. Validity of the questionnaire was supported in a study of university students.

Racial and Ethnic Identity

A vital dimension of the developing person is that of racial and ethnic identity. In American society, many adolescents must deal with being members of racial or ethnic minority cultures. Thus they must forge an identity out of their experiences and perceptions of the culture of society at large and of their specific ethnic or racial group. In a review of the literature pertaining to ethnic identity and mental health outcomes in African American and Hispanic adolescents, Greig (2003) found that adolescents who strongly identified with their own ethnic culture had higher levels of self-esteem and stronger indicators of mental health than those who were less strongly identified. She also found some evidence that ethnic identity may be a protective factor for health-risk behaviors such as substance abuse.

Ethnic identity has been conceptualized in many different ways and has been studied by scholars from many different disciplines. The concept has meaning "only in situations in which two or more ethnic groups are in contact over a period of time" (Phinney, 1990, p. 501). If a society is racially and ethnically homogeneous, the concept has no meaning. Ethnic identity thus reflects a social construction that permits groups of people to share an identity with others and to use these others as a reference for their own behavior (Niemann, Romero, Arredondo, & Rodriguez, 1999). The term *ethnic identity* has sometimes been used interchangeably with *acculturation*, but these are two distinctly different concepts. The former refers to how much an individual retains and reflects the major values of her or his own ethnic culture, whereas the latter refers to how much an individual adapts to and reflects the major values of the dominant culture. Both of these concepts are dynamic, suggesting transitions or changes that occur over time and in response to contexts. Ethnic identity consists of one's identity as a member of a specific ethnic group, feeling a sense of belonging and commitment to that group, having shared values and traditions, and sharing a language and various other customs associated with that ethnic group (Phinney & Rosenthal, 1992). A stage approach to ethnic identity formation views the progression from an unexamined identity through a process of exploration, and culminating with a committed identity (Phinney, 1990; Phinney & Kohatsu, 1997).

Racial/Cultural Identity Development Model

In addition to the models of human identity development described earlier, adolescents from minority racial and ethnic groups must also engage in a process of self-identity that incorporates their racial or ethnic culture. As Sue and Sue (1990) assert, many such models of identity begin with the experience of oppression from the larger society. These scholars propose a five-stage model called the Racial/Cultural Identity Development Model. Each stage is characterized by attitude toward self, attitude toward others of the same minority group, attitude toward others of different minority groups, and attitude toward the dominant group. Stage 1 is *conformity:* The minority person is characterized by a solid preference for the dominant culture over his or her own. In this stage, the person's attitude toward self is often self-deprecating; taking on the values and beliefs of the minority culture is viewed with disdain, and adherence to those of the majority culture is sought. In this stage, the person also tends to view individuals from other minority cultures negatively and acts as if the dominant culture is superior. In Stage 2, *dissonance,* individuals are increasingly aware that an attitude of racism exists. In this stage, they begin to develop an appreciation for their own racial or ethnic culture, as well as for those of other minority groups. Moreover, they also become increasingly aware that many of the values and beliefs of the dominant culture are not advantageous to themselves.

Stage 3 is called the stage of *resistance and immersion.* Individuals begin to appreciate their own developing attitudes and beliefs and their historical roots. They begin to have a stronger sense of identity with their cultural group and develop empathy for individuals from other cultural minorities. Their view of the dominant culture is marked by increasing distrust and dislike. In Stage 4, *introspection,* individuals begin to experience discomfort with the rigidity of views espoused in Stage 3. They begin to search for an individual identity rather than a group identity. In this stage, individuals may experience peer pressure to remain loyal to the minority culture even if it means going against their personal perspective. In this stage, they begin to display concern with ethnocentrism and the tendency to use this in judging others; they also begin to reevaluate their view of the dominant culture. In the final stage, *integrative awareness,* minority adolescents reconcile the positive and negative aspects of both minority and dominant cultures. Attitudes and beliefs toward the self are positive and include racial pride as well as a strong sense of autonomy; they become bi- or multicultural. They take pride in their own racial, ethnic, or cultural group; appreciate the beliefs and values of other minority groups; and are open to constructive components of the dominant culture. Sue and Sue (1990) reiterate that identity development is a dynamic process, and a person may not proceed through the process in a predictable, linear fashion.

Optimal Theory Applied to the Identity Development Model

The process of self-identity typically begins with a child's acceptance of stereotypes held by mainstream society (Sevig, Highlen, & Adams, 2000). Such stereotypes reflect biases and prejudices held by both majority and minority racial and ethnic groups, including biases and prejudices between minority groups. The Optimal Theory Applied to Identity Development (OTAID; Myers et al., 1991) is based on a holistic view of the unity of matter and spirit and the inherent value of persons. This theory asserts that development within the American culture contributes to feelings of low self-worth because of prevailing attitudes such as racism, ageism, and sexism. The developing human being must deconstruct an internalized hierarchical system of prejudices through expansive processes of self-discovery and self-knowledge (Sevig et al., 2000).

According to the OTAID, people are born with an absence of conscious awareness: They do not feel a separate sense of self. Through a process of individuation, developing children experience themselves as separate yet connected to the basic tenets of society. With subsequent experiences of exclusion or discrimination, the developing person begins to feel a sense of dissonance or alienation, particularly if the person is a member of a minority population. Over time, individuals internalize their subgroup's identity into their own self-concept. With optimal identity development, the individual is aware of the social constraints of American culture and chooses to embrace differences. Through a process of transformation, the developing individual consciously recognizes the interrelatedness of life, and the self is defined in a holistic sense (see Myers et al., 1991).

Empirical Referent

The Self-Identity Inventory was developed to measure identity development in oppressed groups and in those with multiple identities (Sevig et al., 2000). Items were generated to fit the OTAID model. The inventory consists of two parts. Part I asks respondents to describe their identities. Part II consists of 195 items, with a six-point, Likert-type format (1 = *strongly disagree*, 6 = *strongly agree*). Construct validity was supported by confirmatory factor analysis, goodness-of-fit indexes, and correlations among subscales. Cronbach alpha coefficients of reliability ranged from .72 to .90 for the subscales.

Identity and Health-Risk Behaviors

The relationship between a sense of personal identity and health-risk behaviors has not been studied a great deal. Stein, Roeser, and Markus (1998) studied the relationships between risky behaviors and three dimensions of the self-concept: the popular, the conventional, and the deviant. The sample consisted of 160 adolescents recruited from one public junior high school in a suburban area. The mean age of the participants was 13.5 ± 0.6 years, 50% were female, 13% were African American, 83% were White, 3% were other races not specified, and 1% did not provide this information. Data were gathered in two waves, 1 year apart. Participants were in eighth grade for the first wave and ninth grade for the second wave. The ninth-grade sample consisted of 137 participants, owing to attrition. Among eighth graders, scores on all self-schema and possible selves were significantly correlated with the composite of risky behaviors (alcohol and tobacco use, sexual intercourse, and poor school performance). Conventional and corresponding possible self-schema were negatively correlated with risky behaviors, whereas deviant and popular self-schema, along with their corresponding possible selves, were positively correlated. Among ninth graders, patterns of relationships were similar in direction and magnitude except for the possible self component of the conventional self-schema. Through multiple correlational analyses, Stein and colleagues demonstrated that the relationship between self-concept and risky behaviors was bidirectional. They concluded that not only do the various self-schemas and possible selves predict future risky behavior, the risky behaviors predict self-concept, such that it has a more permanent structure.

Orem's Self-Care Theory

Origins

One theory of self-care had its origins in the discipline of nursing in the late 1950s and 1960s when Dorothea Orem described the human being's universal requirement for self-care action (Orem, 1971, 1980, 1985, 1991, 2001). The concept of self-care may also be found much earlier in the writings of Florence Nightingale (1946), who is celebrated as the founder of modern professional nursing. Nightingale believed in the ability of human beings to take care of themselves and to cooperate with nature in the healing process. Even in the preface to her classic work *Notes on Nursing: What It Is and What It Is Not,* Nightingale penned these words: "I do not pretend to teach her [every woman] how, I ask her to teach herself, and for this purpose I venture to give her some hints." In the conclusion to her small masterpiece, she noted, "And what nursing has to do in either case, is to put the patient in the best condition for nature to act upon him" (p. 75). In detailing her comments about the management of the ill, Nightingale wrote,

> Whatever a patient *can* do for himself, it is better, i.e. less anxiety, for him to do for himself. . . . It is evidently much less exertion for a patient to answer a letter for himself by return of post, than to have four conversations, wait five days, have six anxieties before it is off his mind, before the person who is to answer it has done so. (p. 22)

Orem's conceptualizations were influenced by Kurt Lewin's (1951) field theory. She found this theory applicable to nurses' understanding of human development and functioning within the social and cultural contexts in which persons lived. Her theory also reflected Helson's (1964) theory of adaptation and Allport's (1955, 1965) approach to personality development. Orem developed three interrelated theories: theory of nursing system, theory of self-care deficit, and theory of self-care. The theory of nursing system subsumes the theory of self-care deficit, which subsumes the theory of self-care (Orem, 1991, 2001). Only the theory of self-care will be presented here because it has the most general application to understanding adolescent health and health-risk behavior.

Purpose

The purpose of Orem's theories of self-care was to define nursing's phenomena of concern and to explain how nurses address human limitations by serving others, providing care that they are unable to give themselves, and promoting their health and self-sufficiency (Orem, 1991).

Meaning of the Theory

Orem observed that in the process of developing, maturing persons learn how to act toward themselves and toward the environment in ways that enable them to survive and thrive. The term *self* has a holistic meaning, as it refers to the person's "*whole being*" (Orem, 1991, p. 117). The theory of self-care is based on four presuppositions:

1. All things being equal, human beings have the potential to develop intellectual and practical skills and maintain the motivation essential for self-care and care of dependent family members.

2. Ways of meeting self-care requisites are culture elements and vary with individuals and larger social groups.

3. Self-care and care of dependent family members are forms of deliberate action, dependent for performance on individuals' action repertoires, and their predilection for taking action under certain circumstances.

4. Identifying and describing recurring requisites for self-care and the care of dependent family members lead to investigating and developing ways to meet known requisites and to form care habits. (Orem, 1991, p. 69)

Self-care is defined as "the personal care that individuals require each day to regulate their own functioning and development" (Orem, 1991, p. 3). Self-care is also conceptualized as a deliberate or purposeful action taken with some measure of effectiveness or success. The concept of self-care means not only to care for and about oneself but to give care to oneself. Over time, the actions taken by a person to maintain health are understood as a self-care system. Self-care behavior is influenced by the person's self-concept and stage of development or maturity. Moreover, it is affected by culture, by position within the family, by social position, and by scientific knowledge about health (Orem, 1991, 2001).

Self-care agency refers to the power and motivation a person has to regulate those factors that influence healthy functioning and development and engage in self-care behaviors. A self-care agent may also provide care to another person who depends on them (e.g., an infant, a young child, or a disabled person unable to meet his or her own needs). A self-care agent uses knowledge, skills, and resources that are learned within the context of a culture such as family, community, or scientific discipline. Self-care actions reflect the habits and beliefs of these various cultures, which also influence the motivation to continue behaviors that promote survival and development. The self-care agent also engages in investigation and decision making (Orem, 1991, 2001).

Self-care requisites are the actions required of persons to maintain life and health. There are three types of requisites: universal, developmental, and health deviation. Assumptions are that (a) persons have common needs for survival (e.g., air, food, water), (b) persons require conditions to promote healthy development through the life span, and (c) genetic and other deviations from normal human structure and function may be prevented or regulated through human action. There are eight universal self-care requisites:

1. Maintaining sufficient intake of air

2. Maintaining sufficient intake of water

3. Maintaining sufficient intake of food and nutrients

4. Provision for elimination and excrement

5. Maintaining balance between physical activity and rest

6. Maintaining balance between social interaction and solitude

7. Preventing hazards to life, functioning, and well-being

8. Promoting life and development within society and within the limitations and potential of the individual. (Orem, 1991, p. 126)

Developmental self-care requisites are of two types: (a) promoting and maintaining life processes and development and (b) providing care when conditions exist that can adversely affect development (e.g., terminal illness, loss of significant others, educational or social deprivation). The first developmental self-care requisites are those required during fetal development, infancy, and stages of later development. Health-deviation self-care requisites are those that exist for persons who have suffered an injury, illness, or disability (Orem, 1991, 2001).

Therapeutic self-care demand is a calculation of the relationship between a person's needs and capabilities in surviving or maintaining health. The demand is greatest when the person is unable to meet the basic needs for survival (e.g., unable to breathe or to obtain water, food, or shelter). The demand is least when the person is able and motivated not only to meet basic needs for survival but to engage in behaviors that promote health and well-being (Berbiglia, 1997). Self-care practices are therapeutic only when they support life and normal functioning; maintain healthy growth and development; prevent injury, disease, and disability; and promote well-being.

Self-care deficit occurs when a person's capacity for self-care behavior is not sufficient to meet her or his therapeutic self-care demand. This deficit status may be partial or complete, displaying a continuum of variation.

> [Dependent-care agency] is the complex acquired ability of mature or maturing persons to know and meet some or all of the self-care requisites of adolescent or adult persons who have health-derived or health-associated limitations of self-care agency, which places them in socially dependent relationships for care. (Orem, 1991, p. 175)

This concept has particular application to persons who have chronic or disabling conditions.

Scope, Parsimony, and Generalizability

Orem's self-care theory has relatively few concepts and addresses many of the health-related needs and behaviors of both healthy and unhealthy persons. It is generalizable to a variety of children, adolescents, and adults. The theory represents Western values on self-responsibility and therefore may have limited ethnic and cultural generalizability.

Logical Adequacy

Orem's self-care theory is a system of interrelated presuppositions, concepts, and propositions developed for the purpose of describing how persons regulate their own behavior or require assistance with this regulation for healthy development and well-being. These structural components make sense, particularly to nurses who practice in settings where their interactions promote such behaviors. Figure 4.6 displays the relationships among the major concepts.

Usefulness

Orem's self-care theory has served as a framework for nursing curricula and the administration of a variety of nursing services (Berbiglia, 1997). It

Concept	Self-Care Agency (SCA)	Self-Care Requisites (SCR)	Therapeutic Self-Care Demands (TSCD)	Self-Care Deficits (SCD)	Dependent-Care Agency (DCA)
SCA	=	+	+	–	–
SCR		=	+	+	+
TSCD			=	+	+
SCD				=	+
DCA					=

Legend: =, same concept; +, positive relationship; –, negative relationship; ±, the relationship can be positive or negative.

Figure 4.6   Relationships Among Major Concepts of Orem's Self-Care Theory

has been useful in the study of children (McNabb, Quinn, Murphy, Thorp, & Cook, 1994) and adolescents with diabetes (Christian, D'Auria, & Fox, 1999; Frey & Denyes, 1989; Frey & Fox, 1990; Shilling, Grey, & Knafl, 2002). It has also been used to study the health behaviors of children (Moore, 1995) and adolescents (McCaleb & Cull, 2000). The theory has been used to guide health promotion intervention research in adolescents (Deatrick, Angst, & Madden, 1998; Denyes, 1988), self-care practices of adolescents (Slusher, 1999), and in a study of pregnant, low-income adolescents (Warren, 1998).

Testability

Partial support for Orem's theory was found in an aggregate sample of 369 adolescents in which several propositions were tested (Denyes, 1988). Frey and Denyes (1989) tested and found support for Orem's theory of self-care in a sample of adolescents with insulin-dependent diabetes mellitus.

Empirical Referents

The Denyes Self-Care Agency Questionnaire. The Denyes Self-Care Agency Questionnaire was developed to operationalize self-care agency. The instrument contains 35 items, with a seven-point, Likert-type response format. Alpha coefficients of reliability have been reported as .86 to .89 (Denyes, 1981, 1988).There is evidence of content, concurrent, and construct validity through factor analysis of the instrument.

The Denyes Self-Care Practice Instrument. The Denyes Self-Care Practice Instrument is a 22-item, self-report measure with a response scale of 0 to 100. Coefficients of internal consistency range from .84 to .92 (Denyes, 1988; Frey & Denyes, 1989).

The Child and Adolescent Self-Care Practice Questionnaire. The Child and Adolescent Self-Care Practice Questionnaire is a 35-item, self-report scale with a five-point, Likert-type response format (1 = *never*, 5 = *always*). Content validity was determined by a panel of experts, and construct validity was determined through factor analysis with factors that corresponded to Orem's conceptualizations. Coefficient alpha was reported as .83 (Moore, 1995).

Related Research

Using Orem's theory as a framework, Canty-Mitchell (2001) surveyed 202 adolescents (85% African American and 55% female) who attended inner city high schools in Miami. There was a significant correlation between hope and self-care agency but no significant correlation between life-change events (stressors) and self-care agency. After multiple regression analyses, the researchers concluded that adolescents in this sample were more likely to engage in self-care if they scored high on a measures of hope and perceived health status and were not attending alternative schools. These researchers suggested that hope serves as a protective factor.

Low-Income Pregnant Adolescents.

In a study of 36 pregnant, low-income adolescents, 18 of whom had a history of abuse or neglect and 18 of whom did not have such a history, Warren (1998) found significant differences between the groups in terms of how they valued and paid attention to their health. Self-care theory is based on the premise that health care is an individual responsibility, that individuals select health goals related to their personal needs, that they can participate in their own care, that they are capable of changing their behaviors, and that it fosters "autonomy, social justice, independence, and self-esteem" (p. 31).

Chapter Summary

William James's early conceptualizations of a sense of self with both objective and subjective dimensions formed the backdrop for examining the progression of thinking and theory development about human identity. Harter drew heavily on this work to describe the construction of the self as a function of cognitions and socialization. Erikson, Marcia, Grotevant, Berzonsky, and Kerpelman expanded on Erikson's description of identity development and extended our understanding of this process. Aspects of identity that profoundly affect adolescents include those of gender, race, ethnicity, and sexual orientation. Orem's theory of self-care is a description of how a sense of self is related to the ability to care for and about oneself with implications for health-promoting behaviors.

Suggestions for Further Study

Further study is needed, particularly to test the identity process models. It is really unknown how much identity changes during adolescence, why, and who is most likely to experience such changes. The relationship between identity construction and health-risk behaviors is also unknown and worthy of exploration. Identity may be an important variable in constructing interventions to enhance health-promoting and limit health-compromising behaviors. Harter's elaboration of the differences in self-representations as children move from concrete to abstract thinking is salient to the development and testing of interventions, and this needs to be considered when planning for behavioral change interventions.

To study identity formation as a developmental process, we need to conduct prospective longitudinal studies of adolescents from various racial and ethnic backgrounds. It is important to include the social environment as context for such development. When integrating the knowledge we have about adolescent development in various domains (i.e., physical, psychological, social, and spiritual), it would be helpful to know how these domains reflect the process of identity formation.

Grotevant (1997) suggests that future research in identity should include narrative approaches. That is, identity should be approached as a personal narrative or story. He suggests that this approach would allow the scientist to understand how different domains of identity are chosen versus those that are assigned and how the different domains are related to one another. Details about the purpose and method of narrative analysis are described in detail in chapter 11. This and other qualitative approaches could also illuminate what identity and the process of its development mean to adolescents. It is also important to discover how the process varies by gender, race, and ethnicity.

Orem's theory of self-care has been tested with adolescents who have chronic illness. Further study could be done to explore the meaning of self-care to adolescents from various ecological niches. In fact, my grounded theory study of homeless adolescents (Rew, 2003), reported in detail in Chapter 11, could be replicated with many different groups of adolescents to develop a more comprehensive understanding of what self and self-care mean to adolescents.

Related Web Sites

Children of Lesbian and Gays Everywhere (COLAGE): http://www.colage.org

Erik Erikson's 8 Stages of Psychosocial Development (Summary Chart): http://facultyweb.cortland.edu/~ANDERSMD/ERIK/sum.html

Family Pride Coalition: http://www.familypride.org

Gay & Lesbian Advocates & Defenders: http://www.glad.org

Gay and Lesbian Medical Association (GLMA): http://www.glma.org

Gay, Lesbian and Straight Education Network: http://www.glsen.org

Gay Parent magazine: http://www.gayparentmag.com

International Foundation for Gender Education (IFGE): http://www. ifge.org

James Marcia: http://www.2.sfu.ca/psychology/groups/faculty/marcia

National Coalition for Gay, Lesbian, Bisexual & Transgender Youth (OutProud): http://www.outproud.org

PFLAG: National Federation of Parents and Friends of Lesbian and Gays: http://www.pflag.org

ProudParenting.com: http://www.proudparenting.com/

LGBT Family and Parenting Services (Fenway Community Health, Boston): http://www.fenwayhealth.org/services/family_flash.htm

True Colors, Inc. Sexual Minority Youth and Family Services of Connecticut: http://www.ourtruecolors.org

Youth Guardian Services: http://www.youth-guard.org/youth/

Suggestions for Further Reading

Harrison, T. W. (2003). Adolescent homosexuality and concerns regarding disclosure. *Journal of School Health, 73*, 107-112.

Lewis, M. (1997). *Altering fate: Why the past does not predict the future.* New York: Guilford.

Perrin, E. C. (2002). *Sexual orientation in child and adolescent health care.* New York: Kluwer Academic/Plenum.

Pfund, R. (2000). Nurturing a child's spirituality. *Journal of Child Health Care, 4*, 143-148.

White, J. (1996). Education, spirituality and the whole child: A humanist perspective. In R. Best (Ed.), *Education, spirituality and the whole child* (pp. 30-42). New York: Cassell.

Zaff, J. F., Blount, R. L., Phillips, L., & Cohen, L. (2002). The role of ethnic identity and self-construal in coping among African American and Caucasian American seventh graders: An exploratory analysis of within-group variance. *Adolescence, 37*, 751-773.

5

Theories of Stress and Coping

The concept of stress is familiar to everyone—children, adolescents, and adults alike. In the science of physics, stress is defined as a body's internal resistance to the application of a force that strains that body. Theories of stress and coping offer valuable frameworks for studying how the interaction between individuals and their environment affects behaviors and, subsequently, health. In this chapter, the pioneering work of Hans Selye, who first introduced the terms *stress* and *stressor* into the everyday vocabulary, are presented. Selye contributed primarily to our understanding of the physiological changes that take place when a person experiences a stressful situation or event. Further work by Lazarus and Folkman shifted the focus to the cognitive domain, indicating that a person's cognitive appraisal of a situation or event becomes an integral component of the stress and coping paradigm. Lazarus and others expanded not only on the cognitive aspect of stress and coping but elaborated on the emotions that accompany such experiences. Other scholars have chosen to focus on the environmental aspects of stress and coping, and two of those models will be examined as well. The relationship of stress to physical and mental health status, as well as the enactment of health-risk behaviors in adolescents, make these theories and models an important resource for further study of these phenomena.

Selye's Conceptualization of Stress

Origins

Hans Selye, often recognized as the father of the family of theories on stress in physical and mental illness, was born in Vienna in 1907. He received both a doctor of medicine degree and a doctor of philosophy degree from the German University in Prague. His first published description of what later became known as the *General Adaptation Syndrome* was in 1936 and was titled "A Syndrome Produced by Diverse Nocuous Agents" (Selye, 1978, p. xi).

Selye's conceptualization of stress was influenced by the works of Claude Bernard, Walter B. Cannon, Charles Darwin, Sigmund Freud, and Albert Einstein, among others. Bernard, at the Collège de France in Paris, and Cannon, at Harvard University in Boston, advanced the concept that human beings maintained an internal balance of chemicals and physiological processes despite drastic changes in their environments. Cannon used the term *homeostasis* to refer to this ability for the human to remain static or the same under conditions of a continuously changing environment (Selye, 1978).

As a medical student, Selye (1974, 1978) was struck by a similarity among many of the first patients he met who, in spite of having different diseases, showed many of the same symptoms. He questioned why diseases such as measles and scarlet fever produced many responses that were the same as those to exposure to allergens and drugs. He began to consider the idea of a general syndrome of being ill or having a disease rather than focusing on the diagnosis of a single disease entity. A few years later, he was working on a series of experiments in which he injected rats with a variety of hormones and watched for changes in their internal organs. Although these experiments did not lead Selye to the discovery of a new sex hormone, which had been his goal, they did lead him to the identification of the General Adaptation Syndrome (GAS). The GAS consisted of an initial alarm reaction followed by a state of adaptation, which he called the stage of resistance. With additional or prolonged exposure to the causative agent, a stage of exhaustion was reached.

In identifying an accurate term for the GAS, Selye (1978) recorded that he "stumbled upon the term *stress,* which had long been used in common English, and particularly in engineering, to denote the effects of a force acting against a resistance" (p. 45). He reasoned that the nonspecific manifestations associated with the GAS were parallel to responses that had been observed in nonhuman materials exposed to stress. However, because English was not Selye's first language, he had failed to distinguish between the concepts of *stress* and *strain.* The term *stress* had begun to mean both cause and effect. Thus he created a new term, *stressor,* to refer to the cause of the outcome he then identified as stress.

Purpose

The purpose of Selye's work was to identify the biological underpinnings of the human being's adaptation to an ever-changing internal and external environment. This work includes a description of his discovery of the stress concept, evidence of its effect on the body, diseases and processes associated with stress, and his search for a unifying theory to explain the body's nonspecific response to any demand made on it (Selye, 1978, p. 55).

Meaning of the Theory

Selye (1978) described stress as "essentially reflected by the rate of all the wear and tear caused by life" (p. xvi). More specifically, he defined stress as "the state manifested by a specific syndrome which consists of all the nonspecifically-induced changes within a biologic system" (p. 64). In addition to the GAS, Selye noted that there was a local adaptation syndrome (LAS), which occurred at the specific site where the human body experienced a stressor (e.g., the inflammation that occurs around the site of a puncture wound such as a mosquito bite). According to Selye, the human body's response to stress consists of three parts: (a) a direct effect on the body, (b) an internal defensive response that destroys offending mechanisms, and (c) an internal response that leads to tissue destruction from excessive defense mechanisms.

Other terms that are critical in this theory are as follows:

- *Alarm signals:* Chemicals released at the site of stressed tissues that send messages to the nervous system
- *Adaptive hormones:* Anti-inflammatory, glucocorticoid hormones and mineralocorticoid hormones produced by the adrenal glands
- *Adaptation energy:* The body's use of stored fuel as it continues to adapt
- *Diseases of adaptation:* Diseases that result from stress or from the body's inability to adapt, particularly those that result from either too little or too much of the body's defense mechanism (Selye, 1978, pp. 83, 169); examples of such diseases include hypertension, inflammatory conditions of all types, and cardiovascular disease
- *Resistance:* The stage in the GAS of the body's response to a stressor during which fat is released
- *Exhaustion:* The stage in the GAS during which the body loses the fat droplets that accumulated during the resistance stage
- *Adaptation:* The ways in which the human body changes in response to demands from the environment, "a balanced blend of defense and submission" (Selye, 1978, p. 169)
- *Distress:* Unpleasant or harmful effects of stress on the body
- *Eustress:* Pleasant or good effects of stress on the body
- *Stressor:* A thing or event that produces stress

Selye showed that various stimuli produced the same stress response (GAS) within the body. He described a triphasic course of activities that comprise the response syndrome (see Figure 5.1). The body's first response to a stressor (alarm reaction) is to discharge fatty acids containing stress hormones (alarm chemicals) from the adrenal cortex. When the body accumulates a large number of fatty acids and stress hormones, it goes into a stage of resistance, and when it depletes these substances, it goes into a stage of exhaustion.

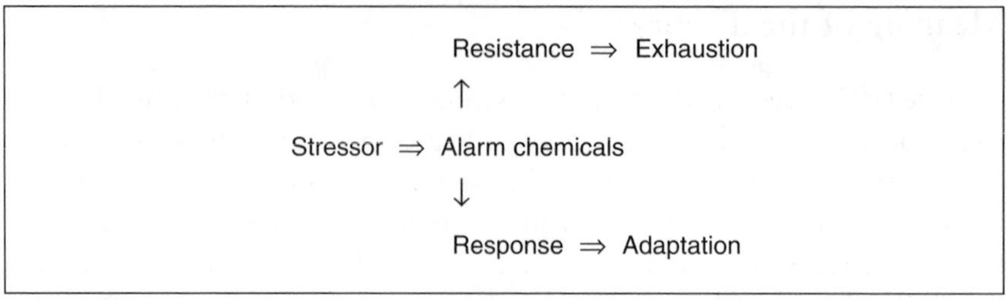

Resistance ⇒ Exhaustion

↑

Stressor ⇒ Alarm chemicals

↓

Response ⇒ Adaptation

Figure 5.1   Selye's General Adaptation Syndrome

Much of Selye's early work focused on the process of inflammation that occurred at the site of local injury or disease to a specific part of the body (e.g., infection in the tonsils, or inflamed tonsils, known as tonsillitis). He went on to show that the same type of response from the pituitary and adrenal glands occurred in response to cognitive and emotional events such as worry, fear, and pain. Eventually, he showed that the GAS involved the entire body.

Scope, Parsimony, and Generalizability

Because Selye's model refers to the nonspecific response of the body to any demand placed on it, it has a very wide scope of influence. It has been the foundation for further exploration, and the terminology from this theoretical perspective has found its way into everyday language and discourse. The theory contains only a few major concepts and therefore is parsimonious.

This theory applies to individuals across the life span and explains person-environment interactions independent of cultural or geographic influences. Moreover, the stress response described by Selye has also been generalized to the relationship between other animals and their environmental demands (Institute of Medicine, 2001).

Logical Adequacy

Selye's work was primarily descriptive and thus does not lend itself to making predictions, other than the predictable outcome of the GAS as a response to any demand made on the person. There has been much agreement among scientists about the foundations laid down by Selye. Scientists in medicine, nursing, psychology, education, and social work agree that the processes and concepts Selye identified are germane to our understanding of human health and behavior.

Usefulness

Selye's conceptualization of stress has had an enormous influence on the development of medicine and psychology. It has formed the framework for the development of a whole new scientific discipline: psychoneuroimmunology, which focuses on the interactions among emotions, the nervous system, and immune response in the body. Subsequent theories of coping have also been found useful in understanding how to reduce the adverse effects associated with the daily stress of living. Although his formulation does not currently have a direct effect on our understanding of stress and coping in adolescence, his work has been useful in encouraging other scientists to think about the phenomenon of stress and its relationship to human behavior.

Testability

Selye's conceptualization of the stress response and general adaptation syndrome has spawned several lines of inquiry in both animal and human sciences. However, defining stress as a "nonspecific response" has made it difficult to define components of the model in operational terms. As Lyon (2000) put it, "the generality of the definition as the sum of all nonspecific reactions of the body obscures the more specific response patterns of psychophysiological responses" (p. 6). In addition, the conceptualization of a nonspecific response does not allow for individual differences or variation in coping styles (Lyon, 2000).

Empirical Referents

A variety of physiological measures has been used to measure stress response in humans. These include the production of antibodies; plasma and urinary levels of cortisol; and heart rate, respiratory rate, and blood pressure (Lyon, 2000). In addition to heart rate, respiratory rate, and blood pressure, several other stress responses occur with activation of the autonomic nervous system. These include the release of neurotransmitters; norepinephrine, which is responsible for increases in heart and respiratory rates; pupil dilation; blood pressure; oxygen consumption by the heart; and glucose levels, all of which can be measured. Valid measures of these empirical indicators depend on the use of appropriate laboratory procedures and reagents along with reliable instruments that can be calibrated (White & Porth, 2000).

_____ Cognitive Appraisal, Coping, and Emotion

Origins

The cognitive appraisal theory of Lazarus (1966) and, later, Lazarus and Folkman (1984) originated in sociology and psychology. These theorists trace the history of their conceptualization through the works of Marx, Weber, and Durkheim in sociology as well as the influence of Freud's emphasis on the role of anxiety in the etiology of psychopathology. They also note that the work of researchers who studied the effects of World War II, the Korean War, and the Vietnam conflict was based on Selye's theory of stress and did much to advance our understanding of physiological and psychological consequences of traumatic events. Lazarus and Folkman also identified other factors that influenced and shaped their thinking about the cognitive appraisal and response to stress. In particular they recognized a renewed interest in psychosomatic medicine that emphasized the centrality of emotion in the creation of physical symptoms, the increase in behavioral therapies to assist persons in coping with or managing stress, the emphasis in developmental psychology on the relationship between person and environment, and the increased focus on social ecology in individual adaptation.

Lazarus (1991a, 1999) modified this theory of cognitive appraisal and coping to become the cognitive-motivational-relational theory of emotion. He referred to the influence of other theorists, such as Albert Bandura and Magda Arnold, on his modified theory. Moreover, he harkened back to Aristotle's treatment of emotions and built on Selye's work in describing the general adaptation syndrome and outlining the physiological processes of the central nervous system and endocrine system in mediating the person's response to a stressor (Lazarus, 1999).

Purpose

The purpose of the original theory of cognitive appraisal and coping was to define concepts and relationships among concepts, including cognitive processes, so that social scientists could explain and predict individual differences in adaptation. It was clearly Lazarus's intent to provide a formulation that went beyond description (Lazarus, 1966; Lazarus & Folkman, 1984). In the revision of the theory, which now includes the concept of emotion, Lazarus (1999) claims that emotion is included to explain further how persons struggle to adapt.

Meaning of the Theory

A major premise of the cognitive appraisal and coping theory is that individuals constantly evaluate their relationship with the environment and that this relationship, which is reciprocal, has implications for their well-being (Lazarus & Cohen, 1977; Lazarus & Folkman, 1984). The theory derives from a phenomenological tradition in psychology, which means that how a person attaches meaning to an event or situation influences both emotional and behavioral responses. The theorists' focus on cognitive appraisal takes into account the thought processes that occur between the stimulus experience of a stressor and the emotional and behavioral responses of the person. Sources of stress come from the environment or from within the individual. The following concepts are central to this model:

- *Stress* is viewed as "a special kind of *transaction* or relationship between two systems, person and environment, or between two or more intraindividual systems (e.g., id, ego, and superego processes) as in the psychoanalytic approach to conflict" (Lazarus & Cohen, 1977).
- *Cognitive appraisal* is the process individuals use to evaluate their transactions with the environment and to determine whether these transactions are stressful.
- *Stress appraisals* are of three types: perceived harm or loss, threat, or challenge.
- *Harm or loss appraisal* means that the person has already experienced damage of some kind (e.g., illness or injury) or has lost something or someone of importance to him or her.
- *Threat appraisal* means that the person has not experienced a harm or loss but anticipates that this could happen. Such an appraisal calls for coping.
- *Challenge appraisal* means that the person has not experienced a gain of some kind but that a gain may be anticipated. This type of appraisal also calls for coping.
- *Psychological stress* occurs when individuals appraise a transaction between themselves and the environment as greater than their resources and therefore a threat to well-being.
- "*Coping* is the process through which the individual manages the demands of the person-environment relationship that are appraised as stressful and the emotions they generate" (Lazarus & Cohen, 1977, p. 19, italics added). Coping is further defined as "constantly changing cognitive and behavioral efforts to manage specific external and/or internal demands that are appraised as taxing or exceeding the resources of the person" (p. 141).
- *Primary appraisal* refers to a person's categorizing a stressor in regard to how it may affect her or his well-being: irrelevant, benign-positive, or stressful.
- *Irrelevant appraisal* occurs when a person perceives the environment as having no effect on well-being.
- *Benign-positive appraisals* occur if the person thinks that the outcome of a transaction is positive or has the potential to improve well-being.
- *Secondary appraisal* includes the person's evaluation of what is at stake in an encounter with the environment and what can be done about it (Lazarus & Cohen, 1977, p. 35).
- *Reappraisal* means that individuals changes their appraisal after receiving more information from the environment.
- *Psychological vulnerability* refers to a person's lack of resources for response to demands from the environment and "by the relationship between the individual's pattern of commitments and his or her resources for warding off threats to those commitments. Indeed, vulnerability can be thought of as *potential* threat that is transformed into active threat when that which is valued is actually put in jeopardy in a particular transaction" (Lazarus & Cohen, 1977, p. 51).

The degree of stress and the emotional response that accompanies it are determined by the interaction between primary and secondary appraisals of the stressor or environmental stimulus. In more recent works, Lazarus (1999) asserts that the term *appraisal* "stands for the evaluative product" (p. 200), whereas "*appraising*, which refers to the act of making an evaluation" (p. 199), is now the preferred term in this theory. The evolving and revised formulation of this theory emphasizes process rather than product.

Lazarus and Folkman (1984) identified characteristics within the person that influence appraisals. These characteristics are commitments and beliefs. They influence the person's appraisal by allowing him or her to identify what is salient for well-being in a given situation, promoting an understanding of the situation, and furnishing a way to evaluate the outcomes of the situation. Commitment is a motivational factor that reflects what is important or meaningful to an individual. Commitment influences one's appraisal of the environment by leading the person toward or away from situations that represent harm or loss, threat, or challenge. Commitment also influences one's appraisal of the environment through *cue sensitivity,* which refers to the weight the person assigns to various aspects of a transaction with the environment. Beliefs are the individual's perceptions about the meaning of the environment. An important type of belief in this theory is the belief about personal control or the feeling that one has mastery and control over a situation. Existential beliefs (e.g., belief in fate or God) may also influence one's appraisal of a situation. Appraising a situation as under one's control may either reduce the experience of stress or increase the perception of threat. Appraisal of control, in turn, influences both affective and coping responses. For example, a person's sense of self-confidence or efficacy can determine whether the person is more likely to appraise the situation as a threat or challenge (Lazarus, 1999). Individuals who are more confident of their ability to manage a situation are more likely to feel challenged rather than threatened.

Factors within the situation or environment also influence the individual's appraisal. Lazarus and Folkman (1984) identify seven situational factors that influence appraisal: novelty, event certainty, imminence, duration, temporal uncertainty, ambiguity, and timing of stressful events. Situations characterized by novelty mean that the person has had no previous experience with the event and thus has no reason to appraise it as harmful or threatening. When a particular situation has a high probability of leading to a specific outcome (predictable), there is event certainty, which is less stressful than events characterized as uncertain. The situational factors of imminence, duration, and temporal uncertainty refer to the timing of appraisal and coping responses. When an event is imminent, it evokes a more intense and urgent response. The duration of a stressful event or anticipation of such an event may permit the person to develop adaptive coping strategies or it can heighten threat and lead to exhaustion. Temporal uncertainty means that the person does not know when a stressful event or situation might occur. Both ambiguity and timing of stressful events throughout one's life can influence the type of appraisal an individual makes of these events. Ambiguous events may be appraised as challenging at one time and threatening at another time, depending on other circumstances operating in the person's life at a given time.

Coping is conceptualized as a process rather than an individual trait. Coping serves to allow the individual to manage or alter a problem and regulate the emotional response to that problem. Two types of coping are recognized: emotion focused and problem focused. Coping both emerges from emotion and affects reappraisal (Lazarus, 1991b). Coping is influenced by the person's beliefs, resources, and environmental constraints. Appraisal of events and coping processes affect adaptation outcomes, which Lazarus and Folkman (1984) describe as "functioning in work and social living, morale or life satisfaction, and somatic health" (p. 181). In more recent writing, Lazarus (1991a) states that there is overlap between cognitive coping and appraisal in that coping is "what a person thinks and does to try to manage an emotional encounter; and appraisal is an evaluation of what might be thought or done in that encounter" (p. 113). Furthermore, Lazarus (2000) writes, "an appraisal is the result of a coping process when it constitutes a motivated search for information and the constructed meaning on which to act under stress" (p. 206).

In the revised model, Figure 5.2, additional personal and environmental antecedents are depicted as forming the person-environment relationship in which appraisal occurs through a process of relational meaning. Coping is viewed as a way of revising the relational meaning of person-environment, leading to the outcomes of emotions and their effects: morale, social functioning, and health. In this reformulation, Lazarus (2000) suggests that there are at least 15 emotions that may occur as a result of the stress, appraisal, and coping process. These 15 emotions are anger, anxiety, compassion, envy, fright, gratitude, guilt, happiness, hope, jealousy, love, pride, relief, sadness, and shame.

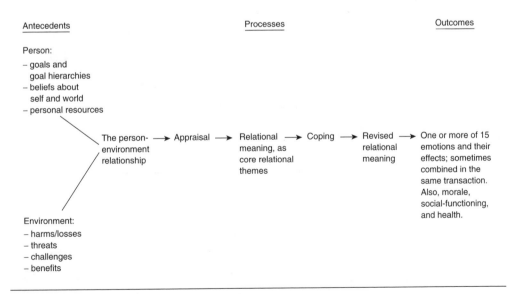

Figure 5.2   A Revised Model of Stress and Coping

SOURCE: Lazarus (1999, p. 198). © 1999 Springer Publishing Company, Inc. Reprinted by permission.

Scope, Parsimony, and Generalizability

This relational theory of stress and coping is broad in scope, contains relatively few concepts, and is generalizable to adolescents and adults in the United States and other industrialized countries. Because the cognitive processes of appraisal are central to the theory, it cannot be generalized to infants or very young children. It is applicable to coping with diverse stressors.

Logical Adequacy

The major concepts of the theory are presented in a matrix, Figure 5.3, showing the proposed relationships among them.

The matrix indicates that there is a relationship between person and environment, and from the theory, one could predict that the relationship between these two concepts may be positive or negative. Similarly, concepts of appraisal or appraising, coping, stress, vulnerability, and reappraisal are related to the person and to the environment. That is, the relationship between individuals and their environment is a function of both appraising and coping (Folkman et al., 1991). Vulnerability has a negative sign because it is defined as the person's lack of resources; thus one could predict that the fewer resources a person has, the more vulnerable she or he is to the negative effects of stress. Appraisal or appraising may be positively or negatively related to coping, stress, vulnerability, or reappraisal, depending on how the person appraises the demand from the environment. Coping may be negatively or positively associated with stress, vulnerability, and reappraisal because it may or may not be effective in facilitating the person's adaptation.

	(P)	(E)	(A)	(C)	(S)	(V)	(R)
(P)	=	±	±	±	−	−	±
(E)		=	±	±	±	±	±
(A)			=	±	±	?	±
(C)				=	±	±	±
(S)					=	+	±
(V)						=	±
(R)							=

Figure 5.3   Relationships Among Concepts in Cognitive Appraisal and Coping Theory

NOTE: P indicates person; E, environment; A, appraisal; C, coping; S, stress; V, vulnerability; R, reappraisal; =, same concept; −, negative relationship between concepts; +, positive relationship between concepts; ±, the relationship can be either positive or negative; ?, the nature of the relationship is unknown.

Stress is positively related to vulnerability, and both of these variables may be positively or negatively related to reappraisal, depending on whether they are recast as a threat or a challenge.

The use of this model by scholars in various disciplines is another criterion of logical adequacy because these scientists agree that the concepts and statements make sense. A number of disciplines have been advanced by Lazarus's model of cognitive appraisal, coping, and emotion. For example, nursing has found agreement with this model of stress and coping and has extended it with the construct of quality of life as a way to cope with chronic illness (Backer, Bakas, Bennett, & Pierce, 2000).

Usefulness

Lazarus and Folkman's theory of cognitive appraisal and coping has been cited in hundreds of studies of stress. It has served as the framework for an intervention for persons with AIDS (Folkman et al., 1991). It has also provided the foundation for Lazarus's (1991a, 1993, 1999, 2000) more recent development of a theory of emotion, which he calls the cognitive-motivational-relational theory. The theory has had many applications to deriving midrange practice theories within the discipline of nursing (Backer et al., 2000).

Testability

This theory has been tested in numerous studies of adults and adolescents (Feldman, Fisher, Ransom, & Dimiceli, 1995; Jalowiec, 2003; Lazarus, 1993, 1999). For example, Folkman and colleagues (1991) translated the theory into a brief intervention for HIV-positive gay males. Outcomes supported the effectiveness of this theory as a framework to provide coping effectiveness training.

Empirical Referents

Several instruments have been developed that operationalize some of the major concepts in this theoretical formulation. In particular, coping can be measured using any of the following valid research instruments.

Ways of Coping Checklist

The Ways of Coping Checklist, Revised (Lazarus & Folkman, 1984) is a self-report scale that contains 67 items with a 4-point, Likert-type response format (0 = *not used,* 1 = *used somewhat,* 2 = *used quite a bit,* 3 = *used a great deal*). The scale can also be administered by interview. The items on the scale represent domains of "defensive coping, information seeking, problem solving, palliation, inhibition of action, direct action, and magical thinking" (pp. 156-157). Factor analysis supported problem-focused coping (e.g., problem solving and formulating a plan of action) and emotion-focused coping (e.g., seeking social support and avoidance).

A 19-item shortened form of the Ways of Coping Checklist is also a self-report scale with a 4-point, Likert-type response format (0 = *not at all*, 3 = *most of the time*). Respondents indicate how often they use a particular coping response when dealing with what is most stressful in their life. This form measures six types of coping: self-control or keeping feelings to oneself, escape or avoidance, distancing oneself, planning and problem solving, seeking social support, and positive reappraisal. Alpha coefficients for the six subscales range from .53 to .69 when used with males 19 to 63 years old (Folkman, Chesney, Pollack, & Phillips, 1992).

Adolescent Coping Orientation for Problem Experiences

The Adolescent Coping Orientation for Problem Experiences (Lewis & Brown, 2002) was designed to measure coping behaviors in adolescents, and it consists of 54 items with a five-point, Likert-type response format (1 = *never*, 5 = *most of the time*). Nine items are reverse scored, and a total score results from summing all items. Twelve subscales have been identified, with alpha coefficients ranging from .50 to .75 (McCubbin & Thompson, 1991).

Adolescent Coping Scale

The Adolescent Coping Scale was originally developed in Australia for use with adolescents between 12 and 18 years old (Frydenberg & Lewis, 1991, 1993). There are long (80 items) and short (19 items) forms of the scale. The long form has both general and specific forms that reflect the conceptual difference between coping in general and coping with a specific stressor. Validity of the scale has been supported through factor analysis, and there is limited evidence of reliability (Humberside Partnership, n.d.). The short form of the scale has evidence of validity through factor analysis and three subscales with reliability coefficients of .50 to .61 (Frydenberg & Lewis, 1993a).

Jalowiec Coping Scale

Based on Lazarus and Folkman's (1984) conceptualization of coping, Anne Jalowiec (2003) developed the Jalowiec Coping Scale, initially in 1977. The scale was developed to measure coping behaviors in a variety of physical, emotional, and social situations. It has been used in studies by researchers in a variety of disciplines and in a number of other countries, including China, Iceland, Thailand, and Turkey. Although initially developed for adults, the instrument has been found to be appropriate for use with adolescents.

The Jalowiec Coping Scale consists of 60 items with a 4-point rating scale (0 = *never used*, 1 = *seldom used*, 2 = *sometimes used*, and 3 = *often used*) that measures the types of coping methods used by the person. The scale also asks the respondent to indicate how helpful each coping method used has been in dealing with a specific stressor. Responses follow a 4-point, Likert-style format (0 = *not helpful in reducing stress*, 1 = *slightly helpful*, 2 = *fairly helpful*, and 3 = *helpful*). The scale is at the sixth-grade reading level and has evidence of content, construct, concurrent, and predictive validity. Reliability estimates based on Cronbach alpha coefficients computed for the total scale used in 25 studies ranged from .57 to .97, with a mean of .85 (Jalowiec, 2003). Permission to use the scale must be obtained from the author: Anne Jalowiec, RN, PhD, FAAN, at jalo@prodigy.net or ajalowiec@yahoo.com.

Conservation of Resources Theory

Origins

The conservation of resources (COR) theory was developed out of concern about the limitations of Lazarus and Folkman's (1984) model of stress and coping. The concern was that previous models of stress and coping put the most emphasis on the individual and ignored the influence of environment (Hobfoll & Schumm, 2002).

Purpose

The purpose of the theory is to describe how the resources of the individual and the community can be used to promote health and health behaviors that contribute to the public health.

Meaning of the Theory

The COR theory focuses on preventing the loss of resources, maintaining available resources, and obtaining resources that are needed to engage in a healthy lifestyle. Resources are conceptualized as "objects, personal characteristics, conditions, or energies" (Hobfoll & Schumm, 2002, p. 287). Conditions that serve as resources include social statuses such as marriage. Resources are also viewed as interrelated, meaning that a change in one or more of them can affect other resources. Whereas loss of resources leads to psychological distress, gaining resources mitigates the negative effects of loss of resources. Losing resources is seen as more powerful than gaining resources, and resources need to be invested to prevent loss or to gain new resources.

Persons are viewed within a social context. A person behaves in ways that "protect and preserve the self and the attachments that establish self in social context relationship" (Hobfoll & Schumm, 2002, p. 287). When a person perceives a threat of loss of resources from the environment, that person experiences psychological distress. This perceived threat may interfere with the person's ability to cope with future challenges from the environment. Psychological distress may also be experienced when a person fails to gain further coping abilities after investing existing resources.

Scope, Parsimony, and Generalizability

The scope of COR theory is limited by its general nature. This makes it applicable to many populations and a variety of stressful situations in which individuals gain or lose resources. However, this is also a limitation because it does not specify what type of resources are applicable to various domains of stress and health (Hobfoll & Schumm, 2002). The theory consists of only a few concepts and propositions and therefore meets the criterion of parsimony.

Logical Adequacy

Figure 5.4 depicts the relationship among concepts in the COR theory. The relationships among concepts are clear, and there are no apparent logical fallacies. Independent of the content of the theory, predictions can be made. Other scientists have agreed that these concepts and relationships make sense for health promotion interventions.

Usefulness

The COR theory has been used as a framework for safer sex interventions for pregnant inner-city women and for the study of post-traumatic stress disorder in veterans of the Vietnam conflict (Hobfoll & Schumm, 2002).

Concept	A	B	C	D	E
A	=	±	±	±	±
B		=	±	±	±
C			=		−
D				=	+
E					=

Figure 5.4 Logical Adequacy of the Conservation of Resources Theory

NOTE: A indicates person; B, environment; C, resources; D, threat of loss; E, distress; =, same concept; −, negative relationship between concepts; +, positive relationship between concepts; ±, the relationship can be either positive or negative.

Testability

The theory is, at least, testable in principle, but valid empirical referents are not available.

_____ Moos's Model of Context, Coping, and Adaptation

Recently, Moos (2002) proposed an integrated framework for expanding stress and coping theory to include contextual and socialization factors related to adolescent health and well-being. This model, Figure 5.5, consists of five panels. The first of these panels contains the *environmental system* and represents the social climate (e.g., family), which includes both daily life stressors and social resources. This panel reflects relative stability of ongoing elements in an adolescent's life. The second panel contains the *personal system*,

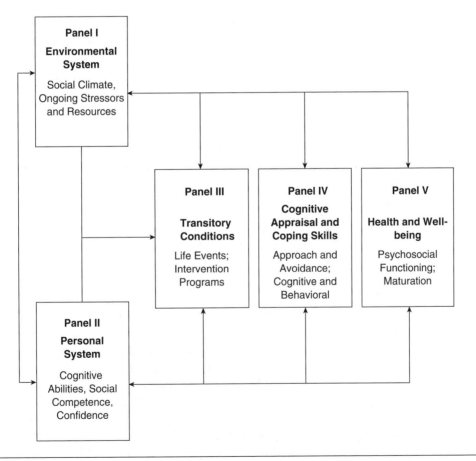

Figure 5.5   Moos's Model of Context, Coping, and Adaptation in Adolescence

SOURCE: Moos (2002, p. 23). © 2002 Society for Adolescent Medicine. Reprinted by permission.

including biological and genetic characteristics of the individual (e.g., cognition, intelligence, social competence, and self-confidence). The third panel includes what Moos calls *transitory conditions,* such as life events. The fourth panel contains the cognitive appraisal and coping skills of the individual, which are shaped by the relationships among the environmental system (Panel I), the personal system (Panel II), and transitory conditions (Panel III). The outcome of interrelationships among all four panels in the model is the fifth panel, *health and well-being.* That is to say, the health and well-being of the adolescent reflect feedback to each of the other components of the model.

In Figure 5.5 it is clear that relationships between each of the major concepts (panels) are delineated. The bidirectional arrows indicate the reciprocal feedback loops. The major contextual factor in this model is the family climate (Panel I) in which the adolescent's development unfolds. Moos (2002) further conceptualizes this environment by identifying three dimensions: (a) relationships of cohesion, expressiveness, and conflict; (b) personal growth in independence, achievement, recreation, intellectual culture, morality, and religion; and (c) system maintenance of organization and control (pp. 23-24).

From studies based on this framework, Moos concludes that to understand the psychosocial adaptation of adolescents, we must consider family climate, social resources in various domains, and the coping responses of approach and avoidance. Among adolescents who have chronic diseases or disorders, family support and structure contribute to more successful adaptation. Moreover, adolescents are at greater risk for problem behaviors and depression when they experience acute and chronic stressors, but they have fewer problems and more self-confidence when they have increased social resources and coping skills characterized by approach rather than avoidance (Moos, 2002).

Research Application

Perceived stress and maladaptive coping strategies have been linked with several health-risk behaviors in adolescents. In a population-based sample of 1769 high school students, Steiner, Erickson, Hernandez, and Pavelski (2002) found that the use of avoidance coping strategies was associated with health-risk behaviors but approach coping was not. Using Moos's dichotomous conceptualization of approach (i.e., facing the problem directly) versus avoidance (i.e., diverting one's attention away from the problem) coping, this research team found that avoidance coping was statistically significantly correlated with general risk-taking behaviors, sexual health-risk behavior, and behaviors that increased risk for nutritional problems. The research team concluded that the style of coping used by an individual in midadolescence is clearly associated with health outcomes and that interventions were needed to assist these youth in developing more approach-type coping styles.

Commonsense Model
of Illness Representation

Origins

The Commonsense Model of Illness Representation is a self-regulation model of behaviors related to health and illness. The model was developed in response to studies of communications intended to invoke fear to motivate people to change their behaviors (Leventhal, 1970).

Purpose

The purpose of the model was to explain a parallel process observed when people responded to a fear message by developing an action plan.

Meaning of the Model

The Commonsense Model is based on four assumptions (Leventhal, Nerenz, & Steele, 1984):

1. Behavior is constructed by an internal information-processing system that integrates information about an incoming stimulus with memories and emotional and coping responses.

2. Information processing involves parallel processes of representation of the health threat and representation of the emotion that accompanies that threat. These two pathways interact to process symptoms and sensations.

3. Information processing operates in three stages (i.e., representation, coping, and appraisal), as depicted in Figure 5.6.

4. The information-processing system is assumed to be arranged in hierarchical order, from simple or automatic responses to those that involve judgments based on synthesis of information.

In the Commonsense Model, a person is viewed as an active problem solver. This problem-solving process occurs as parallel responses to a stimuli: threat and emotional response to the threat. A person is motivated to minimize health risks by taking action to reduce the threat of illness. A person's behavior, or response to a stimulus, is constructed by an information-processing system within the person that allows the person to interpret her or his experiences and emotional responses to them. Coping responses are then constructed based on the appraisal of this system of information processing.

The first of the two parallel pathways of response to a stimulus is a cognitive representation of the threat to health; the second pathway of response is

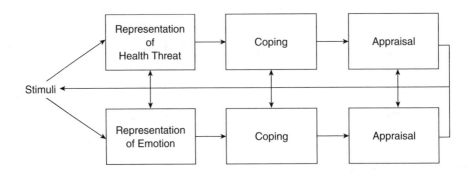

Figure 5.6   Commonsense Model of Illness Representation

SOURCE: Reynolds and Alonzo (2000, pp. 484). © 2000 Sage Publications, Inc. Reprinted with permission.

emotional. The cognitive pathway, which is based on knowledge, includes procedures learned for coping with a health problem. The emotional pathway is more automatic and is embedded in memories of personal experiences and associated perceptions and somatic sensations. Many of these memories and experiences are related to fear and automatic responses of attempting to get away from the stimulus. The two pathways interact to influence the way a person interprets symptoms of stress or disease. External cues from the environment as well as internal cues from memories, emotions, and somatic sensations trigger a cognitive effort to appraise and cope with the threat. The process begins with the person's representation and interpretation of the threat and the accompanying emotion. This process may include identification of a situation and awareness of its cause, how it will unfold, whether the person can control it, and what its consequences might be. The process continues with coping that is based on the meaning ascribed by the person to the threat of illness and the emotional response. The last part of the process is appraisal, in which the person evaluates how well the coping strategy worked.

The model is dynamic, although the figure makes it look static and linear. Individuals process information from the environment and from within their own cognitive and emotional structures to provide feedback for each step of the process. The hierarchical structure of the processing system suggests that some responses to stimuli are automatic and occur without thinking (e.g., removing one's finger from a hot surface), whereas others are more complex, involving considered judgments about the best course of action to take (e.g., deciding to have a surgical procedure to remove a painful stimulus when the chances of permanent paralysis from the surgery are 50-50).

Scope, Parsimony, and Generalizability

The model is very broad in scope, contains few concepts, and is generalizable to people who have intact cognitive and emotional structures. It can apply to people of various ages and cultures.

Logical Adequacy

There is agreement among scientists that the model makes sense. In fact, its name implies that this is so.

Usefulness

The model has been useful in studying adults with hypertension, diabetes, cardiovascular disease, chronic pain, and schizophrenia. It has also been useful in identifying those people who will seek health-care services and those who adhere to treatment guidelines. The model has also been used to guide the development of interventions (Reynolds & Alonzo, 2000).

Testability

Most of the tests of the model have focused on only one or two dimensions rather than on the whole model (Reynolds & Alonzo, 2000).

Empirical Referents

Illness representations have been measured through open-ended and semistructured interviews. A specific example of such an interview is one developed by Hampson, Glasgow, and Toobert (1990) to measure personal representations of diabetes.

Coping has been measured with the Ways of Coping Checklist described under "Cognitive Appraisal, Coping, and Emotion."

Stress and Coping Related to Health and Health-Risk Behaviors

Much of the literature pertaining to adolescent stress and coping is concerned with mental health (Rudolph, 2002; Rudolph et al., 2000). For example, Holahan, Valentiner, and Moos (1995) found that psychological adjustment (defined as happiness and well-being) in adolescents (N = 214) was associated directly with high social support from parents and indirectly through high levels of approach coping. Less has been done to examine the direct associations among stress, coping, and health-risk behaviors in adolescents. More specifically, the experience of post-traumatic stress disorder has been found to be highly associated with anxiety and depression (Murphy, Moscicki, Vermund, Muenz, & the Adolescent Medicine HIV/AIDS Research Network, 2000; Runyon & Kenny, 2002; Turner &

Lloyd, 1995). Stress has also been implicated in the genesis of chronic autoimmune disorders, such as lupus erythematosus and juvenile arthritis in adolescents (McEwen & Dhabhar, 2002; Moos, 2002: Schwartz, 2002).

DiClemente and colleagues (2001) examined the relationship between psychological distress and health-risk attitudes and behaviors among 522 African American adolescent females. Using the Center for Epidemiologic Studies–Depression Scale, with a score of >7 as an indicator of psychological distress, they found that nearly half (48%) of the participants were psychologically distressed. Moreover, those who were distressed engaged in more health-risk behaviors than those who were not distressed. That is, the distressed participants were more likely than the nondistressed to engage in unprotected vaginal intercourse or in sexual activity with multiple partners, fail to use contraceptives, experience dating violence, and have lower self-efficacy in negotiating condom use. The investigators suggested that the relationships between perceived psychological distress and sexual risk behaviors might continue to cause problems for these young women over time owing to feelings of powerlessness in sexual relationships. They strongly suggested that early interventions with adolescent females be developed to decrease the likelihood of adverse health outcomes, including exposure to HIV/AIDS.

Stress, Coping, and Smoking

The relationship between stress, coping, and health-risk behaviors in adolescents has been demonstrated in a number of studies. For example, Siqueira, Diab, Bodian, and Rolnitzky (2000) conducted a cross-sectional study of 954 adolescent clinic patients who were between 12 and 21 years old. Participants in the study were primarily from ethnic minority groups (47% African American, 46% Hispanic, 2% Asian or Pacific Islander, and 5 % White) and female (82%). The purpose of the study was to examine the association among stress, coping, and smoking status in an inner city population of adolescents. Using a stress and coping framework, these researchers hypothesized the following:

1. Smokers, compared to those who never smoked or those who only experimented with smoking, would report more negative life events (stressors).

2. Current smokers would perceive the highest levels of stress, and those who never smoked would perceive the least.

3. Smokers would report that stress was the most common reason for progressing through stages from not smoking to smoking.

4. Those who never smoked would report using more positive coping methods than those who became smokers.

5. Smokers would use more negative coping methods than those who never smoked.

Data were collected through a written questionnaire completed at the medical clinic. The Perceived Stress Scale, the Scale of Negative Life Events, and the Coping Measures Scale were used to operationalize the major concepts of perceived stress, negative life events (stressors), and coping methods. Findings were that 34% of the participants had never smoked, 32% had experimented (i.e., smoked a few times in the past), and 26% currently smoked. Current smokers began smoking at an average age of 13.3 years. Those experimenting with smoking had delayed initiation of this health-risk behavior until an average age of 15.5 years. After adjusting for demographic variables, the researchers found that negative life events, such as having a serious accident, and perceived stress were highest in the group of current smokers and lowest in those who had never smoked ($p < .001$). Using stepwise logistic regression techniques, they also found that the following factors were significantly related to smoking status in this sample: negative life events; perceived stress; frequent use of negative coping methods, such as feeling helpless; and less frequent use of positive coping strategies, such as problem solving and seeking parental support.

All directional hypotheses were supported. Both the number of negative life events (stressors) and perceived levels of stress were highest among smokers, moderate among experimenters, and lowest among nonsmokers. Participants indicated that stress relief was the most common (72%) reason for progressing from experimenting with smoking to becoming a smoker. Nonsmokers used more positive coping methods (e.g., seeking parental support), whereas smokers used more negative coping methods (e.g., throwing things and screaming) for stress relief.

Although the study has limitations, including a subject base of primarily female, inner-city minority adolescents and a reliance on self-report measures, it does provide support for a theory of stress and coping. Hypotheses derived from the theory were supported by empirical evidence. Moreover, as the researchers concluded, early interventions could be developed to assist adolescents to recognize stressful events in their lives and to learn and practice positive coping methods for managing stress. Thus, application of this theoretical framework has the potential for controlling a health-risk behavior in adolescents.

Stress, Coping, and High-Risk Sexual Behavior

In a study of 398 gay and bisexual males 19 to 63 years old (mean age, 35.7 years), Folkman, Chesney, Pollack, and Phillips (1992) found no significant relationship between stress and unprotected anal intercourse. Sex was used as a way to cope with stressful events more often by those men who engaged in unprotected intercourse than those who did not report unprotected sex. Unprotected anal intercourse was also associated with negative coping strategies such as hiding one's feelings. These researchers concluded that a stress and coping model was useful to understand health-risk behavior in vulnerable populations.

Stress, Coping, and Weapon Carrying

Wood, Foy, Layne, Pynoos, and James (2002) conducted two studies in which they (a) compared youth in juvenile detention centers with those in high schools and (b) examined within-group differences among the incarcerated youth. The primary hypotheses of the two studies was that adolescents who experienced higher levels of exposure to violence within their families and communities, along with higher levels of post-traumatic stress symptoms, would also report more delinquent behaviors (e.g., gang involvement and carrying weapons). Findings from the study showed significant differences between the comparison groups in the first study: Youth in juvenile detention centers had experienced more violence and had more symptoms of post-traumatic stress than the youth attending high schools. In the second study, youth who had higher levels of exposure to violence also reported higher levels of post-traumatic stress disorder symptoms, but levels of delinquent activity were not significantly related to these independent variables. However, in the second study, females who had experienced physical punishment were significantly more likely than other females to carry weapons. The authors suggested that further study is needed to identify the trajectories that lead to adolescent delinquent behavior, particularly the role played by early victimization and the stress associated with such experiences.

Stress, Coping, and Attempting Suicide

Coping with stress has also been associated with other extreme health-risk behaviors, such as suicide attempts. Wilson and colleagues (1995) compared 20 adolescents who attempted suicide with 20 comparison youth (13 females, 7 males, all between 14 and 17 years old). The group that had attempted suicide reported more experiences of severe life stress than the group that had never made suicide attempts. Those who attempted suicide also revealed inaccurate appraisal of the amount of control they had over the stressful events they experienced. Although those who attempted suicide could generate as many adaptive coping strategies as the comparison group, they were less likely to actually use them.

Stress and Autoimmune Disorders

Rabin (2002) recently discussed the role of stress in the development of the autoimmune disease multiple sclerosis. The disease is characterized by muscle weakness, impaired vision, and paralysis related to lesions in the brain and spinal cord. The conduction of nerve impulses is interrupted when the myelin sheath that surrounds nerve fibers is destroyed by macrophages and lymphocytes. Rabin argues that although stress is generally associated with reduced functioning of the immune system, in the case of multiple sclerosis, stress would be associated with increased functioning. Further, he points out that additional research is needed to determine the components of the immune system that are functionally altered by stress and how alterations in the immune system are related to damaged tissues (p. 74).

Gender and Ethnic Differences in Adolescent Coping

How adolescents cope with stressful events in their lives varies not only with the type of stressor but also with gender and ethnic differences. Psychological and physiological responses to stress have been found to vary by gender in adolescence (Chase, Treboux, & O'Leary, 2002; Frydenberg & Lewis, 1991, 1993b; Munsch & Wampler, 1993; Steiner, Ryst, Berkowitz, Gschwendt, & Koopman, 2002; Stevens, Murphy, & McKnight, 2003; Thoits, 1991). For example, Steiner et al. (2002) studied heart rate and self-reports of positive and negative affect in 133 adolescents who completed a speech task. The participants (73 females and 60 males) were 14 to 18 years old and were invited to speak uninterrupted for 10 minutes into a tape recorder about the most stressful life event they had ever experienced or to speak spontaneously for 10 minutes with no particular topic requested. The presentation of these two tasks was randomized, and baseline measures were taken in addition to measures immediately following each of the speech tasks. Measurements included heart rate, the State-Trait Anxiety Inventory (Spielberger, 1983), and a Visual Analogue Arousal Scale (Folkman & Lazarus, 1985). The researchers found that approach or problem-solving coping was negatively correlated and avoidance coping was positively correlated with health-risk behaviors and health problems.

Feldman and colleagues (1995) conducted a longitudinal study of a random sample of 166 adolescents (84 females and 82 males). Data were collected at two times: first when participants were adolescents and second when they were young adults. The average time between the two measurements was 5.8 years. The purpose of the study was to examine gender differences in the relationship between coping in adolescence and adaptation in adulthood. Three hypotheses were tested:

1. Adolescent coping behaviors will predict adult adaptation for both females and males.

2. Some links between adolescent coping and adult adaptation will be gender specific.

3. Coping behaviors congruent with female gender role (i.e., using religion and consulting with others) will predict poor adaptation for male but not for female adults.

Findings were that main effects of both gender and coping predicted adaptation at Time 2. Adolescent coping behaviors predicted adult adaptation as hypothesized, but the correlations were modest ($r = .14$, $p < .10$ to $r = .48$, $p < .001$). Also as predicted, coping behaviors congruent with a female gender role predicted adaptive outcome for young women but not for young men. Among females, those who displayed coping responses of turning to religion and consulting friends at Time 1 had low levels of anxiety and depression and high measures of self-esteem at Time 2. However, males who displayed these same coping responses in adolescence did not show adaptation to work satisfaction and romantic attachment as young adults.

Other researchers have shown that stressful experiences early in life predict depression later in life. In a study of fourth and fifth graders (n = 174), Broderick (1998) found that girls more often than boys reported endorsement of a ruminative approach in dealing with stressors associated with school, family, and peers. This approach focuses on emotions turned inward, with attention given to negative thoughts and feelings.

In a study of 378 adolescents (104 females and 274 males) enrolled in drug treatment programs in a southern state, Stevens et al. (2003) found significant gender differences in levels of traumatic stress and in engaging in health-risk behaviors of substance use and HIV-risk behaviors. Specifically, they found that both males and females with acute symptoms of traumatic stress engaged in more problematic substance use and HIV-risk behaviors (e.g., multiple sexual partners, inconsistent use of protection during sexual intercourse) than did those with lower levels of traumatic stress. Moreover, females more often than males reported significantly more substance use problems and HIV-risk behaviors. Females and those with acute levels of traumatic stress also reported more physical and mental health problems than males and those with low levels of traumatic stress.

Rudolph (2002) recently proposed a model for understanding gender differences in interpersonal stress and emotional distress in adolescents. Major concepts of this model are *stress exposure, stress reactivity,* and *emotional responses.* Stress exposure refers specifically to the individual's perception of stress experienced in response to negative interpersonal events. Stress reactivity refers to the consequences of experiencing psychological distress in response to events. Emotional response refers to symptoms of anxiety and depression. Rudolph's hypotheses were as follows:

1. During adolescence, females are exposed to higher levels of interpersonal stress than males are.

2. Females display greater negative emotional reactions (i.e., anxiety and depression) to interpersonal stress than males do.

3. Both a heightened exposure to stress and greater reactivity to interpersonal stress account for differences between males and females in showing symptoms of anxiety and depression.

4. Females have higher levels of interpersonal sensitivity than males, which accounts for some of the gender differences in anxiety, depression, and stress reactivity.

Rudolph (2002) also claimed that gender differences in peer relationships are intensified during adolescence for two reasons: (a) peers become the primary context for one's emotional experience and socialization, and (b) gender roles become more important. For females, changes in friendship circles and in roles result in higher levels of stress than in males. Also, females experience greater stress from the awareness that interpersonal conflict may threaten a friendship. This may be due in part to the relatively greater importance of relationships in self-definition for females than for males. Moreover, females are more likely than males to generate stress within relationships (Rudolph, 2002, p. 11). Because females experience greater emotional responsiveness or reactivity to stress, they are also more vulnerable to anxiety and depression as a consequence of stress.

Some health-risk behaviors, such as smoking and expressions of violence, may actually be coping strategies employed by adolescents to cope with perceived stressors in their lives. Recent evidence suggests that not only do males and females cope differently with stress but that minority youth differ from youth of the dominant culture in the style of coping they use when facing specific stressors. Cultural differences affect attitudes and beliefs about life's experiences. Diverse ethnic groups may have very different perceptions of self, family, community, acceptable and unacceptable behaviors, health and illness (Huff & Kline, 1999a). These shared beliefs and norms also affect how life's experiences and transitions are perceived, what is felt as stressful, and what is considered normal or adaptive in terms of coping. For example, Kobus and Reyes (2000) interviewed 158 Mexican American high school students (62% female; average age 16.4 ± 0.6 years) to determine what they perceived as major stressors in their lives and what strategies they employed to cope with these stressors. The majority of participants (55%) in this study identified family stressors as the most difficult aspect of their lives while in high school. Other major stressors were friends (22%), school (16%), and personal factors (7%) such as getting into trouble with the police, spending time in jail, personal injury or illness, and failing to make an athletic team. Family stressors were identified more than twice as often by females as by males. Friend stressors were also much more common among females than males. School stressors were slightly more common among males than females, and personal stressors were nearly three times as common among males as females.

In Kobus and Reyes's (2000) study, active coping, which included seeking information, decision making, problem solving, and taking direct action, was used more frequently (22.5%) than any other strategy. Family social support (13.9%), self-reliance (13.5%), and behavioral avoidance (11.1%) were also used relatively often by the participants in this study. Coping strategies used less commonly in this sample were friend social support (8.6%); venting emotions (8.2%); distraction (7.8%); mental avoidance or denial (7.4%); other social support (e.g., from professionals such as teachers or counselors; 3.7%); and rebellious activity such as acting out, engaging in violence, or engaging in antisocial activities (3.3%). Family social support was characterized as talking with family members for advice or support. Self-reliance coping meant that the adolescent dealt with the stressor autonomously by dealing with it alone, passively accepting the situation, and maintaining a positive outlook. Behavioral avoidance coping meant that the adolescent actively withdrew or avoided the stressor. There were statistically significant gender differences in coping strategies of family social support $[X^2 (1244) = 4.3, p < .05]$ and in venting emotions $[X^2 (1244) = 4.3, p < .05]$. Females reported using these strategies more often than males.

Kobus and Reyes (2000) also asked participants in their study to identify how helpful they perceived their coping strategies to be. Participants perceived that friend support was the most helpful $[t (38.77) = 4.21, p < .001]$ and that problem-focused strategies were more helpful than emotion-focused ones $[t (239) = 5.66, p < .001]$. The researchers concluded that active coping strategies were used most frequently by these Mexican American youth and that the participants recognized such strategies as being more effective than avoidance or emotional coping. They also noted that gender differences were greater in this sample than in other studies of majority youth.

The interaction of gender and ethnicity on coping was studied in a sample of 244 ninth graders. Multiple analyses of variance reflected significant differences in coping by gender $[F(13, 220) = 14.24, p < .0001]$ and ethnicity $[F(13, 220) = 3.196, p < .0002]$, but there was no significant difference in the interaction between these attributes $[F(13, 220) = 0.759, p < .70]$. Females scored significantly higher than males on four coping strategies: proactive orientation, catharsis, positive imagery, and self-reliance. In contrast, males scored significantly higher on three coping strategies: problem avoidance, physical diversions, and passive diversions. Hispanic participants were more likely than Anglos to use coping strategies of social activities and seeking spiritual support (Copeland & Hess, 1995).

Arguing that school is often a stressful environment for many students, Munsch and Wampler (1993) studied seventh graders in two junior high schools $(N = 464)$ to determine if there were differences in ethnic groups in (a) prevalence of stressful events at school, (b) coping strategies used to address these stressors, and (c) perceived social support from other people. Owing to small numbers of American Indians, Asian Americans, and those of mixed heritage, only three groups were compared: African Americans, Anglo Americans, and Mexican Americans. A total of seven school-related stressful events were compared, and both the African American and Mexican American groups were significantly more likely to have experienced these stressful events than was the Anglo group. The seven events were in-school suspension, difficulty getting along with teacher, failing a test, being sent to detention, being hassled by other students, failing a class, and making poor grades. The Anglo participants were more likely to have experienced a positive stressful event of being chosen for an important activity.

Perceptions of these events as stressful were not significantly different among groups except in two areas: (a) Anglo and Mexican American participants gave being chosen for an important activity a more positive rating than African Americans [$F(2, 296) = 4.93, p < .01$], and (b) Anglo American participants rated *not* being chosen for an important activity as more stressful than the African American participants [$F(2, 138) = 5.26, p < .01$]. Of the six types of coping responses used, there were significant ethnic differences in only two: (a) cognitive avoidance [$F(2, 381) = 3.34, p < .05$] and (b) seeking alternative rewards [$F(2, 381) = 6.76, p < .01$]. Cognitive avoidance was defined as "attempting to avoid thinking realistically about a problem," and seeking alternative rewards was defined as "attempting to get involved in substitute activities and create alternative sources of satisfaction" (Munsch & Wampler, 1993, p. 637). Post hoc analysis (Scheffé's test) did not detect differences by ethnic group for cognitive avoidance coping. African American participants, however, used seeking alternative rewards as a coping strategy significantly more than Anglo participants (Munsch & Wampler, 1993).

In terms of social support, Mexican and African American participants were more likely to seek and receive social support from adult relatives (not parents) than were Anglo participants, but the total number of people named as providers of social support did not differ significantly. African and Mexican American participants were more likely than Anglo participants to receive problem-solving help. African American participants more than Anglo or Mexican Americans reported that they engaged in risk-taking behavior with their social support network (Munsch & Wampler, 1993).

These researchers also found gender differences in the total number of people contacted for social support. Males contacted significantly fewer supportive people than did females [$t(432) = -3.48, p < .001$]. Females reported receiving more emotional support than did males [$F(1, 1597) = 16.04, p < .001$], whereas males reported receiving more instrumental support [$F(1, 1597) = 4.46, p < .05$], more problem-solving support [$F(1, 1597) = 6.61, p < .01$], and more distraction support [$F(1, 1597) = 5.25, p < .05$] than females. Males also reported engaging in more risk-taking behaviors with people who provided social support than did females [$F(1, 1597) = 35.54, p < .001$].

The researchers concluded that the ethnic differences found in this study had important implications for cultural differences in adolescent coping with school stressors. They suggested that the greater perception of events as stressful along with some of the coping strategies of minority groups might alienate them from school and prevent them from being connected in protective ways. They further suggested that programs to enhance coping skills should be sensitive to cultural differences (Munsch & Wampler, 1993).

Research Applications

Hardin, Carbaugh, Weinrich, Pesut, and Carbaugh (1992) described the stressors and coping strategies of 195 high school students who had survived Hurricane Hugo in South Carolina. Participants in this study identified 207 stressors associated with their experiences relative to the hurricane. The top two stressors identified were issues related to concerns about boyfriend or girlfriend and threats to self. Using three different theoretical approaches to dimensions of coping, the researchers categorized the adolescents' responses and found that the majority used positive strategies, such as social support and distraction. Few of them (11%) relied on negative coping strategies, such as aggression and withdrawal.

Stewart and colleagues (1992) developed and evaluated the efficacy of a cognitive social support group intervention for adolescents who had experienced Hurricane Hugo in 1989. The purpose of the support group was to mitigate the experience of disaster stress. The investigators defined disaster stress as "a human response with characteristic feelings, behaviors, and coping mechanisms following a disaster; these responses include both immediate reactions and long-term consequences, which are mediated by coping mechanisms and support" (p. 110). The psychoeducational intervention was designed to help adolescents understand and use social support as an adaptive coping mechanism for dealing with disaster stress. It was 155 minutes in length, was administered by professional therapists, and consisted of both small- and large-group activities. Overall, 96% of rural and 79% of suburban students rated the small-group activities as either "very good" or "excellent." Eighty-five percent of rural and 69% of suburban students rated the large-group activities as either "very good" or "excellent."

Chapter Summary

The concept of stress has been applied to our understanding of how people adapt to a changing environment. Selye's work provided a foundation for examining the effects of stressors on physiological responses that serve to protect the organism but that can, over time, lead to illness. Lazarus and colleagues' work on the relationships among cognitive appraisal, coping, and emotion in response to stressful events has expanded our understanding of the complex dynamics that shape a person's behavior in response to the environment. Coping and emotion are seen as processes rather than traits. The conservation of resources approach focused on the importance of viewing the environment to determine whether or not it contained adequate resources to assist a person in coping successfully and adapting to stress. Moos articulated the importance of the environment on coping responses in the adolescent, particularly the role of the family and its use of social resources. Other models of stress and coping were shown to highlight differences in the way male and female adolescents and those of diverse ethnic groups respond to social stressors and how perceived stress affects health-risk behaviors.

Suggestions for Further Study

The biological, social, and psychological models of stress and coping have shed some light on our awareness of the effects of stress and coping on adolescent health and health-risk behaviors. However, much more could be done to enhance this awareness. Whereas previous research has focused on perceived stress or stressors as causative factors, they may also be viewed as mediators between developmental stage and health-risk behaviors. Longitudinal studies should be conducted to determine how perceptions of stress and coping skills are developed over time and how these are related to other competencies in early and late adolescence. Selye's model provides a framework for examining the physiological changes that occur over time as the individual experiences various stressors. Combining physiological measures with cognitive appraisals, emotions, and observations of the resources within the environment would require theory synthesis and would lead to a more holistic understanding of how stress affects the whole person.

In his expansion of the conceptualizations of stress and coping to include the process of emotion, Lazarus (1999) suggests the use of narrative analysis rather than traditional quantitative methods of research. He further argues that each stressor is unique and presents a variety of threats, demands, challenges, and opportunities for the person who experiences the stressor. He also asserts that a narrative approach is the preferred method for examining a systems approach to stress, coping, and adaptation. A narrative approach would require sophistication in regard to analyzing and interpreting qualitative data. A combined narrative and qualitative approach to the study of stressful life events as well as traumatic stress would be particularly useful in developing interventions appropriate for various developmental stages.

More work is needed to clarify the concept of distress and its relationship to coping, to health-risk behaviors, and to mental health outcomes. Unfortunately, such concepts have been used to study adolescents without being framed by theory. This atheoretical approach to knowledge development leads to equivocal findings that impede progress in the science of adolescent health.

Differences by gender and ethnicity in both the perception of stress and the coping strategies used to manage them also should be studied in more detail. Again, longitudinal studies could be designed to identify how gender and ethnicity interact over time to influence the physiological, cognitive, and emotional responses to stressful environments and experiences. The findings of these studies could provide a foundation for developing anticipatory guidance interventions to offset the risk for adverse outcomes related to perceived stress.

The Commonsense Model of Illness Representation may be a useful framework for studying the interaction of cognitive and emotional responses to stressful stimuli in adolescents. The inclusion of personal representations of the threat of a stimulus and one's emotional response to it as part of an information-processing system is worthy of further investigation, particularly as it relates to health-risk behaviors in adolescents.

Related Web Site

Stress and Disease: The Contributions of Hans Selye to Neuroimmune Biology: http://home.cc.umanitoba.ca/%7Eberczii/page2.htm

Suggestions for Further Reading

Ahmad, A., Sundelin-Wahlsten, V., Sofi, M. A., Qahar, J. A., & von Knorring, A.-L. (2000). Reliability and validity of a child-specific cross-cultural instrument for assessing posttraumatic stress disorder. *European Child & Adolescent Psychiatry, 9*, 285-294.

Foa, E. B., Johnson, K. M., Feeny, N. C., & Treadwell, K.R.H. (2001). The Child PTSD Scale: A preliminary examination of its psychometric properties. *Journal of Clinical Child Psychology, 30*, 376-384.

Greenwald, R. (2002). Motivation-adaptive skills-trauma resolution (MASTR) therapy for adolescents with conduct problems: An open trial. *Journal of Aggression, Maltreatment & Trauma, 6*(1), 237-261.

Huerta, R., & Brizuela-Gamino, O. L. (2002). Interaction of pubertal status, mood and self-esteem in adolescent girls. *Journal of Reproductive Medicine, 47*(3), 217-225.

Kanner, S., Hamrin, V., & Grey, M. (2003). Depression in adolescents with diabetes. *Journal of Child and Adolescent Psychiatric Nursing, 16*(1), 15-24.

Lerman, C., & Glanz, K. (1997). Stress, coping, and health behavior. In K. Glanz, F. M. Lewis, & B. K. Rimer (Eds.), *Health behavior and health education: Theory, research, and practice* (2nd ed., pp. 113-138). San Francisco: Jossey-Bass.

Rice, V. H. (Ed.). (2000). *Handbook of stress, coping, and health: Implications for nursing research, theory, and practice*. Thousand Oaks, CA: Sage.

6

Risk, Vulnerability, and Problem Behavior

In the previous chapter, we saw how events and circumstances in the environment place demands on the individual. In general, as perceived stressful experiences increased, those persons with few adaptive coping resources were likely to engage in behaviors such as early smoking or sexual relationships. Engaging in these behaviors carries with it a predisposition or vulnerability for adverse health outcomes. In this chapter, we will take a closer look at the concepts of risk and vulnerability and how they are manifested in the behaviors of and related health outcomes in adolescents.

Risk and Vulnerability

The concept of *risk* has long been associated with the insurance industry and represents the amount of money the company stands to lose if an insured person has an accident or dies. The chance that the insurance company will profit by insuring someone with low risk is contrasted with the chance that the company will lose money by insuring someone with high risk, thus accounting for differences in the prices of insurance policies. This concept is well known to parents who purchase insurance for the family car when there is an adolescent of driving age in the family. Because adolescents are involved in more serious motor vehicle accidents than middle-aged adults, the cost of insuring the family car increases dramatically when one or more adolescents obtain a driver's license. In the eyes of the insurance company, a family with a teen driver is a greater risk than a family without such a driver. The insurance company stands to lose more money from insuring this family because of the increased likelihood of a motor vehicle crash; also, the insurance company stands to lose more money from an accident involving the young driver than it receives in payment for the insurance policy.

Garmezy (1985) traced the concept of risk back to the field of marine insurance. Hundreds of years ago, when going to sea was much more dangerous, bargains were struck to determine the cost for travel or shipment by boat. The consumer and provider had to consider the possibility of success versus failure of the venture and what factors (e.g., mechanical, human, weather) needed to be considered in calculating the chances of success versus failure.

In epidemiology, the term *risk* is concerned with identifying factors that increase one's possibility of developing a disease. More specifically, "risk is a statement of the probability or chance that an individual will develop a disease over a specified period, conditioned on that individual's not dying from any other disease during the period" (Friis & Sellers, 1996, p. 76). Risk ranges from zero to one; statements of risk require a specific reference period. Risk can be estimated as the cumulative incidence of a particular disease or the proportion of the specified population that acquires the disease within a specified period of time (Friis & Sellers, 1996). Applied to the social morbidities and mortalities of adolescence, the term has come to represent those factors, particularly behaviors or processes, that increase an individual's or population's chances of experiencing adverse health outcomes.

The term *vulnerability* is used to reflect a person's susceptibility or sensitivity to a disease or injury. High vulnerability is generally thought of in terms of a lack of resources or lack of accessibility to resources that would protect one from adverse health outcomes or minimize their effects (Flaskerud & Winslow, 1998). For example, children growing up in poverty are vulnerable to poor health outcomes because their families may have too few resources to ensure that they eat nutritionally balanced meals. The family may lack knowledge of health-care providers who might furnish guidance about healthy development or low-cost care when a child is ill. Also, poor families are likely to lack health insurance, which can prevent children from receiving recommended immunizations and regular healthy child examinations. All of these factors increase a child's vulnerability to poor health status.

Many factors can contribute to a person's vulnerability by increasing the risk for specific outcomes. For example, children of alcoholics are vulnerable to adverse health outcomes owing to their parents' inability to pay sufficient attention to their child's health and safety. The parents' modeling of a health-risk behavior (i.e., alcohol abuse) also increases children's risk for abusing alcohol or other substances, either as adolescents or as adults (Chassin, Pitts, DeLucia, & Todd, 1999). There is even evidence that substance abuse in fathers is related to a reduction in cortisol production in adolescent boys, which reduces the adolescent's ability to cope with stress, thus making him more vulnerable to engaging in health-risk behaviors as a coping strategy. A study of 300 adolescent males between 10 and 12 years old was conducted to test hypotheses that (a) cortisol levels would be lower in boys whose fathers had a substance abuse problem and (b) that the cortisol underreactivity would be related to the sons' drug use. Results were that the boys whose fathers had a substance use disorder did, in fact, have lower cortisol levels than boys whose fathers did not have such a disorder. And these lower cortisol levels were related to regular cigarette smoking and marijuana use in adolescence (Moss, Vanyukov, Yao, & Kirillova, 1999).

Factors that increase adolescents' risk for adverse health outcomes exist within the context of social changes that affect the individual, the family, and the community (Dryfoos, 1992). Adolescent development takes place within complex ecological niches that are heterogeneous. For example, the health risks associated with living in inner city neighborhoods are much greater than those associated with living in socially and financially advantaged suburban neighborhoods. Inner city minority youth, in particular, are exposed to neighborhoods where violence and drug use are common. Daily experiences with drug peddlers and persons with short tempers may adversely affect an adolescent's physical and mental well-being. A sample of 522 female African American students 14 to 18 years old was surveyed and interviewed to determine history of gang involvement and health risk behaviors. Logistic regression analyses showed that, compared to participants who did not report a history of gang involvement, those who did were more than three times as likely to have been expelled from school ($OR = 3.6$), have a nonmonogamous sexual partner ($OR = 2.4$), test positively for marijuana ($OR = 2.6$), test positively for *Trichomonas vaginalis* ($OR = 2.2$) or *Neisseria gonorrhoeae* ($OR = 3.6$), be a binge drinker ($OR = 3.3$), and have been involved in at least three fights during the previous 6 months ($OR = 3.8$) (Wingood et al., 2002).

Another ecological niche that carries a high risk for adverse health outcomes is that of disadvantaged, poverty-stricken rural areas. Whereas most impoverished inner city adolescents are ethnic or racial minorities, the majority of poor rural adolescents are White. The necessities of helping with the work associated with rural living force many adolescents to grow up before their time. Many drop out of school because of the demands to work in support of the family. This early transition into adult responsibilities often exposes these youth to early involvement in adult behaviors such as sexual relationships and alcohol use (Crockett, 1999).

Adolescent Risky Behavior

Throughout recorded history, adults have expressed concern about the behaviors displayed by adolescents. Each new generation finds a way to question and challenge the status quo. Over time, the behaviors that were labeled as risqué by adults in a particular historical and sociocultural setting become normative, and the next group of youngsters must find new ways to express its growing independence.

The decades of the 1960s and 1970s in the United States were characterized by dramatic social changes. Adults expressed great concern about the behaviors of that generation's youth. Adolescents were outspoken about the Vietnam conflict and experimented with alternative lifestyles that made their parents and grandparents cringe. Specifically, adults were concerned about the rising numbers of youth involved in political activism and social protest, use of illicit drugs, and relaxation of social norms for sexual behaviors. At the same time, technological advances in basic sciences had nearly eradicated the life-threatening diseases of the previous generations. It was in this context that social and behavioral scientists became interested in systematic examination of the various behaviors of youth that threatened their health and their very lives. Problem-behavior theory, proposed by Jessor and Jessor (1977), provided a coherent conceptualization of a phenomenon worthy of scientific attention. Classified as a midrange theory because of its delimited scope on specific behaviors, it provided an important road map for understanding the social morbidities and mortalities of individuals in the second decade of life.

Problem-Behavior Theory

Origins

Richard and Shirley Jessor began their conceptualization of deviant behavior (i.e., heavy alcohol use) in a rural community in the Southwest. They were interested in examining differences in three ethnic groups within this community. The original model was revised, with particular changes made in concepts within the personality system and the environment system. This revision was made to provide for the potential for understanding youth development (Jessor & Jessor, 1977). Jessor and Jessor were strongly influenced by Kurt Lewin's field theory and Rotter's (1966) conceptualization of locus of control.

Purpose

The theory was constructed to allow social and behavioral scientists to assess and explain deviant social behaviors of adolescents. The original conceptualization was in response to heavy alcohol use in a rural community (see Figure 6.1). This framework was then expanded to address other behaviors (i.e., marijuana and alcohol use, sexual intercourse, political activism, and general deviance from social norms). Further extension of the theory was done to include risk taking while driving, termed risky driving (Jessor, 1987).

Meaning of the Theory

Assumptions of the problem-behavior theory are that specific behaviors exhibited by adolescents cause problems for those adolescents and those in the environment around them. Individuals are characterized as having a set of cognitive attributes (e.g., attitudes, beliefs, values, expectations) that are derived from social interaction and have social meaning. The environment influences, supports, models, and controls the individual. The environment is defined by how it is perceived by the individual. Behavior is the outcome

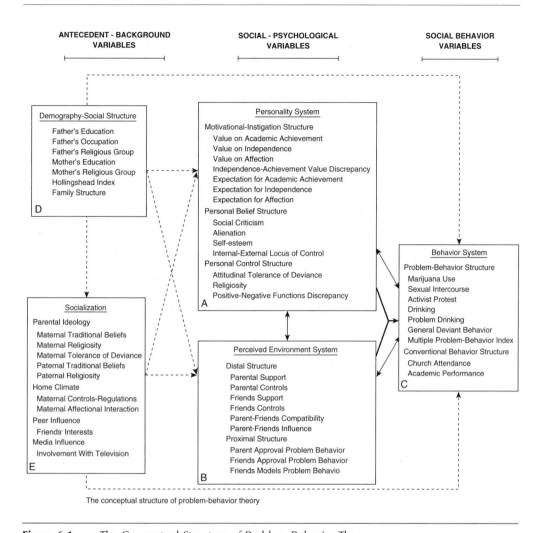

Figure 6.1   The Conceptual Structure of Problem-Behavior Theory

SOURCE: Jessor and Jessor (1977, p. 38). © 1977 Elsevier Science. Reprinted with permission.

of the interaction between personality and environment (Jessor & Jessor, 1977). Jessor and Jessor claim that the use of the term *problem behavior* is value free. That is, they note that any behavior may be perceived as benign or problematic depending on the personal meaning, social definition, context, and time in history at which it occurs.

Other specific assumptions underlying the theory include the following:

1. The value placed on academic achievement reflects an individual's orientation toward conventionality (Jessor & Jessor, 1977, p. 23).

2. The value placed on independence reflects an individual's orientation away from conventionality and from regulation and control by adults (Jessor & Jessor, 1977, p. 24).

3. Problem behavior is purposive and instrumental in attaining goals (Jessor, 1987).

4. Explaining problem behavior in adolescence depends on the psychosocial and behavioral attributes of the individual adolescent, the situation, and the larger society in which the behavior takes place (Jessor, 1987, 1991).

Concepts of the theory represent three domains or systems: environment, personality, and behavior. These major components of the theory are described as systems because of the organization and relationships within and among them that lead to a dynamic state in which problem behavior is more or less likely to occur.

The major variables within the personality system are described as structures and consist of a motivational-instigation structure, a personal belief structure, and a personal control structure. According to Jessor and Jessor (1977), these three structures constitute the nature of persons. The *motivational-instigation structure* refers to those goals and pressures that lead to the urge to engage in a particular behavior.

The motivation to engage in a particular behavior depends on the value an individual places on the goal and his or her expectation that the goal can be obtained. A proposition derived from the theory is that a high value on a goal implies higher likelihood of action toward achieving the goal. In other words, when a person places a higher value on one goal than another goal, there is a greater likelihood that the person will take action toward achieving the goal with the higher relative value. Three psychosocial goals are salient to adolescent problem behavior: (a) academic achievement, (b) independence, and (c) peer affection. Seven variables in the motivational-instigation structure are value on academic achievement, value on independence, value on affection, independence-achievement value discrepancy, expectation for academic achievement, expectation for independence, and expectation for affection. Each of these variables influences the individual in taking action toward achieving a goal. Each of these also has consequences for developing problem behaviors.

Problem behavior is defined as those activities that are "socially defined as a problem, a source of concern, or as undesirable by the norms of conventional society and the institutions of adult authority, and its occurrence usually elicits some kind of social control response" (Jessor & Jessor, 1977, p. 33). Later, Jessor (1982) wrote, "To speak of *problem* behavior, therefore, is not to identify something intrinsic to the act itself, but to emphasize the social and personal *meaning* the behavior has in relation to the actor, the setting, the culture, and a given point in history" (p. 296).

The *personal belief structure* of interest here is constructed of those factors that prevent the individual from engaging in problem behavior. This structure contains four variables: social criticism, alienation, self-esteem, and internal-external locus of control.

Social criticism refers to society's general acceptance or rejection of specific values and behaviors. If the adolescent accepts society's norms about such things as social justice, education, and personal fulfillment, that acceptance becomes a powerful control over engaging in behaviors not condoned by that society. *Alienation* is defined as "a sense of uncertainty about self, a concern about the meaninglessness of one's daily roles and activities, and a belief that one is isolated from involvement with others" (Jessor & Jessor, 1977, p. 21). This definition implies that the individual lacks purpose in life that stems from a lack of social connectedness. *Self-esteem* may be defined as the degree to which individuals evaluate themselves in a positive light; a high amount may prevent an individual from engaging in deviant behavior. *Internal locus of control* "reflects a commitment to the ideology of the larger society, a relatively conventional perspective that, unlike an external orientation, functions to safeguard conventional behavior and to protect against nonconformity" (Jessor & Jessor, 1977, p. 21). *External locus of control,* in contrast, "eliminates the very notion of appropriate behavior since whatever happens is cognitively 'untied' from one's behavior and depends instead upon forces outside oneself" (p. 21). A proposition here is that these four variables are related to each other and covary; relationships among social criticism, alienation, self-esteem, and locus of control produce a patterned set of beliefs that regulate behavior. None of the these personal beliefs relates directly to problem behavior, but each has indirect influences on behaviors.

The *personal control structure* of the personality system is more directly related to problem behaviors. Three concepts comprise this structure: attitudinal tolerance of deviance, religiosity, and discrepancy between positive and negative functions.

Attitudinal tolerance of deviance refers to the individual's disposition toward behaviors that go against society's norms (e.g., lying, stealing). When individuals are intolerant toward deviance, they have direct control over engaging in problem behaviors. *Religiosity* is an individual's involvement in the activities and beliefs associated with religion, particularly those moral sanctions that exist within organized religious ideologies. "Religiosity as a personal control against problem behavior follows from the moral beliefs and the conventional perspectives that are inherent in religious involvement" (Jessor & Jessor, 1977, p. 22). *Positive and negative functions* are the attributes of good and bad that may exist simultaneously in a given behavior (e.g., the positive function of engaging in sexual intercourse is that it can make one feel grown-up and accepted; the negative function of the same behavior is that it can make one vulnerable to unplanned pregnancy and sexually transmitted infections).

The personality system of the adolescent contributes to problem behavior by representing a balance between *instigations,* or the urge to engage in a particular behavior, and *constraints* against engaging in that behavior. Based on the specific assumptions already identified, adolescents who value academic achievement are motivated to participate in conventional activities, whereas when such a value is low and when the value on independence is high, they are more likely to engage in behaviors that are less socially acceptable, such as skipping school. Further, the personal belief structure that emphasizes social criticism and alienation leads to looser controls by an individual and, therefore, a greater likelihood of engaging in problem behaviors. Finally, adolescents with low self-esteem, external locus of control, little religiosity, low expectations for academic achievement, tolerance for deviance, and who place greater importance on positive rather than negative aspects of problem behavior are more likely to engage in those behaviors than adolescents with opposite attributes (Jessor & Jessor, 1977, p. 26).

The structure of the *perceived environment system* is based on the premise of perception—that is, "the environment as it has meaning for an actor, the social-psychological rather than the physical, geographic, or social structural, or demographic environment" (Jessor & Jessor, 1977, p. 27). This is not an objective environment, and it has both distal and proximal structures. The *distal structure of the perceived environment* is the social context in which the individual is located and is somewhat remote in relation to the actual performance of a problem behavior. Examples include parents and friends whose expectations are congruent for a specific adolescent. A hypothesis of the theory is that when an adolescent is located in the parental context, she or he is less prone to engage in problem behavior than when located in a peer context. Six variables comprise the distal structure: perceived support from parents, perceived support from friends, perceived controls from parents, perceived controls from friends, parent-friends compatibility of expectations, and relative influence of parents and friends.

Perceived support means that the individual feels that support and encouragement from parents or friends will be forthcoming when needed. *Perceived controls* means that the individual feels that significant others (i.e., parents or friends) have standards for behavior and would sanction or disapprove of specific behaviors. A hypothesis is that youth in an environment perceived as high in support and controls would be protected from engaging in problem behavior—especially if the support is from parents. The congruency or consensus between parents and friends concerning the youth's behavior is known as *compatibility of expectations* and leads to a sense of certainty for the individual about how to act. The hypothesis here is that low compatibility between parents and peers leads to greater likelihood of problem behavior. *Relative influence of parents and friends* refers to the perception of greater or lesser impact of parents versus friends on an individual's behavior. Parental influence is assumed to be more conventional and of longer duration than that of friends. The hypothesis is that an adolescent who is not currently exposed to conventional standards and who is more involved with peers is more likely to engage in problem behavior.

The *proximal structure of the perceived environment* consists of those factors or persons directly involved in the individual's behaviors (e.g., number of close friends who are also engaging in sexual intercourse). The theoretical definitions of distal and proximal structures are related specifically to the problem behaviors rather than being static phenomena.

Factors in the proximal structure of the perceived environment are generally more powerful than those in the distal structure. Three factors comprise the proximal structure of the perceived environment: friends' approval or disapproval of behavior, parents' approval or disapproval of behavior, and friends' models for problem behavior.

The perceived environment of the adolescent who is prone to problem behaviors is characterized by

> low parental support and controls, low peer controls, low compatibility between parent and peer expectations, and low parent versus peer influence [in the distal structure]. In the proximal structure, it would be characterized by low parental disapproval of problem behavior and by high friends models and approval for engaging in problem behavior. (Jessor & Jessor, 1977, p. 32)

The structure of the behavior system concerns "actions of youth that are considered by the larger society to be inappropriate or undesirable, to depart from widely shared and institutionalized legal or social norms, and to warrant the exercise of social controls" (Jessor & Jessor, 1977, p. 34). General deviant behavior includes lying, stealing, destroying property, and behaving disruptively or aggressively. Six areas of problem behavior were identified in the original model: activism, alcohol use, alcohol abuse, drug use, sexual intercourse, and general deviance. Engaging in problem behavior is a way for the adolescent to achieve certain goals that might not otherwise be attainable. It may also be a way to rebel against adult authority and the conventions of society, or it may represent a way of coping with frustration and failure. Problem behavior may also be a way for the adolescent to identify with peers and to establish a sense of personal identity. Finally, engaging in problem behavior may be symbolic of marking a developmental transition, an attempt for the adolescent to fill the role of adult within the society. Engaging in problem behaviors may also represent a syndrome or cluster of behaviors that enhances this developmental transition (Donovan & Jessor, 1985; Donovan, Jessor, & Costa, 1988; Jessor, 1982, 1991).

In contrast to problem behavior, *conventional behavior* is that activity of which society generally approves and that is expected of individuals within a specific age range. This construct consists of two specific variables: religious involvement and academic performance. Both of these variables are viewed as conventional institutions for socializing youth. The dynamics within the behavior system of the model are obvious. Engagement in one type of behavior (e.g., conventional behavior) precludes engagement in the other (i.e., problem behavior). Moreover, problem behaviors have a tendency to cluster together (e.g., there is a link between heavy drinking and weapon carrying; Bailey, Flewelling, & Rosenbaum, 1997) and to have meaning for youth.

Within each of the three systems of psychosocial influence (i.e., personality, environment, and behavior), explanatory variables include either the *instigations* to engage in the behavior or *controls* against such engagement. Together, these variables comprise a dynamic state of *problem behavior proneness,* or an individual's propensity for engaging in multiple behaviors that are not sanctioned by society (Jessor, 1987). This concept of problem behavior proneness is similar to, if not synonymous with, the terms *risk, risky behavior,* and *psychosocial risk factors* (Jessor, 1992).

In addition to the problem behaviors identified in Jessor and Jessor's original model, Jessor (1987) later included risky driving as a problem behavior. Analyzing data on driving behaviors of 1800 junior and senior high school students, they found that 60% of males and 33% of females reported that they had engaged in risk taking while driving one or more times in the previous 6 months. This behavior was highly correlated with other deviant behaviors in the previous 6-month period. When correlated with the specific domains of problem-behavior theory, risky driving was significantly and positively correlated with measures of higher value on independence relative to achievement and negatively correlated with intolerance of deviance for both males ($p < .05$) and females ($p < .01$). In the perceived environment system, risky driving was significantly correlated with friends who modeled problem behavior for both males ($r = .44$, $p < .001$) and females ($r = .38$, $p < .001$). In the behavior system, risky driving was significantly correlated for both males and females with times drunk in the past 6 months, smoking, marijuana use, and, for males only, frequency of sexual intercourse.

Scope, Parsimony, and Generalizability

Although the original formulation of problem-behavior theory focused on specific problem or deviant behaviors identified in a rural community, the model has been revised and expanded to address a broader range of behaviors across sociocultural settings. However, the broad scope is offset by the inclusion of many concepts or variables that are somewhat cumbersome and detract from the parsimony of the theory. The theory has been generalized to a variety of behaviors, ethnic groups, and countries (Pickett et al., 2002), but it has not been tested in other developmental age groups.

Logical Adequacy

The sheer number of concepts and relationships within the theory make it difficult to determine its logical adequacy. However, predictions can be made from the theory independent of its content. For example, the hypothesis that youth in an environment with perceived support and control are not likely to engage in problem behaviors can be diagrammed:

$$Y + SE \rightarrow PB$$

where Y = youth, SE = supportive environment, and PB = problem behavior. In addition, a number of social scientists have agreed that the theory makes sense.

Usefulness

Jessor's Problem-Behavior Theory has been useful in identifying those behaviors that indicate important developmental transitions in the second decade of life. It has also been useful in providing a rationale for why youth engage in behaviors with health risks. The identification of a cluster of behaviors that may be conceptualized as a syndrome also has useful implications for the development of prevention and health promotion programs (Jessor, 1982).

Testability

Jessor and Jessor (1977) proceeded to test the adequacy of their theory through two longitudinal studies with repeated measures conducted in 1969 and 1972. These studies were of adolescents in junior high schools (grades 7-9), high schools (grades 10-12), and those in colleges in the western part of the United States. In the first study, a random sample of 1126 students, stratified by sex and grade level, was recruited for a 4-year, cohort-sequential study. Of this initial sample, 589 participated in the initial data collection, and at the end of the fourth year, 483 (82%) of the original sample were retained and tested for the last time. A final sample of 432 had complete data sets for all 4 years and was designated as the high school developmental sample. This sample was composed of 89% Anglo, 4% Chicano, and 7% unspecified as Black, Native American, or other race or ethnic category. They were primarily Protestant (71%) and middle class (56% of the subjects' fathers had completed college). Thus the sample is not representative of the American society.

The college study used a straight longitudinal design and was done with students who were freshmen in 1970, through 1973, in a large university (enrollment of approximately 20,000 students). A random sample, stratified for sex, was drawn from the enrollment roster of students in the College of Arts and Sciences. A final sample of 276 students was recruited, and 83% were retained over the 4 years, resulting in 226 for whom there were complete data sets.

Through univariate analyses, Jessor and Jessor showed that the conceptual variables in the model were related to problem behavior. They then conducted multivariate analyses (multiple correlations) to test the utility of the model in predicting problem behaviors in youth. Fourteen stepwise regressions were conducted to analyze each of the problem behaviors, as follows:

- Motivational-instigation structure (value on academic achievement, value on independence, expectation for academic achievement, expectation for affection)
- Personal belief structure (social criticism, alienation, self-esteem)
- Personal control structure (tolerance of deviance, religiosity)
- Personality system (independence vs. achievement, expectation for academic achievement, social criticism, self-esteem, tolerance of deviance)
- Distal structure of perceived environment (parental support, parental controls, parent-friends compatibility, parent-friends influence)
- Proximal structure of perceived environment (parental approval, friends approval, friends as models)
- Perceived environment system (parent-friends compatibility, parent-friends influence, parental approval, friends as models)
- Field pattern (independence-achievement value discrepancy, expectation for academic achievement, social criticism, tolerance of deviance, parent-friends compatibility, friends as models)
- Aggregate set—all preceding variables ($n = 16$)
- Positive-negative functions discrepancies (drug disjunctions and sex disjunctions)
- Behavior system (each problem behavior was regressed on all remaining problem and conventional behaviors)
- Behaviors and functions discrepancies
- Socioeconomic background (father's education and occupation, mother's education)
- Overall set (14 personality, environment, behavior, and socioeconomic variables)

Multiple correlation coefficients of .77, .74, .68, and .68 were obtained for the overall set for females and males in high school and college samples, respectively. These coefficients indicate strong support for the theory (Jessor & Jessor, 1977).

Risky driving as a correlate of other problem behaviors identified in problem-behavior theory provides further support for the theory. Risky driving and involvement in motor vehicle crashes has been found to relate to alcohol use, marijuana use, and delinquent behaviors (Williams, 1998).

Further tests of the problem-behavior theory have been performed by Jessor, Turbin, and Costa (1998). Three ethnic groups (White, Black, and Hispanic) of high school students ($N = 1493$) participated in a longitudinal study.

Empirical Referents

To test the efficacy of the theory, Jessor and Jessor (1977) developed operational definitions for all major variables in the model. These measures are described fully in their book and are beyond the scope of this review.

General psychometric properties of the constructs within each of the systems (i.e., personality, perceived environment, and behavior) have respectable reliabilities (i.e., Cronbach alphas of .71–.92). Measures of constructs with lower reliabilities, however (i.e., Cronbach alphas of .28–.61), should be interpreted cautiously. For example, these include the friends controls (.28), multiple problem behavior index (.43), and parent approval of problem behaviors (.53). Reliability coefficients did vary by age of sample.

The Risky Driving Scale (Jessor, 1987) is composed of four self-report items. Three of the items ask about frequency of risky behaviors in the past 6 months. The fourth item simply asks if the respondent fastens his or her seat belt when riding in a car. Scores on this scale correlate significantly with scores on other measures of constructs from problem-behavior theory (e.g., correlation with frequency of marijuana use in past six months, $r = .62$, $p < .001$). Reliability and validity of the scale were not reported.

Theory Revision and Extension

In 1991, Jessor published a manuscript in which he defined the psychosocial concepts of risk, risk behavior, and lifestyle. In this article, he argued that the traditional epidemiological meaning of *risk* was restrictive and that the term should be broadened to include behavior as well as biomedical outcomes. He added that the outcomes of risk also needed to be broadened because some outcomes of risk behaviors, such as smoking, can be positive. That is, smoking may allow the adolescent to be accepted by peers and may contribute to a sense of maturity and independence.

Jessor (1991) cited considerable empirical evidence to support the covariation among risk behaviors within an individual. He termed this phenomenon *risk behavior syndrome,* noting that the evidence was most profound for risk behaviors that were also problem behaviors (i.e., alcohol and drug abuse, sexual precocity, and delinquency). His use of the term *lifestyle* was meant to convey a holistic view of the adolescent. That is, the risk behavior syndrome means that an individual displays "an organized pattern of interrelated behaviors" (p. 600). Jessor further argued that this had implications for interventions that may need to focus on a youth's lifestyle as a whole rather than on a specific problem behavior.

Jessor and colleagues also identified a clustering of problem behaviors that they termed problem behavior syndrome (Donovan & Jessor, 1985; Donovan, Jessor, & Costa, 1988). Identifying a common group of antecedents, Donovan and Jessor (1985) concluded that these behaviors reflected unconventionality both within individuals and in the environment in which they lived. This notion that the clustering of risky behaviors implied a single underlying process was challenged by other researchers, who failed to find consistent support for the mechanisms that explained diverse problem behaviors (Basen-Engquist, Edmundson, & Parcel, 1996; McCord, 1990).

For example, Basen-Engquist and her colleagues tested the problem behavior syndrome theory by using multidimensional scaling and cluster analysis. Results of analyzing data from 5537 surveys completed by a representative sample of high school students in one state indicated that whereas traditional problem behaviors, such as smoking, drinking, and having sexual relations, represented a single factor, other more destructive behaviors, such as engaging in violence, using hard drugs, and attempting suicide, comprised an independent factor. These researchers concluded that although a single dimension of unconventionality to explain problem behavior was a more parsimonious approach, their demonstration of a multidimensional structure was more precise and could be more beneficial when planning interventions to reduce various health-compromising behaviors.

In an effort to extend his earlier work, which focused on psychosocial factors and outcomes of problem behaviors, Jessor (1991) provided a new conceptual framework for adolescent risk behavior (see Figure 6.2). This framework included the antecedents or determinants of risk behaviors as well as outcomes. The revised model includes three major components: (a) risk and protective factors, also called interrelated conceptual domains of risk factors and protective factors; (b) adolescent risk behaviors and lifestyles; and (c) health- and life-compromising outcomes. The first of these components, interrelated conceptual domains of risk and protective factors, constitutes a "web of causation" (Jessor, 1991, p. 601). Although not all direct and indirect effects of these conceptual domains of causation on risk behaviors are depicted in the figure, Jessor asserts that the effects of various risk domains are "mediated through other risk domains" (p. 601). For example, under the domain of social environment, the risk factor of poverty may have an influence on the personality domain, affecting the adolescent's perceived life chances and therefore having both a direct and an indirect influence on the risk behavior lifestyle of the adolescent.

In further explaining the conceptual framework for adolescent risk behavior, Jessor (1991, 1998) added that a limitation of the model is that it is static or cross-sectional and does not reflect the processes of developmental changes that are continuously occurring in all domains. Moreover, Jessor explained that causal influences throughout the model are bidirectional (i.e., top to bottom and bottom to top) or multidirectional, making the term *web of causation* appropriate for his conceptualization.

Jessor's problem-behavior theory has been extended by others to identify a lifestyle profile of risk-taking adolescents. Using data from the National Longitudinal Study of Adolescent Health (Add Health), Zweig, Phillips, and Lindberg (2002) examined profiles of risk behaviors across four domains of individual psychosocial adjustment, including self-worth and decision-making skills; individual daily adjustment, including hobbies and physical activity; school connectedness; and family connectedness, including parental expectations for education. These researchers had two hypotheses:

Interrelated Conceptual Domains of Risk Factors and Protective Factors

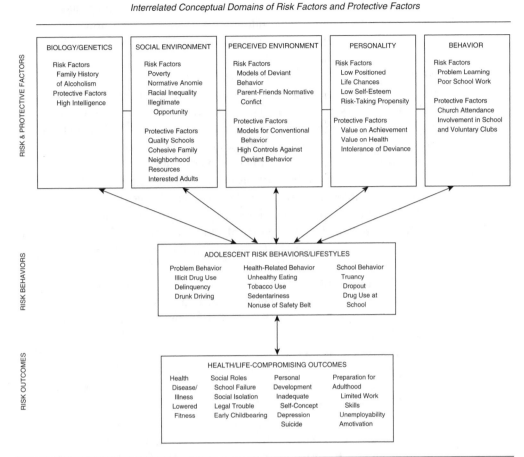

Figure 6.2 A Conceptual Framework for Adolescent Risk Behavior: Risk and Protective Factors, Risk Behaviors, and Risk Outcomes

SOURCE: Jessor (1991, p. 602). © 1991 by Elsevier. Reprinted with permission.

1. Adolescents at lowest risk (i.e., lowest risk profile) would report higher levels of psychosocial adjustment (self-worth, decision-making skills, and positive outlook), individual daily adjustment (hobbies, physical activities, and housework), school connectedness, and family connectedness (parental expectation for education, quality of relationship with parents, and parent-youth closeness) and lower levels of depression than adolescents in other risk profiles.

2. Adolescents at highest risk (i.e., highest risk profile) would report lower levels of psychosocial adjustment, individual daily adjustment, school connectedness, and family connectedness, and higher levels of depression than adolescents in the other risk profiles.

Findings from the study were similar for both males and females. Four distinct profiles differentiated adolescents at higher, high, low, and lower risks relative to vulnerability and protective factors in three of the four domains (i.e., psychosocial adjustment, school connectedness, and family connectedness). In the domain of individual daily adjustment (hobbies, physical activities, and housework), there were few differences by risk profile. The authors concluded that adolescents with high-risk profiles also engaged in many positive behaviors and, consequently, those who plan and provide programs for prevention of health-risk behaviors should understand that recreation alone is not a sufficient intervention.

Influenced by the findings of resilience in the discipline of developmental psychopathology, Jessor, Van Den Bos, Vanderryn, Costa, and Turbin (1995) began to explore the interaction of protective factors with risk factors in predicting adolescent problem behaviors. Using data collected during a longitudinal study of young adolescents in the seventh through ninth grades, Jessor's team found that protective factors, such as positive orientation to school, moderated the relationship between risk factors and problem behavior outcomes. They also demonstrated that protective factors predicted changes in problem behaviors over time. The concepts of protection and resilience will be addressed in more detail in Chapter 7.

Jessor's problem-behavior theory has been extended to address health-related behavior by including concepts of proximal and distal protective factors (Jessor et al., 1998). Proximal protective factors are health specific and are directly related to health behaviors. These factors include an individual's value of health, internal health locus of control, and perceived social support from parents and peers for engaging in health behaviors. Distal protective factors do not have a direct reference to health but nevertheless can serve to protect one from adverse health outcomes. These factors include the individual's personality; perceived social environment; and conventional behaviors such as volunteer work, participation in school and club activities, and involvement with family and church.

Blum, McNeeley, and Nonnemaker (2002) note that the research on vulnerability to adverse health outcomes in adolescents has been complicated by "the lack of a commonly agreed-on language" (p. 28). In particular, they observe that the term *risk* is used to describe risk-taking behaviors such as drinking and smoking, as well as to refer to adolescents who have one or more disadvantages, such as poverty, ethnic minority status, or genetic predisposition to certain diseases. They continue by presenting an ecological model of childhood antecedents of adolescent health-risk behaviors and associated health outcomes. This model is based on concepts of vulnerability, which these researchers define as "an interactive process between the social contexts in which a young person lives and a set of underlying factors that, when present, place the young person 'at risk' for negative outcomes" (p. 28). Blum and colleagues identify two factors that predispose to vulnerability: biologic conditions such as chronic illness and cognitive factors such as how the individual perceives her or his risk. They add that vulnerabilities often result from the effects of disadvantaged environments (such as families in which there is violent and abusive behavior) on an individual as well as the individual's temperament. To offset these vulnerabilities, individuals have resilience, resources, assets, and protective factors emanating from individual, family, and social environments. These scholars also assert that risk behavior is synonymous with problem behavior as defined by Jessor, and these behaviors "jeopardize one or more elements of health or development" (p. 30). This model is an elaboration of Jessor's model and is depicted in Figure 6.3.

In Blum's ecological model, risk and protective factors are identified within the social environment, school, family, peer group, and within the individual. Protective factors will be discussed in greater detail in Chapter 7. Blum and colleagues note that although the risk and protective factors appear to be fixed in the model, they are not, because some factors may increase either risk or protection, depending on developmental stage or on how the terms are defined. The risk and protective factors are depicted as antecedents of health-risk behaviors (i.e., substance use, physical inactivity, eating disorders, violent behavior, and risky sexual activity). Health outcomes of these behaviors include indicators of physical, emotional, and social health.

Risk Perception

Since the introduction of problem-behavior theory, researchers from various disciplines have posed and answered myriad questions about the antecedents, mediators, moderators, and consequences of these behaviors in adolescents. These adolescent behaviors have been identified by a variety of terms, including *risky behaviors, risk-taking behaviors,* and *health-risk behaviors.* An important element, regardless of the term used, is that of the adolescents' own perception of risk in relation to their behavior. The concept of *risk perception* is critical to other theories that may form the basis for interventions such as the Health Belief Model (Rosenstock, 1974a), social cognitive theory (Bandura, 1986, 1997), and the theory of reasoned action and planned behavior (Ajzen, 1985; Fishbein & Ajzen, 1975).

Millstein (2003) proposed a process model of risk perception (Figure 6.4) that consists of three phases. The first phase of the process is *attention,* which is influenced by knowledge about and memory of potential risks. This phase is also influenced by affect, including transient moods as well as affective dispositions such as trait anxiety. Perception of risk, then, begins with paying attention to a real-life situation or cue, having some knowledge about the potential for an adverse outcome, and experiencing some feelings

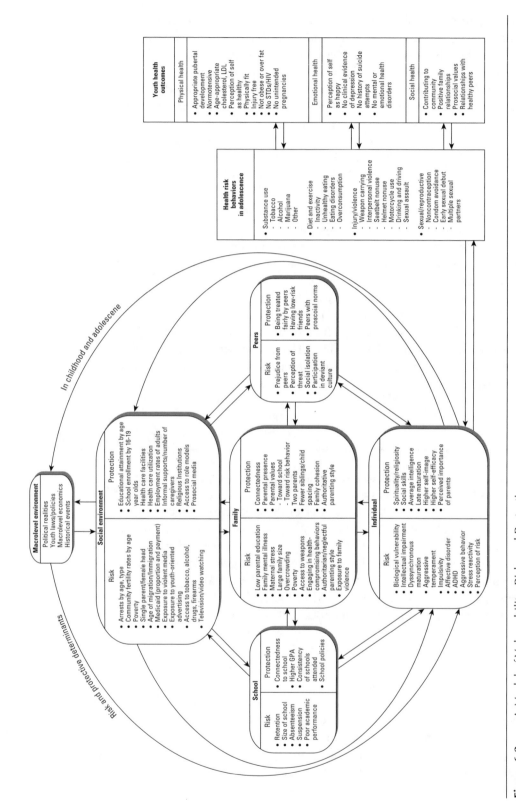

Figure 6.3 A Model of Vulnerability, Risk, and Protection

SOURCE: Blum et al. (2002, p. 37). © Sage Publications, Inc. Reprinted with permission.

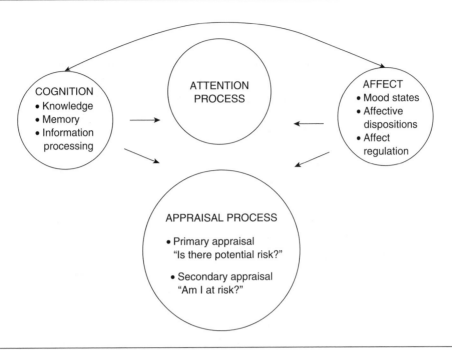

Figure 6.4   A Process Model of Risk Perception: Attention and Appraisal Phases

SOURCE: Millstein (2003, p. 38). © 2003 Sage Publications. Reprinted with permission.

about the situation. The second phase, *appraisal*, consists of primary and secondary levels. The primary appraisal level is more general and focuses on the hypothetical possibility that a risk exists. The secondary appraisal level is more personal and focuses on how likely it is that the person is at risk. Millstein adds that the primary appraisal level is basically cognitive, whereas the secondary appraisal is more emotional.

Risk perception has been the focus of several studies of adolescent health and behavior. For example, between 1975 and 2001, Johnston (2003) demonstrated inverse trends in marijuana and cocaine use relative to perceived risk. Byrnes (2003) notes that not all forms of risk-taking behaviors are harmful. He states, "In my view, all behaviors are performed in contexts and all contexts contain uncertainty because of the inherent probabilistic structure of the world" (p. 13). Moreover, he adds that there are many unintended negative outcomes as a result of virtually everything we do. Thus, there is no way to live without taking risks because all human activity involves some degree of risk. What Byrnes suggests is that adolescents can learn to differentiate between those risks that should and should not be taken. This, he adds, has implications for interventions: Reducing risks for engaging in specific behaviors such as smoking may better be replaced with more comprehensive strategies that focus on developing competencies and health-promoting behaviors.

Related Research _____

Loeber, Farrington, Stouthamer-Loeber, and Van Kammen (1998) have argued against a single underlying syndrome to explain the variety of behaviors that place children and adolescents at risk for adverse outcomes. They have noted that problem behaviors change with age. That is, with increasing age, the frequency, severity, and number of problem behaviors increase. They also have found from their research with males who exhibit delinquent behaviors and conduct disorders that there are different risk factors at different ages for different problem behaviors. These researchers argue that problem behaviors should be extended beyond those identified by Jessor to include symptoms of ADHD, withdrawn and shy behaviors, and depressed mood. Moreover, they provide evidence from a prospective longitudinal survey of 1517 males (initially recruited when they were in first grade, surveyed for a second time in fourth grade, and surveyed a final time in seventh grade) of risk factors for the eight problem behaviors. The eight problem behaviors were (a) delinquency (e.g., minor delinquency was engaging in such things as shoplifting and vandalism; moderately serious delinquency included gang fighting and carrying weapons; serious delinquency included car theft, forced sex, or selling drugs), (b) lifetime substance use, (c) symptoms of ADHD in previous 6 months, (d) symptoms of conduct disorder in previous 6 months, (e) lifetime physical aggression, (f) covert behavior such as manipulation, (g) symptoms of depressed mood in previous 2 weeks, and (h) shy or withdrawn behavior in past year.

Across the three samples (i.e., first grade cohort, fourth grade cohort, and seventh grade cohort), strong associations were found among high scores on the measures of ADHD, conduct problems, covert behavior, and physical aggression. Depressed mood was associated with substance use. However, shy or withdrawn behavior was not. The only risk factor that was related to all eight problem behaviors for all three grade cohorts was low academic achievement. Other risk factors that were related to ADHD, conduct disorder, depressed mood, and shy or withdrawn behaviors were poor supervision within the family and poor communication, particularly in the older cohorts. Risk factors for physical aggression were also related to delinquency and included living in a bad neighborhood, low socioeconomic status, and shy or withdrawn behavior (Loeber et al., 1998).

From this longitudinal study and earlier work, Loeber and colleagues (1998) determined that problem behaviors change with age, but increases in one domain do not necessarily mean that there are increases in all other domains. For example, they found that whereas delinquent behaviors and substance use tended to increase with age, there were gradual decreases by age in disruptive behavioral disorders such as ADHD. They also found that interrelations among the problem behaviors did not vary with age except for the relationship between delinquency and physical aggression, which actually decreased across the grade cohorts. Whereas many risk factors were associated with outcomes at various ages, a few risks were associated with problem behaviors at earlier ages rather than at later ones. For example, being older than one's peers for grade level, having few friends, low academic achievement, and shy or withdrawn behavior were associated with problem behaviors in the youngest cohort but not the older ones. Similarly, family risk factors, including parent substance use, parental anxiety and depression, and parent deviance were associated with more problem behaviors at a younger rather than older age.

Jelalian, Alday, Spirito, Rasile, and Nobile (2000) examined the relationship between demographic (age, gender, race, and grade in school) and behavioral (risk-taking) factors and self-reported injuries from motor vehicle crashes of adolescents attending public high schools. Results of two studies were reported. In the first study, 1576 students in the 9th through 12th grades completed questionnaires concerning their risk-taking behaviors and injuries sustained in the previous 6 months. In the second study, 573 males from an all-male school completed questionnaires concerning their risk-taking behaviors and injuries. Self-reported injuries related to motor vehicle crashes were similar in both studies, with 10% reported by participants in the first study (both males and females) and 16% reported by participants in the second study (only males).

Overall, males reported more risk-taking behaviors and more crash-related injuries than females. In the mixed-gender study, injuries were best predicted by age and risk-taking behaviors. In the males-only study, injuries were best predicted by risk-taking behavior and conduct problems. There were no significant differences in self-reported injuries by race (White vs. non-White). Age was significantly related to use of seat belts and riding with a drunk driver or one who was using drugs. Compared with 16- and 17-year-olds, 14-year-olds were less likely to use seat belts. However, 14-year-olds were less likely than 15-, 16-, and 17-year-olds to ride in a car driven by a person who was drunk or using drugs. In the mixed-gender study, significantly more males than females reported sustaining injuries from riding a moped, motorbike, or snowmobile ($X^2 = 27.74$, $p < .0001$); from driving a car or truck ($X^2 = 8.94$, $p = .004$); and from being hit by a moving vehicle ($X^2 = 5.94$, $p = .02$).

In the males-only study, participants who self-reported injuries related to motor vehicles were significantly more likely to be characterized as having conduct problems [t (620) = 4.56, $p < .001$], impulsivity and hyperactivity [t (621) = 3.16, $p < .001$], problems with inattention [t (621) = 4.30, $p < .001$], and emotional lability [t (626) = 3.39, $p < .001$] than participants who reported no such injuries. Although the research reported by Jelalian and colleagues (2000) did not claim to use problem-behavior theory as a guiding framework, these researchers did cite a previous study by Jessor indicating that risky driving is a problem behavior and that it is related to several other problem behaviors, including substance use. However, two questions from Jessor and Jessor's (1977) Health Behavior Questionnaire that were based on problem-behavior theory were used in the males-only study, and in the discussion section, the research team related their findings to findings from Jessor's previous study (1987) linking adolescent problem behavior with lifestyle.

Co-Occurrence of Health-Risk Behaviors

Brener and Collins (1998), of the Centers for Disease Control and Prevention, reported on the co-occurrence of health-risk behaviors in a nationally representative sample of 10,645 adolescents who were between 12 and 21 years old. Data from the YRBSS from 1992 were analyzed to examine the co-occurrence of multiple health-risk behaviors and to determine if multiple risk behaviors varied by gender, age, or enrollment in school. Younger participants (i.e., 12- to 13-year-olds) were asked if they engaged in the following behaviors in the last 30 days: carrying a weapon, smoking cigarettes, using other tobacco products, drinking five or more alcohol drinks in a row, using marijuana, using cocaine, using seat belts. Older participants were asked these questions as well as whether they had had sexual intercourse in the last 90 days, and the oldest (i.e., 18- to 21-year-olds) were asked if they had used a condom at last intercourse.

Results of the study were that most adolescents who were 12 to 17 years old did not engage in multiple health-risk behaviors; only 8% of 12- to 13-year-olds engaged in two or more of these behaviors, whereas 33% of 14- to 17-year-olds and 50% of the 18- to 21-year-olds engaged in two or more health-risk behaviors. Males reported higher co-occurrence of risk behaviors than females across all age groups. Among the 12- to 13-year-olds, there was no significant difference in multiple health-risk behaviors between those who were not enrolled in school and those who were. However, among the 14- to 17-year-olds and the 18- to 21-year-olds, there was a significant difference ($p < .001$). Among the 12- to 13-year-olds, the most common single health-risk behavior was carrying a weapon or failing to use a seat belt. The older adolescents with only one risk behavior were most likely to report sexual intercourse in the past 90 days (14- to 17-year-olds) and failure to use condoms at last intercourse (18- to 21-year-olds). According to Brener and Collins (1998), the data indicated that engaging in health-risk behaviors varies by age and that both males and those who are not enrolled in school engage in multiple health-risk behaviors much more than most other adolescents. Thus, for males in particular, dropping out of school increases vulnerability to adverse health outcomes by increasing the risk of engaging in behaviors that are detrimental to health or well-being.

Although studies have shown the association of specific health-risk behaviors with one another, there is still considerable speculation about the underlying explanatory mechanisms. Clearly, developmental stage and environmental factors intersect in some ways to increase both vulnerability to poor health outcomes and risk of engaging in health-risk behaviors.

However, other intrinsic and extrinsic factors may also play a key role in the manifestation of these behaviors in adolescents.

Problem Behavior and Adolescent Employment

An investigation of the antecedents, correlates, and consequences of adolescent employment was conducted by Leventhal, Graber, and Brooks-Gunn (2001). These researchers developed a theoretical model that included problem behaviors (e.g., early alcohol and drug use) as an antecedent to adolescent and adult employment among low-income, African American children who had been studied since birth. Leventhal and colleagues found that the participants who repeated a grade in school became employed later in adolescence than their peers and that those who never worked were less advantaged than their peers. The group that was never employed was significantly different from the group that was employed in terms of engaging in problem behavior [$F(1, N = 245) = 6.25, p < .01$]. Employment status may indicate that an adolescent either has or does not have a set of social and behavioral skills necessary to function fully in American society. It may, therefore, be the lack of these skills rather than the employment itself that makes youth more vulnerable to engaging in health-risk behaviors.

Substance Use and Sexual Risk Behavior

The purpose of a prospective, longitudinal study conducted by Tapert, Aarons, Sedlar, and Brown (2001) was to investigate the relationship between substance use and sexual risk taking in late adolescents and young adults. A sample of youth enrolled in substance abuse programs ($n = 105$) and a comparison sample of community-based youth who did not have a history of substance abuse ($n = 77$) were recruited. After baseline data were collected, additional data were collected at 2, 4, and 6 years after the initial collection. Participants were an average of 15.5 years old at baseline and 21.5 years old at the time of the final data collection. Comparisons showed that participants in the substance abuse programs (clinical group) had earlier onset of sexual behaviors, more STDs, more sexual partners, and more inconsistent use of condoms than those in the comparison group. The participants in the clinical group also reported more HIV testing. Females in the clinical group also had higher rates of pregnancy and STDs than those in the comparison group. This pattern of strong association between substance use and sexual-risk behaviors continued over time.

Violence and Parental Influence

In a study of 384 low-income, 10- to 15-year-old African American children attending public schools, Smith, Flay, Bell, and Weissberg (2001) explored the roles of parental and peer influence on children's violence involvement. Violence involvement was defined as self-reported lifetime participation in physical fights, carrying weapons, using weapons, and engaging in verbal aggression. Using a cross-sectional design, survey data were analyzed with descriptive statistics and structural equation modeling to determine the equivalence of preadolescent and adolescent groups. Findings were that all examples of violence involvement were significantly greater for older rather than younger participants and that younger ones felt closer to their parents than older ones. Additional findings were that parental closeness did not have a direct influence on the child's violence involvement, but when there was a close parent-child relationship, the child was more likely to select prosocial friends, and this was directly associated with lower levels of violence involvement.

Disordered Eating

A study to determine the prevalence of disordered eating by gender and ethnicity and to identify risk and protective factors that were specific to gender and ethnicity was conducted by Croll, Neumark-Sztainer, Story, and Ireland (2002). From a sample of more than 81,000 high school students, 56% of the 9th grade and 57% of the 12th grade females and 28% of the 9th grade and 31% of the 12th grade males self-reported disordered eating behavior, including fasting or skipping meals, using diet pills or laxatives, vomiting, smoking cigarettes, and binge eating. With respect to ethnicity, Native American and Hispanic respondents reported higher prevalence rates of disordered eating than African American or White respondents. Among females only, Hispanic and Asian respondents were significantly more likely to engage in disordered eating. Among males only, Native American, Asian, and Hispanic respondents had significantly more disordered eating behaviors than Whites. Risk factors for both females and males included concern about personal appearance and alcohol and cigarette use. Protective factors for both females and males were family connectedness, emotional well-being and self-esteem, and school achievement. There were significant differences in risk and protective factors by ethnicity, particularly among females. The most significant risk factors for Hispanic and Native American females were concerns about appearance and alcohol use, whereas the most significant risk factor for Asian and African American females was cigarette smoking. For Hispanic females, high self-esteem and emotional well-being were protective factors, whereas for Native American females, family connectedness was the most significant protective factor. High emotional well-being was the only significant protective factor for African American females, and several factors were significant in protecting Asian females (i.e., living with both parents, high self-esteem, and emotional well-being).

Problem Behavior and Injury

In a representative sample of 49,461 youth 11, 13, and 15 years old from 12 countries, Pickett and colleagues (2002) examined the relationship between self-reported health-risk behaviors (i.e., smoking, drinking, truancy, bullying, nonuse of seat belts, excess time spent with friends, poor dietary habits, and alienation from school and parents). The study was based on Jessor's problem-behavior theory and was designed to determine whether risk for injury increased with risk and problem behaviors and whether or not this association was reflected across countries. Participants who reported five or more health-risk behaviors also reported medically treated injuries 2.46 times more than those who reported no health-risk behaviors. These findings were consistent among participants in all 12 countries and within demographic groups. Moreover, the associations were more notable for severe, nonsports, fighting-related injuries.

Health-Risk Behaviors and Area of Residence

A survey comparison (Atav & Spencer, 2002) of rural ($n = 497$), suburban ($n = 441$), and urban ($n = 1156$) students in the seventh, ninth, and 11th grades demonstrated that participants from rural areas showed significantly more health-risk behaviors than those in suburban and urban areas. Specifically, rural students were about twice as likely as urban ($OR = 2.27$) or suburban ($OR = 1.97$) students to use tobacco and alcohol (urban: $OR = 2.23$; suburban: $OR = 1.96$). Rural students were more than twice as likely to use other drugs as urban ($OR = 2.33$) or suburban ($OR = 2.08$) participants. The rural participants were also more likely to be engaged in sexual activity than urban ($OR = 2.11$) or suburban ($OR = 1.81$) youth. Participants from rural areas were significantly more likely to carry a knife, club, gun, or other weapon to school and more likely to carry a gun in the community than participants from urban and suburban areas. Although the results of this study are not generalizable, they offer evidence that location of residence may be an important factor in the etiology of health-risk behaviors in youth (Atav & Spencer, 2002).

Peer Influence and Health-Risk Behavior

In a study of 527 adolescents in grades 9 through 12, Prinstein, Boergers, and Spirito (2001) found that, overall, males more than females had significantly more friends who exhibited deviant behavior [$F(1, 525) = 42.50$, $p < .0001$], whereas females more than males had more friends who exhibited prosocial behaviors [$F(1, 525) = 43.78$, $p < .0001$]. In this sample, peer behavior explained a sizable proportion of explained variance in participants' health-risk behaviors. Specifically, participants whose friends engaged in substance use were more likely to use cigarettes and marijuana, engage in episodes of heavy drinking, and engage in physical fighting. Having friends who engaged in deviant behaviors increased the likelihood that a participant engaged in episodes of heavy drinking, marijuana use, and physical fighting. There was also a significant relationship between friends' suicidal behavior and the suicidal behavior of the participants ($p < .001$). Participants whose friends exhibited prosocial behaviors had lower rates of violent behavior, including weapon carrying, physical fighting, and cigarette use. The researchers concluded that owing to the social reinforcement of friends, interventions led by peers could be a reasonable strategy for promoting healthy behaviors.

Steinberg (2003) asserts that most risk-taking behavior in adolescence is a group phenomenon. He notes that, in particular, drinking, delinquent acts, and sexual behaviors are rarely done in isolation from other youth. These behaviors also have an emotional component that may be enhanced when adolescents are with their peers and focusing on the moment. Other scholars also suggest that health-risk behaviors and the decision making that may accompany them are based more on feelings than rationality. The role of affect, for example, plays a key role in advertising, such that an adolescent may be prompted to begin smoking because the images and emotions that are aroused seem more desirable than deliberate analysis of the hard facts (Slovic, 2003).

Long-Term Health Outcomes of Adolescent Risk Behavior

Not only does the adolescent's behavior affect short-term health status, it has been shown to have long-term effects on health-risk behaviors and associated health status into adulthood. For example, Gil, Vega, and Turner (2002) conducted a 10-year longitudinal study of a cohort of sixth and seventh graders. The purpose of the study was to examine the relationship among six domains of risk factors (i.e., family structure, family environment, school factors, psychological factors, drug-use modeling, and delinquency factors) present during adolescence and subsequent alcohol and marijuana abuse or dependence diagnosed in early adulthood. The original sample consisted of 7386 participants who completed questionnaires at wave 1. For the analyses reported here, the sample consisted of 298 African American and 345 European American participants who were 19 to 21 years old at the time of the last follow-up interview.

As young adults, the African Americans in the sample had significantly lower levels of substance dependence than the European Americans ($p < .001$). Only one of the risk factors (family drug use problems) measured at time 1 was associated with alcohol dependence in early adulthood for European Americans. The highest risk factor for alcohol dependence among European Americans was school behavior problems measured at time 3, which was in the third year of this longitudinal study ($OR = 2.7, p < .001$). Other significant risk factors measured at time 3 for European Americans were delinquent behavior ($OR = 2.3$, $p < .01$), disposition to deviance ($OR = 2.1$, $p < .05$), teacher derogation ($OR = 2.1$, $p < .05$), low self-esteem ($OR = 2.1$, $p < .05$), family drug-use problems ($OR = 2.1$, $p < .05$), family derogation ($OR = 2.1$, $p < .05$), symptoms of depression ($OR = 1.9$, $p < .05$), low familism ($OR = 1.9$, $p < .05$), and low family cohesion ($OR = 1.8$, $p < .05$) (Gil et al., 2002).

For African Americans, risk factors in only two domains (i.e., delinquency and family structure) measured at time 1 were not significantly correlated with alcohol abuse in early adulthood. At time 3, the domain of family environment was most strongly related to alcohol abuse. More specifically, low familism ($OR = 9.4$, $p < .001$), parent derogation ($OR = 3.6$, $p < .05$), and family communication ($OR = 4.5$, $p < .01$) were significant predictors. Other risk factors measured at time 3 that were significantly associated with alcohol abuse for African Americans in this cohort were low self-esteem ($OR = 8.6$, $p < .01$), teacher derogation ($OR = 4.7$, $p < .01$), suicide attempts ($OR = 3.8$, $p < .05$), poor school work ($OR = 2.9$, $p < .05$), and family drug-use problems ($OR = 2.6$, $p < .05$) (Gil et al., 2002).

Chapter Summary

In this chapter, the concepts of risk, vulnerability, and risk perception were differentiated. Although human beings will always be vulnerable to loss, injury, and death, learned behaviors can increase or decrease the risk for these undesirable outcomes. The problem-behavior theory was presented in some detail. The revision and extension of this theory was also explored. An ecological model of the antecedents and health outcomes associated with health-risk behaviors was discussed to illustrate the interaction between risk and protective factors. Research related to problem behaviors and health-risk behaviors was described. The chapter ended with an overview of health-risk behaviors in adolescents and the relationship between these behaviors and long-term health outcomes.

Suggestions for Further Study

As the scholar and scientist have more theoretical tools with which to work, increasingly more interesting and complex questions may be posed and answered. As noted in Chapter 1, concept, statement, and theory synthesis strategies may be used to generate new ways of looking at familiar phenomena. Whereas many health-risk behaviors in adolescence have previously been viewed primarily from a perspective of the psychology of behavior, what might we learn if the same behaviors were viewed from a developmental perspective? Longitudinal studies would allow us to consider how these behaviors, or the factors that reflect increased risk for engaging in them, develop over time. In fact, such studies are currently under way in response to the National Institutes of Health's interest in this trajectory. Such studies will allow us to investigate how family, peers, and communities contribute to the development or prevention of such behaviors.

Longitudinal studies that consider the development of the sense of self (identity) could shed new light on how sexual, spiritual, and ethnic identities contribute to increasing or decreasing the risk for specific health-risk behaviors. Loeber and colleagues (1998) noted the need for longitudinal studies to identify how problem behaviors develop over time and how one or more problem behaviors may influence the onset and continuation of other problem behaviors. Longitudinal studies would permit researchers to differentiate profiles of youngsters who have persistent, recurrent, or sporadic problem behaviors and determine how these are related to risk and protective mechanisms. These kinds of studies are also needed to determine the influence of neighborhoods on the developing child's behavior and how moving from one neighborhood to another increases or decreases risks for specific problem behaviors. Findings from these longitudinal studies will have implications for the development and testing of interventions.

Intervention research that is theory driven needs to be conducted. As Byrnes (2003) has pointed out, with respect to health-risk behaviors of adolescents, an integrative approach to theory development and intervention testing may provide the most fruitful results. For example, scholars with opposing viewpoints on risk behaviors comprising a syndrome versus such behaviors each having a unique set of predictors should combine their perspectives to find an explanation of contradictory findings. These findings could then be more instructive for developing interventions that address the real causes of behaviors associated with increased risk for adverse health outcomes.

Future studies of health-risk behaviors must take into account the social, contextual settings and circumstances under which these behaviors occur. Youth in various rural, urban, and suburban settings have varied vulnerabilities to health-risk behaviors and associated short- and long-term health outcomes. Exploration is needed of factors within these geographic settings that increase risk. As Steinberg (2003) pointed out, many of the health-risk behaviors exhibited by adolescents occur under conditions of emotional arousal and in the company of peers, and the interaction of these factors often leads to behaviors that would not be performed under other circumstances. Studies that are closer to real-life situations rather than surveys of hypothetical conditions may yield more accurate models of these behaviors.

Many studies will undoubtedly be done using longitudinal data from the National Longitudinal Study of Adolescent Health (Add Health) to provide answers to multiple questions about the health of adolescents. Studies can be done to determine how different health and health-risk behaviors are related to different environments, how they vary among adolescents exposed to the same environment, and how risk and protective factors vary among adolescents exposed to the same environment (Udry & Bearman, 1998).

Scholars from various disciplines will be able to collaborate on studies using this rich data set, bringing multiple perspectives to bear on the formulation of questions and interpretation of findings.

A final area for further research is that of sexuality and sexual behavior in adolescence. In reviewing the recent state of research on adolescent sexuality, Graber et al. (1998) have noted that we have failed to incorporate the work of scholars in a variety of disciplines. They argue that adolescent sexual behavior is normal but that some disciplines do not consider it in this light, and thus a normal developmental transition becomes identified as a "problem behavior." They also urge scholars to consider adolescent sexuality as a series of events within a developmental context and to move beyond the view that it is just sexual intercourse. Rather, they ask us to frame sexuality "as an interaction of biological and social influences" (p. 291) and to focus on health promotion rather than on preventing intercourse. Clearly this is an area where listening to the words of the adolescents themselves will be instructive to scholars.

Related Web Sites

Problem-Behavior Theory:

(Institute of Behavioral Science Research Program on Problem Behavior, Program Overview) http://www.colorado.edu/ibs/PB/about.html

(Program News) http://www.colorado.edu/ibs/PB/news.html

Suggestions for Further Reading

Doswell, W. M., & Braxter, B. (2002). Risk-taking behaviors in early adolescent minority women: Implications for research and practice. *Journal of Obstetrics, Gynecology, and Neonatal Nursing [JOGNN]*, 31, 2-9.

Jessor, R., Donovan, J. E., & Costa, F. M. (1994). *Beyond adolescence: Problem behaviour and young adult development*. New York: Cambridge University Press.

Perry, C. L., Williams, C. L., Komro, K. A., Veblen-Mortenson, S., Forster, J. L, Bernstein-Lachter, R., et al. (2000). Project Northland high school interventions: Community action to reduce adolescent alcohol use. *Health Education & Behavior*, 27(1), 29-49.

Philbin, J., Richards, M. H., & Crawford, I. (1998). Adolescent alcohol involvement and the experience of social environments. *Journal of Research on Adolescence*, 8, 403-422.

7

Conceptualizations of Resilience and Protection

A s described in the previous chapter, adolescents may be vulnerable to short- and long-term adverse health outcomes owing to their state of development and the stressors they experience throughout their development. They are vulnerable to poor health outcomes, owing to many circumstances that place them at increased risk. Some of this vulnerability stems from their increasing independence from the constraining forces and protective influences of parents and social institutions such as schools and churches. Moreover, many adolescents are vulnerable to health-risk behaviors and associated poor health outcomes because of personal attributes, poverty, and lack of social resources. However, regardless of their lack of access to resources, a significant number of youth seem to be protected from negative consequences and are said to be "invulnerable" to stress, or *resilient* (Rutter, 1980). Factors that explain such resilience, particularly in the face of multiple odds against adaptive development, are known as *protection*.

In this chapter, the concept of resilience is defined in several ways. Although there is no formalized theory of resilience, much research has been done to identify factors that mitigate a person's risk for adverse outcomes. These factors have been termed *protection* or *protective resources*. Such resources are found at the individual, family, and community or society levels. Whereas risk and vulnerability represent the negative or threatening end of the continuum of experience, protection and resilience represent the positive end, as depicted in Figure 7.1.

Resilience Defined

The concept of resilience has evolved from multidisciplinary studies of children who developed social competence and health in spite of great odds against such outcomes. Garmezy and Nuechterlein (1972) were among the first to argue that, in spite of conditions of poverty associated with the development of psychopathology in children, many children growing up under such conditions seemed invulnerable to deleterious outcomes; they were

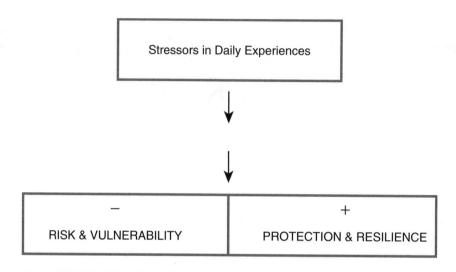

Figure 7.1   Risk-Resilience Continuum of Experience

capable of resisting mental illness. Garmezy and Nuechterlein suggested that parental factors, as well as coping mechanisms and cognitive styles of the children themselves, served to protect them from adverse outcomes. Garmezy (1971) referred to the "invulnerability" of those children who were at high risk for psychopathology owing to the disorganized environments in which they were living but who displayed a number of competencies. These children had positive peer relations, high academic achievement, and were committed to education and other goals. He further referred to these invulnerable children as the "keepers of the dream" (p. 114). He encouraged social scientists to study those factors that enabled these invulnerables not only to survive but to adapt and contribute to society.

Garmezy (1987) also referred to children who were vulnerable to psychopathology but who had emerged unscathed as "stress-resistant" (p. 161) rather than "invulnerable" (p. 164). In summarizing the findings from numerous studies of children who developed psychiatric disorders, Garmezy identified six risk factors: (a) severe marital distress of parents, (b) low socioeconomic status of family, (c) overcrowding of large families, (d) criminality of child's father, (e) psychiatric disorders of child's mother, and (f) placement of child in foster home. He also noticed the cumulative effect of risk factors. Children with only one of these risk factors were no more likely to develop a psychiatric disorder than the general population of children. However, as the number of factors increased from two to six, the progression to a psychiatric condition was geometrical. Under the same set of risk factors, however, some children were protected by factors such as a cohesive family climate with stable support and the opportunity to develop cognitive and social competencies in a nurturing school environment. Soon the search was on for protective factors that could buffer the deleterious effects of stress.

In 1955, Werner and her colleagues began a 30-year longitudinal study of a multiracial cohort of 698 infants born that year on the island of Kauai, Hawaii. The purpose of the study was to document the impact of biological and psychosocial risk factors on development through childhood, adolescence, and early adulthood. One of every three infants born in 1955 was considered to be at risk for poor developmental outcomes owing to their family's poverty status, being raised by a mother with little formal education, experiencing perinatal stress, and living with family discord such as a mental illness or the alcoholism of one or both parents. Two thirds of the at-risk children displayed serious behavior and/or learning problems by the time they were 10 years old. What surprised the research team, however, was that one third of the at-risk group became "competent, confident, and caring young adults" (Werner, 1989, p. 73).

Werner (1989, 2003; Werner & Smith, 1992) found three categories of factors that characterized the resilient children: individual attributes, family characteristics, and factors outside the family. Attributes of the resilient individuals were temperament in infancy that brought the baby positive attention from others and alertness and autonomy as toddlers. In school, these children related easily to their classmates, had many interests, and had good reading and reasoning skills. In adolescence, these individuals had a positive self-concept and an internal sense of control and were nurturant, responsible, and oriented toward achievement. The families of these resilient children provided structure, rules, and expectations for completion of daily chores. The families also contained at least one caregiver who was consistently available during the first year of life. Outside the family, other people provided support and friendship. These children also participated in extracurricular activities and many developed a religious faith. Werner (2003) also found that for those who had coping problems during their adolescence, most had recovered by their 30s.

Resilience in Adolescence

Rutter (1980) refuted earlier conceptualizations of the adolescent stage of development known as "storm and stress." According to Rutter, adolescence as a period of inherent instability, psychological imbalance, or emotional upset (i.e., storm and stress) was initiated by G. Stanley Hall and promoted by psychoanalytic theorists such as Anna Freud. Rutter asserted that normal adolescence should not be characterized in this way. He further asserted that most adolescents continued to have warm relationships with their parents throughout this developmental stage in spite of popular beliefs to the contrary. Rutter noted that several factors influenced an adolescent's behavior: (a) biological factors, including genetics, chromosomal anomalies, sex, nutrition, and physical appearance; (b) family relationships and communication patterns; (c) exposure to media, particularly those presenting violence; (d) school environments; and (e) geographical location and social groups. However, even when children were exposed to the most damaging environments, some children came through such experiences relatively unharmed.

> It is not that they have been unaffected by their experiences; they may well have been left with susceptibilities and inner insecurities of various kinds. But there is still the world of difference between those individuals who become ordinary reasonably well adjusted people in spite of chronic stress and disadvantage and those who become delinquent, mentally ill, or educationally retarded. (Rutter, 1980, pp. 180-181)

Rutter (1980) termed this "the phenomenon of resilience under stress" (p. 183).

Models of Resilience

Three general models of resilience have been proposed (Garmezy, Masten, & Tellegen., 1984). These are the (a) compensatory (simple additive model), (b) challenge (curvilinear relationship between stress and adjustment outcomes), and (c) protective versus vulnerability (interaction between stress and personal attributes).

Compensatory Model

The first of these models is linear and is referred to as the compensatory model, in which a compensatory mechanism neutralizes a person's exposure to risk. Such a mechanism has a direct effect on the outcome. The risk factor, or stress plus a compensatory factor such as self-esteem, combine additively to yield an outcome of competence. Such an outcome is an indicator of resilience in the person (Masten et al., 1988). Using this model in a study of 144 inner city adolescents (62 males and 82 females) who were between 14 and 17.2 years old ($M = 15.3 \pm 0.78$), Luthar (1991) found that ego development was a compensatory mechanism against stress. More specifically, ego development influenced school grades.

Challenge Model

The challenge model of resilience suggests a curvilinear relationship between perceived stress and adjustment such that the experience of stress may either enhance or reduce competence in the individual (Garmezy et al., 1984; Luthar & Zigler, 1991). Although the concepts of eustress and distress are not identified in the model, the conceptualization of stress is similar to these same concepts as defined by Selye (1978). In the challenge model, too little stress is insufficient challenge, but too much stress creates a helpless feeling in the person. Optimal stress contributes to adaptation through the process of challenge, which results in preparation for the next stress encounter (Zimmerman & Arunkumar, 1994).

Protection-Vulnerability Model

A third model, protection versus vulnerability, reflects "a conditional relationship between stress and personal attributes with respect to adaptation, such that personal attributes modulate (dampen or amplify) the impact of stress as a variable" (Garmezy et al., 1984, p. 102). This model "implies an interactive relationship between stress and personal attributes in predicting adjustment" (Luthar, 1991, p. 602). In this conceptualization of resilience, some personal attributes of the individual are viewed as protective if those who have high levels of the specific attribute are relatively unaffected by stress and those who have lower levels of the attribute express less competence in the face of similar levels of stress. In contrast, other personal attributes of the individual are viewed as indicators of vulnerability, and individuals who have high levels of such attributes have poorer outcomes in response to stressors than those with low levels of these attributes. In the study described earlier, Luthar (1991) also tested the protection-vulnerability model and found that internal locus of control and social skills served as protective factors. This model operates in an indirect way to influence resilient outcomes. That is to say, protective factors or processes interact with risk factors to reduce the probability of adverse outcomes (Zimmerman & Arunkumar, 1994). Further development of this approach will be discussed in detail later in this chapter.

Benda (2001) developed a conceptual model of risk-taking behavior based on assets and risks. Using structural equation modeling, he tested hypotheses that demonstrated the following:

- Attachment to caregivers was inversely related to unlawful behaviors, such as drug use and crime, in females.
- Religiosity was inversely related to unlawful behavior more in rural than in urban settings.
- Parental monitoring was inversely related to unlawful behavior more among males than among females.
- Having been abused and caregiver substance abuse was related to unlawful behavior in all groups (male and females in rural as well as urban areas).

Findings from Benda's study suggest that protective factors within the individual and family are related to less engagement in behaviors that lead to poor outcomes.

Stewart, Reid, and Mangham (1997) defined resilience as "The capability of individuals to cope successfully in the face of significant change, adversity, or risk. This capability changes over time and is enhanced by protective factors in the individual and the environment" (p. 22). These scholars further noted that resilience is an important concept in understanding mental and physical health, as well as health behaviors. Moreover, they argued that health behaviors themselves may act as protective resources for psychological well-being and physical health.

Domains of Resilience

Rutter (1993) traced the history of the concept of resilience as a term that replaced *invulnerable* to describe children who escaped serious consequences of adversity. He referred to resilience as "the term used to describe the positive pole of individual differences in people's response to stress and adversity" (Rutter, 1987, p. 316). He referred to the negative pole as vulnerability. The effect of resilience or vulnerability, according to Rutter, is apparent only when viewed in the light of risk. Moreover, he argued that a particular factor or mechanism could act as a vulnerability factor in one set of circumstances and as a protective factor in another. For example, he pointed out that an individual may cope successfully with a particular stressor at one point in her or his life but may be unsuccessful at another time. Rutter added that the concept of resilience is useful for framing questions about the developmental and situational mechanisms involved in protective processes. He noted that it is impossible for a person to display resilience in the face of all types of stressful events, that resilience is not merely a trait of a person. This suggests that a person may be resilient at one period of time and display competencies in some areas of functioning but may not be resilient in other areas or at other times.

If resilience is defined as successful coping and adaptation to the demands or stressful stimuli of the environment, then domains of resilience include the many settings in which adolescents live their lives. This includes home, school, church, community, and any other social group to which the adolescent belongs. Masten and Coatsworth (1998) defined resilience as "manifested competence in the context of significant challenges to adaptation or development" (p. 206). They asserted that to identify resilience, two conditions must be met: (a) the person experiences a serious threat or risk for adverse outcomes, owing to conditions such as poverty or lack of other social resources or to severe trauma such as the death of a parent, and (b) the developmental outcome of adaptation is considered to be good.

Resilience and Maltreatment of Children

The resilience paradigm has been applied to the study of maltreated children for nearly three decades. Findings are that in spite of horrendous experiences that could be expected to produce trauma and stress, many individuals emerge as competent and caring young adults. For example, Zimrin (1986) conducted a 14-year follow-up study of 28 children who had been abused and a matched control group who had not been abused. Among the children who had experienced abuse, two subgroups were identified: survivors and nonsurvivors. The nonsurvivors were characterized by attitudes of fatalism, low self-esteem, aggression, self-destructiveness, difficulty expressing emotions, inability to establish personal relationships, and cognitive difficulties. In contrast, the survivors exhibited feelings of being in control, positive self-esteem, less self-destructiveness, and outstanding cognitive ability. Moreover, members of the survivor group had found an adult who treated them with empathy and encouragement. Subjects in the resilient group also had developed responsibility for caring for someone else who depended on them, such as a younger child or a pet.

Another study of school-age children ($N = 206$; 8-13 years old; $M = 9.58 \pm 1.45$) from low socioeconomic backgrounds who attended a summer camp program was done to examine the resilience framework (Cicchetti, Rogosch, Lynch, & Holt, 1993). The researchers found that children who had been maltreated ($n = 127$) had fewer competencies (e.g., ego resilience, intelligence, adaptive functioning) and environmental resources (e.g., adequate family income, working mother, two-parent family, mother's education) to protect them than the children who had not been maltreated.

Resilience as a Growth Experience

More recently, Polk (1997) defined resilience as "The ability to transform disaster into a growth experience and move forward" (p. 1). Using the strategy of concept synthesis described by Walker and Avant (2005) and presented in Chapter 2 of this text, Polk identified 26 clusters of the phenomena in the literature on resilience. These phenomena were reduced to six types: psychosocial attributes, physical attributes, roles, relationships, problem-solving characteristics, and philosophical beliefs. This classification was reduced to four types by combining roles with relationships and physical with psychosocial attributes. Resilience was then further conceptualized as four patterns that reflected the defining attributes of the concept: dispositional, relational, situational, and philosophical.

The dispositional pattern includes the physical and psychosocial attributes of the person that reflect competence and a sense of self. Temperament, health, feelings of self-worth and self-confidence, autonomy and self-reliance, and intelligence are intrinsic personal phenomena that are characteristic of the resilient individual. The relational pattern consists of roles and relationships. This pattern is characterized by intrinsic skill in finding positive role models, seeking a confidant, and being committed to relationships and intimacy. It is also characterized as an extrinsic value of having a broad social network. The situational pattern involves cognitive skills such as problem solving, creativity, resourcefulness, and flexibility. The philosophical pattern contains personal beliefs such as the belief that one's life has purpose and meaning. Other concepts that are in the model include the energy fields of the person (human) and the environment. Viewed as separate but characterized by dynamic interaction, the person and the environment form the context for resilience wherein the person experiences adverse conditions that become the impetus for change.

Resilience is a term that carries a lot of promise for developing interventions that can promote the health and well-being of adolescents. If we know the variables that are most closely related to health-promoting and health-enhancing behaviors, we can focus on strategies that will ensure that youth develop these behaviors. One approach to this is to minimize the effects of trauma or stress on young people. As Bell (2001) hypothesizes: "If children can be identified immediately after suffering a traumatic stressor and helped to cope with that stressor, they will be less prone to engage in self-destructive behaviors such as drug abuse, school failure, unsafe sex, and violence" (p. 376). Put differently, if children are more resilient, they are less likely to engage in health-compromising behaviors. This conceptualization of resilience is similar to the Developmental Assets Framework described in Chapter 3. To meet the challenges inherent in living, the developing person who has multiple assets or resources, including personal attributes and positive coping strategies, is more likely to develop into a healthy and competent adult than the developing person who is deprived of these assets.

Protection

Resilience may be viewed as a balance between risk factors or stressors and adaptive coping. Factors that decrease the likelihood of adverse outcomes in the presence of factors that increase that risk are referred to as protection or protective factors (Jessor et al., 1995; Werner & Smith, 1992). Put another way, protective factors "moderate the effects of individual vulnerabilities or environmental hazards, so that a given developmental trajectory reflects more adaptation in a given domain than would be the case if protective processes were not operating" (Hauser, 1999, p. 4). Garmezy (1985) continued to search for factors that protected vulnerable children from the deleterious effects of poverty and stress. Specifically, he sought to find protective factors or characteristics of the child or family that contributed to resilience or the "ability of children to meet and to conquer adversity" (p. 228). With his particular focus on the biological children of parents who were diagnosed with schizophrenia, Garmezy (1985, 1987) began to identify stress-resistant or protective factors. Crediting Rutter as the pioneer in identifying protective factors in vulnerable children, Garmezy (1987) concluded that protection was afforded through three general mechanisms: the child's personality or adaptive temperament; a stable, cohesive, and supportive family; and attainment of social and cognitive skills in a nurturing school environment.

Several factors have been identified among children who lived in poverty that served to protect them from negative outcomes that could have resulted from stressors they experienced (Garmezy, 1991). Temperament, a positive response to others, and cognitive skills were identified as individual attributes that served as protective mechanisms in the face of extreme stressors. Another set of mechanisms was the presence of a warm, caring, and responsible adult providing some cohesion to the family. The final set of mechanisms was external supports provided by institutions such as schools and the personnel who worked within them. According to Garmezy, "Protectiveness is not the obverse of vulnerability" (p. 428). Rather, protective mechanisms "operate indirectly, their effects partly a function of their interaction with and their modification of the risk variable" (p. 428).

"Protective factors refer to influences that modify, ameliorate, or alter a person's response to some environmental hazard that predisposes to a maladaptive outcome" (Rutter, 1985, p. 600). Protective factors are not just positive experiences. Positive experiences may have a direct effect on normal development, but protective factors operate in the face of risk factors to modify their otherwise deleterious effects. Protective factors may lead to self-esteem, self-confidence, self-efficacy, and a range of social problem-solving skills through three possible mechanisms: secure and stable relationships, experiences of successful achievement, and gaining emotional distance from a bad situation that one cannot escape.

According to Rutter (1987), "Protection does not reside in the psychological chemistry of the moment but in the ways in which people deal with life changes and in what they do about their stressful or disadvantageous circumstances" (p. 329). He recommended studying processes rather than variables because a factor may be a risk at one time and a protective factor at another time (Rutter, 1993).

There are various processes through which protection acts to mitigate the adverse outcomes from situations that place a person at risk. One protective process includes altering one's exposure to risk. For example, the risk of unplanned pregnancy and STDs may be directly affected by preventing a 14-year-old girl from dating an 18-year-old boy. A second protective process is to interrupt a chain of negative responses to a risk encounter. If, for example, the 14-year-old girl were invited to a party attended by several boys who were 18 years old or older, the presence of adult chaperones who prevented the girl from leaving the party with one of these older boys would serve as a protective mechanism to disrupt a negative chain of events. A third protective process results when an individual learns additional coping skills or behaviors that enhance self-efficacy and self-esteem (Rutter, 1993). To carry the example a step farther, the 14-year-old girl who has a great deal of self-confidence and assertive communication skills may be adequately equipped and motivated to protect herself from a sexual proposition from an older boy.

Protective factors generally fall into three main areas: within the individual, within the family, and within the larger social environment or community. It is now clear that whereas some factors clearly increase risk for adverse outcomes and other factors clearly decrease that risk, many factors can serve to increase both risk and protection. But first, let us turn to those factors identified primarily as protective factors. "Protective factors ameliorate or decrease the negative influences of being at risk, but may also operate independent of risk" (Stewart et al., 1997, p. 22).

Protective Factors Within the Individual

A number of studies have identified several factors within the individual that serve to protect him or her from the adverse effects of extreme or prolonged stress:

- Temperament
- Sense of humor
- Positive self-image
- Prone to engage in self-care strategies
- Beliefs
- Internal locus of control
- Religiosity
- Intolerant of deviance
- Skills
- Early communication
- Competent in academics
- Engaged in extracurricular activities
- Provides care for younger child or pet

In her classic longitudinal study of the 1955 birth cohort on the Hawaiian island of Kauai, Werner (1989) found that the temperament of an individual as an infant was associated with resilience later in life. These babies were easygoing and affectionate and had fewer sleeping and eating problems than other infants. As toddlers, the resilient children displayed more advanced communication and self-care skills. In school, they showed interest in multiple activities and were very engaged. At the time of high school graduation, they were responsible, had a positive self-concept, and were prone to display an internal locus of control. As young adults, the resilient babies had achieved a measure of educational and vocational competence that contributed to their adaptation and success (Werner, 2003; Werner & Smith, 1992).

Temperament is a group of intrinsic traits that shapes a person's responses to events. It accounts for *how* rather than *why* individuals respond to stressors from the environment as they do (Rutter, Birch, Thomas, & Chess, 1962). Temperament is manifested as behavioral style shortly after birth; this style has been shown to have an impact on mother-infant relationships and on the caring response to the child (Medoff-Cooper, 1995). Throughout childhood, differences in individual temperaments reflect the diverse ways in which children respond to their environments and to the people and events in them. As such, temperament may serve as a protective factor against mental health problems or it may serve to increase a child's risk for mal-treatment (Gross & Conrad, 1995). In later childhood, temperament influ-ences the child's interaction in multiple social environments, such as family and school. Whereas children with difficult temperaments, who respond negatively to stimuli or who withdraw from social interactions, are at risk for adverse behavioral and health outcomes, children with more pleasant temperaments, characterized by positive affect and task persistence, are protected from such consequences (McClowry, 1995).

Other individual characteristics that act as protective factors are intellec-tual capacity and engagement in school (Borowsky, Ireland, & Resnick, 2002; Herrenkohl, Herrenkohl, & Egolf, 1994). Gonzales and Padilla (1997) found that Hispanic high school students who felt a strong sense of belong-ing at school were at far less risk for academic failure than those who did not feel as engaged. Several researchers have found that both scholastic ability and competence, along with social skills, foster resilience in children (Garmezy & Masten, 1991; Luthar & Zigler, 1991). In a longitudinal study of 173 adolescents (80 females and 93 males) who were at risk owing to poverty, Carlson and colleagues (1999) found high correlations among early academic achievement (e.g., math, reading, spelling, and general knowledge), emotional health in grade school, and high adjustment during adolescence.

The feeling of hope and a positive self-image were associated with successful coping and survival in a longitudinal study of abused children (Zimrin, 1986). Zimrin also found that those children who cared for some-one else or a pet were more resilient than those who had not had these expe-riences. Herrenkohl et al. (1994) conducted a longitudinal study of 476 children who had suffered abuse and neglect. They found that resilience changes over time and that adaptive functioning at one time is no guarantee of adaptive functioning at another time. In addition to the personal variable of average or above-average intelligence quotient (IQ), the resilient adoles-cents had at least one caring adult throughout their childhood and clear expectations about their academic performance. These researchers added that resilience fluctuates because as an individual develops, there are chang-ing demands from the environment and individuals may be limited in their potential in various areas. Herrenkohl et al. suggested that, for example, an individual who functions well academically might not be socially competent and might lack the skills for developing close interpersonal relationships with others. The researchers concluded,

> The protective process in resilient children may operate by supporting the development of a positive self-image and an internal sense of con-trol, which are expressed in goal-setting and planning behavior and in a determination to be different from disappointing parental models. (Herrenkohl et al., 1994, p. 308)

However, this determination can lead to positive outcomes only when nurtured by support and reinforcement. When the environment fails to provide such support, these children can be overwhelmed and experience less than optimal outcomes.

A sense of humor has also been identified as a personal protective factor that enables individuals to cope with stressors by facilitating social interactions and gaining cognitive mastery of the stressful situation (Dowling & Fain, 1999; Wooten, 1996). Masten (1986) conducted a study of 93 school-aged children (42 males and 51 females) from an urban area. The majority of participants were from lower and middle income families and households with only one parent. The purpose of the study was to explore relationships between three types of humor and three adaptive outcomes (i.e., social, behavioral, and academic competence). Univariate correlations between all three types of humor (appreciation or mirth, comprehension, and production) and academic competence or achievement were significant. The relationship between appreciation of humor and academic competence for females was $r = .33$, $p < .01$ and $r = .35$, $p < .05$ for males. The relationship between comprehension of humor and academic competence was $r = .55$, $p < .001$ for both males and females. The relationship between production of humor and academic competence was $r = .50$, $p < .001$. There were significant negative correlations between high scores on the Sensitive-Isolated Scale of Social Competence and all three indicators of humor ($r = -.30$, $p < .05$ to $r = -.48$, $p < .001$). This finding suggested that those children who were humor challenged lacked social competence. There were also significant positive correlations between the types of humor and teachers' ratings of behavioral cooperation ($r = .52$, $p < .01$ for boys, $r = .23$, n.s. for girls [mirth]; $r = .36$, $p < .01$ [comprehension]; and $r = .41$, $p < .001$ [production]).

In a series of hierarchical regression analyses, Masten (1986) also found that IQ, humor appreciation, and humor production accounted for 33% of the variation in the social competence outcomes of social isolation. With respect to other indicators of competence, humor shared the variance in outcomes with IQ. Overall, however, children who scored high in humor appreciation, comprehension, and production also scored high in academic and social competence. Masten concluded that humor may be an adaptive coping response that protects children from the harmful effects of stress.

Jessor and colleagues (1995) demonstrated that individual protective factors, including positive orientation to school and health, intolerance of deviant behavior, positive relationships with adults, religiosity, and awareness of prosocial friends, were significant predictors of changes in adolescent problem behaviors (e.g., drinking, physical aggression, marijuana use, sexual activity) over time. They also showed that these protective factors were directly related to behavior and behavior change across gender, racial, and ethnic groups.

In the first report of findings from the National Longitudinal Study on Adolescent Health, which included data from a nationally representative sample of 12,118 adolescents in grades 7 through 12, Resnick and colleagues (1997) found that perceived school connectedness and parent-family connectedness provided protection against all health-risk behaviors except pregnancy. Other intraindividual factors that acted to protect adolescents from engaging in health-risk behaviors were high levels of self-esteem and high importance placed on religion and prayer. Similarly, in a study of college students, Stewart (2001) found that spirituality has a moderate protective effect on the decision to use marijuana and alcohol. Wallace and Forman (1998) also found that religion acted to protect adolescents from carrying weapons, fighting, and drinking and driving, and others have found that it protected youth from early sexual activity (Lammers, Ireland, Resnick, & Blum, 2000).

Protective Factors Within the Family

Scholars recognize that families can be a source of stress for children, as in the case of serious neglect and abuse, but they also provide powerful resources that protect children and promote the development of resilience (Calvert, 1997; Patterson, 1995). A number of factors within the family have been identified as significant protective resources in the lives of children and adolescents. These are summarized in Table 7.1. Parents who are caring and connected to their children early in life provide training and support for developing competencies within their children that serve to protect them in the face of increased risks (Carlson et al., 1999; Chewning et al., 2001; Croll et al., 2002; Resnick et al., 1993, 1997). Connectedness, families with two parents, and parents who had high expectations were found to protect adolescents from early onset of sexual activity (Lammers et al., 2000). Other resilient outcomes, such as self-esteem and academic motivation, are also influenced by protective factors of caring and supportive family members (Ryan, Stiller, & Lynch, 1994).

The resilient children of Kauai grew up in families with no more than four children. These children were also at least 2 years older or younger than the next sibling. As infants, they did not experience a prolonged separation from their caregiver, and at least one of their caregivers provided abundant positive attention during the first year of life. Families of resilient children were characterized by structures and rules. These children were expected to perform routine chores during adolescence (Werner, 1989). Often the nurturance of these children came from extended family members, such as aunts, uncles, older siblings, and grandparents. The families of these resilient children also tended to engage in religious activities that provided structure and meaning for their lives (Werner, 2003).

In families with abusive dynamics, Spaccarelli and Kim (1995) found that having a warm and supportive relationship with the nonabusive parent strongly correlated with resilience in sexually abused girls. Similarly, family

Table 7.1   Protective Factors Within the Family That Promote Resilience

Parents who	are caring and connected to children
	are at home at key times of day (e.g., before and after school, dinner, and bedtime)
	have high expectations for academic performance
	disapprove of health-risk behaviors
	have not had prolonged separations from children
Families with	both parents in the home
	fewer than four children
	cohesion and structure

cohesion even when a father drinks excessively was shown to be protective against problem drinking, psychological distress, and deviant behavior in adolescents (Farrell, Barnes, & Banerjee, 1995). Family connectedness has also been found to enhance emotional well-being in adolescents with learning disabilities (Svetaz, Ireland, & Blum, 2000). Parent-family connectedness has been identified as a significant protective factor against perpetration of violence (Borowsky et al., 2002). From the National Longitudinal Study on Adolescent Health (Add Health), Resnick and colleagues (1997) found that for those adolescents whose parents were at home during important times, such as before and after school, at dinner time, and at bedtime, this connectedness provided modest protection against emotional distress and suicidality. Parent-family connectedness and parents' expectations for their child's academic achievement were also identified as weak protective factors for violence. Family connectedness was identified as somewhat protective for cigarette smoking, marijuana use, and alcohol use. Delay of sexual activity among adolescents in the Add Health study was significantly associated with protective factors of parent-family connectedness and parental disapproval of the adolescent's contraceptive use and of the adolescent's participation in sexual activity.

Protective Factors Within the Community

In addition to protective factors within the individual and the family, the resilient children of Kauai sought emotional support through close friends and neighbors. In school, they participated in extracurricular activities, and many of them established friendships with teachers, who also served as positive role models. Some of these resilient children and adolescents were closely connected with adults from churches and youth groups. These were the children who tended to respect and follow the law (Werner, 1989; Werner & Smith, 1992). As young adults, these resilient individuals found support through attendance at community colleges or through enlisting in the military, and some received help from psychotherapy (Werner, 2003).

Other studies have also shown the protective influence of teachers and friends on resilient outcomes in adolescents (Hawkins, Catalano, Kosterman, Abbott, & Hill, 1999; Ryan et al., 1994). A study of 384 African American students in grades 5 through 8 showed that although parental connectedness did not have a direct influence on adolescents' involvement in violent behaviors, it did improve adolescents' ability to choose friends who exhibited prosocial behaviors. Consequently, the selection of this kind of friend was directly related to less violent behavior in youth (Smith et al., 2001). Protective factors within the community may be summarized as follows:

- Caring adults
     Teachers in schools
     Pastors, teachers, other adults at church and recreation centers
- Positive role-modeling by adults
- Peers
- Those who exhibit prosocial values and behaviors
- Value placed on adolescents' contributions to the community
- Access to resources
- Easy access to supportive resources, such as health-care facilities and
     services that are youth-friendly
- Normative expectations
- Clear and consistent boundaries set for adolescents' behaviors

Using an experimental design, Public/Private Ventures, a not-for-profit research corporation, conducted a study of 959 adolescents between 10 and 16 years old who participated in Big Brothers or Big Sisters programs. Half were randomly assigned to a treatment group and the other half to a waiting list. The intervention focused on supplying the participants with a personal mentor who provided three protective resources in their relationships with students: (a) caring, (b) respect and positive expectations, and (c) recognition of risks in the environment, not in the adolescent. Application of these protective mechanisms resulted in lowered incidence of drug and alcohol use, fewer missed days of school, moderate improvements in school grades, and improved relationships with parents and peers (Benard, 2000).

Schools are the one place where most American adolescents spend the majority of their waking hours. Although they are a significant source of stress for many, many adolescents, there are schools that have recognized the importance of their role in fostering resilience in youth. The resiliency wheel model, Figure 7.2, identifies six critical areas in which schools can provide protective resources for children and adolescents. These areas are (a) increasing prosocial bonding; (b) setting and communicating clear and consistent boundaries; (c) teaching life skills that include conflict resolution, cooperation, assertiveness, communication, and decision making; (d) providing caring support and encouragement; (e) setting and communicating high expectations for success;

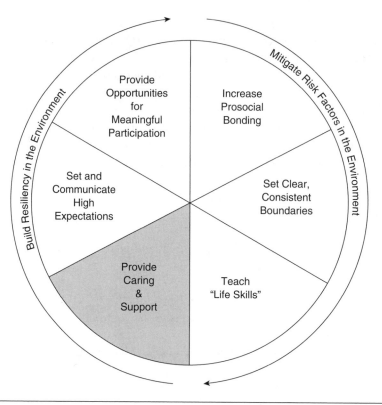

Figure 7.2   The Resiliency Wheel

SOURCE: Henderson and Milstein (2003, p. 12). © 2003 Sage Publications. Reprinted by permission.

Note: The "Provide caring and support" section is shaded for emphasis because, according to the author, "it is the most critical of all the elements that promote resiliency" (Henderson & Milstein, 2003, p. 13).

and (f) providing opportunities for meaningful participation in making decisions and helping others (Henderson & Milstein, 2003).

Specific strategies for meeting each of the six protective resources depicted in the resiliency wheel model are illustrated in Figure 7.3. The model and strategies have been used successfully in transforming the Albuquerque, New Mexico, public school district. As a result of a 3-year, federally funded project, the schools in this district included resiliency in their school vision and mission statements, which reflected an ongoing commitment to the concept of promoting resilience among the students (Henderson & Milstein, 2003).

Hunter and Chandler (1999) conducted a pilot study of 51 adolescents enrolled in an inner city vocational school. They used a triangulated design to collect both quantitative and qualitative data. Participants in the study completed a self-report measure of resilience (Resilience Scale), and they participated in a writing activity and focus groups. These researchers found that resilience had a different meaning to these youth than what was measured

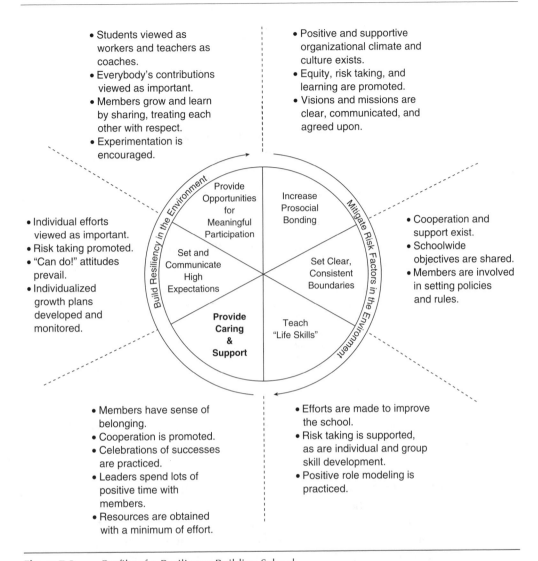

Figure 7.3   Profile of a Resiliency-Building School

SOURCE: Henderson and Milstein (2003, p. 58). © 2003 Sage Publications. Reprinted by permission.

by the Resilience Scale. To these youth, being resilient meant that they were not connected to others, they felt there was nobody to trust, and they were survivors. Hunter and Chandler noted that these youth believed that they needed to be self-reliant and to trust themselves more than others to survive. The researchers focused on these findings as strengths of youth and proposed a model of resilience as shown in Figure 7.4.

In this model, Hunter and Chandler (1999) identify protective factors as those that modify the effects of stress. Outcomes are conceptualized on a continuum from less optimum to more optimum resilience. Those individuals with less optimum resilience have the greatest potential for maladaptation,

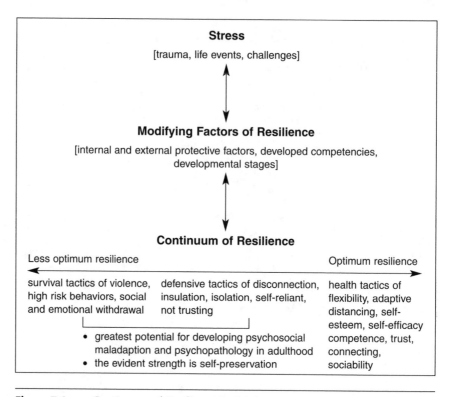

Figure 7.4   Continuum of Resilience in Adolescents

SOURCE: Hunter and Chandler (1999, p. 246). © 1999 Sigma Theta Tau International.
Reprinted with permission.

whereas those with more optimum resilience have the greatest potential for healthy adaptation.

Using the same scale to measure resilience, Rew, Taylor-Seehafer, Thomas, and Yockey (2001) explored the relationships among selected risk and protective factors and resilience in a convenience sample of 59 homeless adolescents. The mean score of the participants on the resilience scale was 4.48 (with 1 as the lowest and 7 as the highest attainable scores). This was similar to the mean of 5.3 reported by Hunter and Chandler (1999). Those participants who scored low on the resilience scale scored high on measures of hopelessness, loneliness, and life-threatening behaviors. Hopelessness and lack of connectedness explained 50% of the variance in the resilience scores. This finding was consistent with the findings of Hunter and Chandler. For high-risk youth, particularly those who lack the usual social connections to family and schools, resilience may indicate an adaptive strategy for survival. Resilience was negatively correlated with life-threatening behaviors (i.e., being suicidal), suggesting that in spite of low levels of connectedness, homeless youth who were resilient felt less lonely and less hopeless than the nonresilient participants.

_____ Interrelationships of Risk and Protective Factors

There is increasing evidence that risk and protective factors are not distinctly different phenomena. Rather than being opposites, they may differ in the impact of their relationship on some health-related outcome. Stouthamer-Loeber and colleagues (1993) have suggested that the relationship between risk and protective factors may actually be nonlinear. They conducted a study of males in the first, fourth, and seventh grades. Approximately 500 boys from each grade cohort were in the study. The purpose of the study was to determine if risk and protective factors co-occur, if they differ in the effects they have on outcomes, and if the effects change with age. Data were collected at two times: initial screening and 6-month follow-up. Findings were that for outcomes of delinquent behavior, protective factors occurred together with risk factors rather than alone, in most cases, and risk effects also occurred in tandem with protective factors more than alone. These researchers found no variable with only or primarily protective effects. There were no clear distinctions in effects of either type of factor on delinquency outcomes. That is to say, protective factors were just as likely to be associated with nondelinquency as they were to suppress serious delinquency. Similarly, the risk factors were just as likely to promote serious delinquency as they were to suppress nondelinquency. The magnitude of risk and protective effects did increase with age, which means that the relationship between risk and protective factors for delinquency became more pronounced with age.

From the model depicted in Figure 6.3 (Chapter 6), Blum et al. (2002) offer three hypotheses about how protective processes function to moderate poor health outcomes in adolescents:

1. "Protective processes span multiple contexts" (p. 32). As found in previous research, protection operates not only at the individual and family levels but also at environmental levels (e.g., peers, schools, churches, neighborhood).

2. "Protective processes vary across domains of functioning" (p. 32). That is, a factor that protects in one domain, such as in academic performance, may not protect in another domain, such as in social functioning.

3. "Protective processes vary across risk processes" (p. 32). Although there is a considerable body of knowledge that identifies common protective processes, the complexity of resilience is such that different types of protection may operate to produce positive outcomes under varied conditions of risk.

Blum and associates used data from Add Health to demonstrate this with violent behavior. Specifically, they found that classroom management climate is a critical protective resource for violence related to weapon carrying but ineffective as protection against cocaine use or sexual intercourse.

Resilience in Maltreated Youth

Children who have experienced abuse or neglect are at high risk for maladaptation, but protective mechanisms have been identified that contribute to resilient outcomes. In a study of 206 children attending a summer camp program, Cicchetti et al. (1993) compared those who had not experienced maltreatment (n = 79) with those who had been maltreated (*n* = 127). Participants in the study ranged in age from 8 to 13 years (*M* = 9.58, *SD* = 1.45 years) and most (69%) were from minority populations. All participants were from a low socioeconomic background. The children who had experienced maltreatment were significantly more likely to exhibit disruptive and aggressive behaviors, social withdrawal, and internalizing symptoms such as anxiety and depression or somatic complaints than were their unabused peers.

In a small study of 43 sexually abused girls who were 10 to 17 years old (median age = 14 years), Spaccarelli and Kim (1995) found that resilience was correlated with a warm and supportive relationship with a nonoffending parent. Other factors associated with resilience in this sample were low levels of stress related to the abuse, few cognitive appraisals of the abuse situation, and few aggressive coping strategies.

It has been well documented that although adolescents who have been maltreated and put in foster care engage in the same health-risk behaviors as adolescents who have not been maltreated, the maltreated ones engage in these behaviors earlier, more often, and with more intensity (Taussig, 2002). This is particularly true for sexual risk behaviors (e.g., greater number of sexual partners, inconsistent use of contraceptives, exchanging sex for food or drugs), alcohol and other drug use, self-destructive behaviors such as suicide, and violent or delinquent behaviors. To determine what factors contributed to health-risk and destructive behaviors and what factors were protective, Taussig developed a working model (Table 7.2) in which risk behaviors were identified in four domains (delinquency, self-destructiveness, substance use, and sexual activity) and served as the outcome variable. Demographics of age, ethnicity, and gender, types of maltreatment, behavior problems, and cognitive and adaptive behavioral functioning were seen as control variables, and psychosocial predictors were social support and self-perception.

Time 1 control and psychosocial predictors (social support and self-perception) significantly predicted time 2 behaviors (outcomes). Physical abuse was related to delinquency, and neglect was significantly related to substance use.

Table 7.2   Taussig's Working Model of Risk and Protective Factors in
                  Maltreated Youth in Foster Care.

Demographic Factors	Psychosocial Factors	Risk Behaviors
Age	Social Support	Delinquency
Gender	Self-perception	Self-destructiveness
Ethnicity	Scholastic competence	Substance use
Maltreatment type	Social acceptance	Sexual risk activities
Behavior problems	Athletic competence	
Behavioral functioning	Physical appearance	
	Behavioral conduct	
	Global self-worth	

Empirical Referents

The concepts of resilience and protection have not only been defined in various ways theoretically, the operational definitions are also quite diverse. A few scales, however, have been developed that might be useful in measuring these phenomena directly.

Resiliency Questionnaire for Children and Adolescents

The Resiliency Questionnaire for Children and Adolescents is a 25-item inventory that focuses on temperament and self-esteem, family environment and interactions, support from outside the family, and previous response to stress. The questionnaire is administered by interview and is designed for use by school and institutional counselors (Rak & Patterson, 1996). A limitation of the instrument is the lack of published evidence of reliability and validity.

Resilience Scale

Wagnild and Young (1993) developed the Resilience Scale for the purpose of identifying resilience as a positive personality characteristic that contributes to individual adaptation. The scale was originally developed for use with older women but was also intended for use by both sexes and across a wide range of ages. Elements of resilience that were identified through qualitative analyses of 24 women interviewed in the first stage of instrument development were "equanimity, perseverance, self-reliance, meaningfulness, and existential aloneness" (p. 167). These elements were validated through a review of the literature, thus establishing content validity. A 25-item, 7-point Likert-type response scale was then developed (1 = *disagree*, 7 = *agree*). The Cronbach alpha coefficient of internal consistency was found to be .89 in a sample of undergraduate nursing students and .91 in a sample of community-dwelling older adults. Test-retest reliability was reported with significant ($p < .01$) correlations ranging from .67 to .84. A principal components analysis was done and resulted in a satisfactory two-factor solution that explained 44% of the variance in scores. The two factors are personal competence (17 items; e.g., "I have self-discipline") and acceptance of self and life (8 items; e.g., "It's okay if there are people who don't like me"). Concurrent validity was supported by significant positive correlations with measures of life satisfaction, high morale, and physical health and by significant negative correlations with a measure of depression.

The Resilience Scale was also used in a study of 59 homeless adolescents (Rew, Taylor-Seehafer, Thomas, & Yockey, 2001). The researchers found that resilience was significantly related to measures of social connectedness (respondents believed that people cared about them), hopelessness, loneliness, and life-threatening behaviors. There were no significant differences in resilience or its correlates by gender or sexual orientation. Using stepwise multiple regression analyses, we found that hopelessness and connectedness explained 50% of the variance in resilience. Participants who scored high on the Resilience Scale felt less lonely and hopeless than those who scored low on this measure. In addition, participants who scored high on resilience reported fewer life-threatening behaviors than those who scored low on the Resilience Scale.

Self-Reported Ego-Resiliency

The Self-Reported Ego-Resiliency Scale was developed to measure a person's "general capacity for flexible and resourceful adaptation to external and internal stressors" (Klohnen, 1996, p. 1067). The scale consists of 29 items and has coefficients of internal consistency that range from .81 to .88 in samples of university students. There is also evidence to support construct, convergent, and divergent validity (Klohnen, 1996). A limitation of the scale is that it is based on resilience as an intraindividual or personality construct.

Resilience and Health-Risk Behaviors

Jessor's problem-behavior theory (see Chapter 6) has been extended to address health-related behavior by including concepts of *proximal* and *distal* protective factors (Jessor et al., 1998). Proximal protective factors are health specific and are directly related to health behaviors. These factors include an individual's value of health, internal health locus of control, and perceived social support from parents and peers for engaging in health behaviors. Distal protective factors do not have a direct reference to health but nevertheless serve to protect one from adverse health outcomes. These factors include the individual's personality; perceived social environment; and conventional behaviors, such as volunteer work, participation in school and club activities, and involvement with family and church.

Using Jessor's problem behavior theory as a framework, Chewning and colleagues (2001) conducted a written survey study of 484 Native Americans attending five rural schools, four of which were on Indian reservations. Participants were in grades 6 through 12, but their ages were not reported. The purpose of this study was to identify protective factors in four sexual domains: timing of sexual debut, reduction of sexual intercourse in past 3 months, increased use of contraception in past 3 months, and increased use of condoms in past 3 months. Forty-nine percent of the sample had already experienced sexual intercourse, 79.6% of the girls and 69.7% of the boys had not had sex in the last 3 months, and 68% of those who had had used birth control most or all of the time. Factors that protected against the risk of early intercourse (i.e., never having had sex) were (a) perception that friends did not use drugs, (b) perception that parents had not discussed sex with adolescent in the past year, and (c) lower grade in school. Valuing academic achievement was a protective factor for girls but not for boys and also was a protective factor in not having had sex in the past 3 months. For both boys and girls, having parents who knew the adolescent's friends and activities outside of school was a protective factor for not having had sex in the past 3 months. Protective factors for consistent birth control use were perceptions that friends were not having sex and that mother was supportive. Perception that friends were not having sex and self-efficacy were associated with condom use.

A longitudinal study of 1512 students (734 females and 780 males) in two junior high schools was conducted to compare resilient and nonresilient adolescents with respect to their relative likelihood of engaging in health-risk behaviors (Rouse, Ingersoll, & Orr, 1998). The average age of participants was 13.13 ± 0.8 years. Resilient participants were defined as those who were predicted to score above a standardized mean on health-risk behaviors (on the self-administered Health Behaviors Questionnaire) but who scored below the mean; nonresilient participants were defined as those who were predicted to score above this mean and actually did. A low-risk (normal) comparison group was defined as those who were predicted to score below the mean and who actually did. At 1-year follow-up, the individuals defined as resilient were less likely than those defined as nonresilient to engage in health-risk behaviors such as substance use, running away, having sex, being arrested, or being suspended from school. These resilient youth were, however, more likely than the normal comparison youth to engage in these health-risk behaviors. The researchers concluded that the relatively lower rates of initiating health-risk behaviors among the resilient versus nonresilient youth reflected the resilient participants' competence in the face of adversity. Similarly, the relatively higher rates of initiating health-risk behaviors among the resilient versus normal youth reflected the influence of adverse conditions on the resilient youth.

Chapter Summary

In this chapter, the concepts of resilience and protection were defined. The literature that supports these conceptualizations was presented, and several models of resilience were described. Outcomes of longitudinal studies of children provide ample evidence that in spite of extreme vulnerabilities related to poverty and other social disadvantages, many individuals develop into capable and caring adults. Protective factors were identified as present in three domains: within the individual, within the family, and within the larger community. The chapter ended with a focus on the relationship between resilience and health-risk behaviors in adolescence. Individual, familial, and societal protective resources have been identified as moderators of health-risk behaviors such as alcohol, cigarette, and marijuana use; physical aggression and weapon carrying; and unprotected and promiscuous sexual activity. The identification of protective factors at these three levels has implications for interventions that could enhance their protective powers.

Suggestions for Further Study

Blum and colleagues (2002) have hypothesized that we need to examine risk and protective mechanisms at all levels (i.e., individual, family, environment, and society). In particular, complex designs might answer questions about how protective factors in all three domains interact to provide maximum protection. Blum's research team also suggested that protective processes should be examined across domains of functioning and across risk processes. Again, more complex designs with multivariate analyses are warranted. The Add Health data set provides data from all three levels, making such analyses feasible.

Zimmerman and Arunkumar (1994) suggest that a resilient process "may operate differently at different phases of development" (p. 10). They also suggest that it differs along domains. Thus, again, exploring these mechanisms in various domains of competence (e.g., scholastic, social) across time may help us to understand how protection works throughout adolescent development. The inclusion of qualitative data may also help to illuminate what adolescents think is protective in their lives and how important these mechanisms are to them.

Much more work needs to be done to establish theoretical models of resilience. The lack of consistence in the use of terms is compounded by the lack of conceptual models in which these terms can be placed. The study of vulnerability, risk and protective processes, and resilience is further hampered by the lack of valid instruments to measure these constructs. Theory construction and methodological studies are needed to remedy these shortcomings. Heller, Larrieu, D'Imperio, and Boris (1999) also suggest that further studies should include both cross-sectional and longitudinal data about resilience in children who have been maltreated.

There is very limited evidence that taking care of pets or a family member (see Zimrin, 1986) and having a sense of humor (see Masten, 1986) can act as buffers against the adverse outcomes associated with stress. We know very little about how a sense of humor is developed or how it can be nurtured to enhance its protective properties. We don't know if maximum protection is afforded through the appreciation, comprehension, or production of humor or whether it is a combination of all three. Examination of these and other less usual phenomena would broaden our understanding of what works in the lives of early and late adolescents. Masten also suggested that humor should be examined across ages and across domains of competence. Is it a protective mechanism that can be enhanced through intervention? What kind of intervention might work, and at what age and in what setting could it be optimally delivered? Answers to these and related questions require creative thinking.

It would be interesting to know if the development of self-identity serves in any way as a protective factor. Interventions that facilitate the development of an individual's identity as a competent person could then be developed and tested. A recent study of self-image and self-esteem in African American preteen girls suggests that lowered levels of these phenomena contribute to early sexual activity and increased risk for sexually transmitted diseases and unplanned pregnancies. An intervention that focuses on promoting health and fostering a strong self-image could serve as an important protective process (Doswell, Millor, Thompson, & Braxter, 1998).

We need to continue to examine multiple pathways to competence. Children and adolescents grow up in multiple contexts, some of which may be sources of either protection or risk. We need to identify why the same factor sometimes increases vulnerability but at other times offers protection. We need to examine how brain development relates to the development of competencies. Longitudinal studies are needed to explore how trauma alters the course of development and, ultimately, behavior. We need to conduct studies that integrate biological, psychological, social, and spiritual development to address the health needs and behaviors of holistic persons.

Related Web Sites

ERIC Digest: http://www.ed.gov/MailingLists/EDInfo/Archive/msg 00049.html

Hardwired to Connect: http://www.americanvalues.org/html/hardwired .html

Jordan Institute for Families: http://ssw.unc.edu/jif/

School Violence Prevention: Resilience (working paper): http://www .mentalhealth.org/schoolviolence/5-28Resilience.asp

Resiliency in Action (books, training, and a newsletter): http://www .resiliency.com

Suggestions for Further Reading _____

Dyer, J. G., & McGuinness, T. M. (1996). Resilience: Analysis of the concept. *Archives of Psychiatric Nursing, 10,* 276-282.

Henderson, N., Benard, B., & Sharp-Light, N. (Eds.). (1999). *Mentoring for resiliency.* San Diego, CA: Resiliency in Action.

Monasterio, E. B. (2002). Enhancing resilience in the adolescent. *Nursing Clinics of North America, 37,* 373-379.

Resnick, M. D. (2000). Protective factors, resiliency, and healthy youth development. *Adolescent Medicine: State of the Art Reviews, 11*(1), 157-164.

Smith, R. S., & Werner, E. E. (1998). *Vulnerable but invincible.* New York: Adams, Bannister, Cox.

Smith, R. S., & Werner, E. E. (2001). *Journeys from childhood to midlife.* Ithaca, NY: Cornell University Press.

8

Theories of Social Cognition

During adolescence, the developing person's cognitive abilities change in dramatic ways. Unlike children, adolescents are no longer bound to thinking about what is real and concrete; they develop the ability for abstract thinking. Adolescents also develop the ability to think in multiple dimensions simultaneously and are able to consider things as relative. Unlike children, adolescents are capable of metacognition, or the ability to think about thinking itself. These changes in cognitive ability have enormous implications for behavior in general and health behavior in particular.

Social cognition refers to the ways in which individuals make sense of their social setting and the relationships within it. Theories of social cognition thus focus on how a person's thoughts or thinking processes mediate between observable stimuli from the environment (social setting) and behavioral responses, many of which are health behaviors (Conner & Norman, 1996). Social cognitive theory (SCT) is an outgrowth of social learning theory, which originated in the early 1940s with the work of Miller and Dollard (1941). These cognitive psychologists sought to explain both human and animal behaviors as an outcome of learning in social situations. Subsequent development of both social learning theory and SCT was based on the notion that human cognition moderates, in numerous ways, the relationship between a stimulus from the environment and a behavioral response from the person. This moderation allows individuals to have control over the way in which they respond to environmental stimuli.

Social Cognitive Theory

Origins

Bandura (1986) noted the limitations of Freud's psychodynamic theory and Skinner's behaviorism.

In the social cognitive view people are neither driven by inner forces nor automatically shaped and controlled by external stimuli. Rather, human functioning is explained in terms of a model of triadic reciprocality in which behavior, cognitive and other personal factors, and environmental events all operate as interacting determinants of each other. (p. 18)

Purpose

The purpose of social cognitive theory is to explain and predict human behavior. SCT also explains and predicts how behavior can be changed or modified.

Meaning of the Theory

The assumptions of Bandura's SCT are as follows:

1. People learn by watching other people.

2. Learning is an internal process, and it may or may not alter behavior.

3. Behavior is goal directed.

4. Self-regulated behavior is initiated, monitored, and evaluated by a person in pursuit of his or her own goals.

5. Reinforcement and punishment have both direct and indirect effects on behavior.

According to Bandura (1986), human behavior is not merely instinctual, nor is it a response to external stimuli. In simplest terms, human behavior can be explained as an interaction among cognitive and other personal factors, influences from the environment, and the behavior itself. A model of triadic reciprocity, or *reciprocal determinism*, illustrates the mutual action between three causal elements: person (cognitions, affect, beliefs, expectations), environment (social setting, other individuals, groups, media messages), and behavior (observable, intentional, and goal-directed actions; required skills). The three elements interact to determine each other, as depicted in Figure 8.1. The reciprocal nature of the relationships among these major elements does not imply symmetry in the strength of the influences on each other. The relative influence of each of the elements varies by individual for different activities and under different circumstances. Bandura further asserts that the reciprocal nature of the relationships does not mean that the influences are necessarily simultaneous. Rather, the mutual effects occur sequentially over time. Patterns of behavior continue as individuals select those environments that reinforce the behavior pattern and produce or alter such environments to be congruent with the behavior pattern.

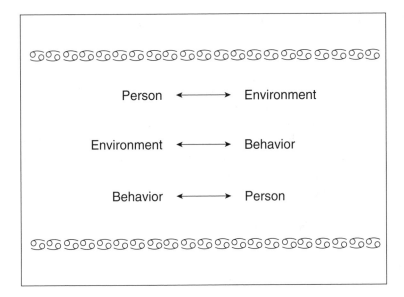

Person ←——→ Environment

Environment ←——→ Behavior

Behavior ←——→ Person

Figure 8.1   Relationships Among Concepts of Reciprocal Determinism in
                   Social Cognitive Theory

The arrows between each of the three constructs in the triadic model are bidirectional to indicate the reciprocal nature of the relationships. The person's biological makeup, feelings, and thoughts all influence her or his actions. This is reflected in the person-behavior interaction. In carrying out an action, one's thoughts and emotions are also influenced. Beliefs, expectations, and competencies are influenced by social circumstances, which is reflected in the environment-person interaction. In turn, individuals influence the makeup of the social environment. People both produce and are products of their environments, and thus there is a reciprocal relationship between environment and behavior. Behavior influences how the person experiences the environment through a process of selective attention. The environment itself is influenced by the person as she or he creates a situation with positive or negative characteristics (Bandura, 1989).

Persons are viewed as having five types of capabilities that affect behavior: symbolizing, forethought, vicarious, self-regulatory, and self-reflective.

A person's *symbolizing capability* is a major way in which that person adapts to or changes the environment. Symbols allow the person to produce mental images or internal models that give form and meaning to lived experiences. This capability also allows the person to store and retrieve information from transient situations for future use. Use of symbols permits the person to communicate and to imagine possible outcomes of circumstances. The symbolic activity of the person forms the basis for the capability of forethought. Also known as future time perspective, *forethought capability* is evident in a person's ability to anticipate the outcomes of behavior. This capability permits a person to have the motivation to carry out intentional and purposive acts. *Vicarious capability* means that a person can learn how to act by observing how another person acts and seeing the consequences of that action. "The capacity to learn by observations enables people to acquire rules for generating and regulating behavioral patterns without having to form them gradually by tedious trial and error" (Bandura, 1986, p. 19).

Self-regulatory capability permits the person to engage in behaviors that are motivated and tempered by internal standards. The existence of internal personal standards allows the person to evaluate his or her performance against these standards, thus leading to greater personal control over behavior. This capability reflects the person's ability to substitute internal controls for external controls of behavior. The *self-reflective capability* is closely related to self-regulation and means that a person has the capacity to evaluate and modify thinking. The capacity to reflect on oneself can result in a judgment about one's personal behavior that is accurate or inaccurate. An important type of self-reflection that is critical to SCT is that of *self-efficacy,* which is a person's judgment about her or his ability to perform a specific act (Bandura, 1986, 1997). Each of these capabilities is discussed in more detail later.

Modeling, as a way to convey attitudes, values, thoughts and behavior patterns, is a construct of central importance in SCT. Related to the first assumption, that people learn by watching or observing others, modeling is the process by which a person internalizes rules of conduct that serve to guide behavior. Modeling is not the same as imitation or mimicry. In SCT, modeling is characterized by its ability to produce novel behaviors by observing skills and rules that can be transformed into something new and unique. When individuals learn through modeling, they observe the structure and rules of the person engaging in the desired behavior and form a mental conception of a particular skill or behavior. Modeling also serves to overcome behavioral inhibitions previously learned, to prompt a previously learned behavior that has not been consistently performed, or to arouse emotion that can alter behavior. Learning occurs as a cognitive process involving the ability to form abstract, reflective, and generative thoughts. Learning is analyzed "in terms of the cognitive competencies necessary for acquiring knowledge and performance skills" (Bandura, 1986, p. 128).

Environment influences behavior through a process of symbol use. A person forms a conception or symbol of appropriate behavioral responses by observing patterns in rules and decisions made by others. A process of conception matching known as *enactive learning* is one of several modes of learning social behavior. A conception integrates the rules of action and specifies how a particular behavior is enacted. When individuals learn by enacting the behavior directly, they form a conception based on the effects of their own actions as opposed to the conception formed through modeling. This feedback is critical to mastering complex behaviors. "Learning proceeds most rapidly when outcomes follow actions immediately, regularly, and without other confusing occurrences" (Bandura, 1986, p. 129). The relationship between behavior and outcomes is probabilistic and depends on a variety of factors that may or may not be under the control of the individual (Bandura, 1986).

Beliefs also influence learning and behaviors. In particular, one's beliefs about the rewards associated with a behavior may affect that person's behavior more than the outcome of the behavior itself. In SCT, "People regulate their level and distribution of effort in accordance with the effects they expect their actions to have. As a result, their behavior is better predicted from their beliefs than from the actual consequences of their actions" (Bandura, 1986, p. 129). An important type of belief is that of *outcome expectations,* or the perceived results (either positive or negative) associated with a given behavior. In general, there are three types of outcomes: physical, social, and self-evaluative. Physical outcome effects include positive or negative sensations (e.g., pleasure vs. pain) or health consequences (e.g., weight loss vs. increased discomfort) associated with a particular behavior. Social outcome effects include change in status; rewards, such as approval from family and peers; and public recognition. Self-evaluative effects are either negative or positive internal responses that occur as a result of performing the behavior. Examples of self-evaluative effects include the feeling of disappointment versus the feeling of self-satisfaction (Resnicow, Braithwaite, & Kuo, 1997).

Two other personal factors that are important in SCT are skills and goals. Skills are specific abilities that a person must develop to perform a specific behavior or sequence of behaviors. For example, assertive communication involves developing the proficiency to use language in a way that protects oneself against domination by another person. Goals may be short or long term and refer to specific behaviors or outcome effects that increase a person's motivation to engage in a particular type of behavior (Resnicow et al., 1997).

Social cognitive theory addresses the learning that occurs not only in the individual but also in social groups. The concepts of *innovation* and *diffusion* are salient in explaining how new behaviors are spread within or between social groups. Any idea or activity that people perceive to be new is an innovation, and the process of spreading the idea or activity within a social community is diffusion. In SCT, the social diffusion of innovative ideas or practices involves two distinguishable processes: acquisition of knowledge about the innovation and adoption of the innovation. In the process of acquiring knowledge about the innovation, the primary mechanism of modeling, discussed earlier, is operative. Through modeling, people observe the new behavior and its associated outcomes. They are not only informed of new ideas and behaviors but may also be motivated to perform them. If an innovation is satisfying and functional, it is easily and readily diffused. Other factors that determine whether people will adopt a new idea or behavior include incentives that are tangible. In making the decision to adopt an innovation, people act "on the basis of anticipated benefits and possible detriments" (Bandura, 1986, p. 148). If a person perceives greater benefit than harm from an innovation, he or she is more highly motivated to adopt it. Individuals are also more likely to engage in the innovation if they see other knowledgeable people engaging in the same practice. In summary, an innovation is more likely to be adopted when it leads to "prompt, observable benefits and when the causal relationship between new practices and results can be easily verified" (p. 162).

Two types of motivators for behavior are described in SCT. These motivators are biological and cognitive. Biological motivators include physiological processes such as the pain response to an aversive stimulus or the pleasure response to a sexually arousing stimulus. Cognitive motivators occur through expectations about the future. Such expectations may include material, sensory, or social rewards. Other types of cognitive motivators include one's internal standards and self-evaluation of personal performance. Intrinsic motivation occurs when a person engages in an activity or exhibits a behavior with no apparent external reward. Many human endeavors, such as training for an athletic event, are maintained by anticipating long-term rather than short-term or immediate outcomes. In contrast, extrinsic motivation occurs when rewards or contingencies are applied arbitrarily to the performance of a behavior. Extrinsic motivators are not natural consequences of the action but are applied as a penalty or reward by another person or object. When new skills are being learned, as in the case of a child learning to solve arithmetic problems, external rewards in the form of praise, gold stars, and special privileges may serve to motivate continuation of the behavior (Bandura, 1986).

Self-regulation is the process employed by individuals to make and maintain changes in their behavior. According to Bandura (1986), self-regulation occurs as the result of three subfunctions: self-observation, judgment, and self-reaction. Self-observation is the process of paying attention to one's behavior. Specifically, people tend to pay close attention to some of their behaviors and ignore others. Self-observation provides information for setting performance standards that are realistic and for assessing progress in changing behaviors. The judgmental subfunction is the process of establishing internal standards against which one can judge one's behavior. In this process, people may also consider a number of other referents for comparison. For instance, individuals may compare their performance to that of others who are (a) perceived as representing a normative group or (b) perceived as being associates. Similarly, people may compare their performance at a given time to a previous performance, thus making a self-comparison. The subfunction of self-reaction can be either positive or negative. Such reactions occur primarily with regard to activities that have significance for a person and vary according to how that person perceives the determinants of particular activities or behaviors (Bandura, 1986).

Self-efficacy is a person's judgment about her or his capability to perform a specific activity at an acceptable level. Such a self-judgment is one aspect of determining how the person will act. Self-efficacy is also task-specific, which is to say that it is not a personality trait but that individuals make a judgment about how confident they feel that they can perform a specific task. This sense of efficacy or confidence can develop through one of the following sources: performance mastery, arousal or other psychophysiological state, verbal persuasion, or vicarious observation. The greatest efficacy effects are derived from performance mastery, in which the task is perfected through practice. Arousal or other psychological or physiological states such as fear or pleasure can have a negative or positive effect on the person's judgment of confidence in performing a task. Verbal persuasion through another person's encouraging words can also affect an individual's motivation to perform a task. When a person can see another person perform the behavior either directly or through an instructional type of media presentation, vicarious observation occurs and can lead to self-efficacy (Resnicow et al., 1997). Self-efficacy can be debilitating when individuals are overwhelmed with doubts about their capacity to perform particular behaviors (Bandura & Jourden, 1991).

In summary, social cognitive theory purports to explain and predict human behavior through the reciprocal relationships of person, environment, and behavior. Of central importance is the cognitive capacity of the person for symbolizing, forethought, vicarious observation of others, self-regulation, and self-reflection. The environment in which a person behaves consists of other persons, groups, and situations that influence a person's actions by providing rules for action as well as contingencies in the form of rewards and punishments. Motivations for behavior are both cognitive and behavioral, intrinsic and extrinsic. Behavior is goal directed, intentional, and observable; it requires skills and is regulated by a person through self-observation, judgment, and self-reaction.

Scope, Parsimony, and Generalizability

Bandura (1986) asserts that the scope of SCT is broader than its title; it helps to explain motivation and self-regulation in learning and in other processes. SCT has had considerable impact on the diffusion of health practices for society at large. Bandura states, "People's health is largely in their own hands rather than in those of physicians" (p. 178). Although there are many processes described in the theory, the three major concepts in the model of triadic determinism provide a parsimonious framework on which the details of the theory are placed. The theory is generalizable to most behaviors across the life span and within various cultures.

Logical Adequacy

The triadic model of reciprocal determinism, which forms the core of social cognitive theory, reflects its fundamental logical adequacy. This is

Concept	Person	Environment	Behavior
Person	=	±	±
Environment		=	±
Behavior			=

Legend: = indicates same concept; ±, concepts may be either positively or negatively related.

Figure 8.2   Logical Adequacy of Three Core Variables in Social Cognitive Theory

illustrated in Figure 8.2. Relationships between person and environment, person and behavior, and behavior and environment are reciprocal. The meaning of each concept is clear, and there are no logical fallacies in the general statements that can be made about the relationships.

There is agreement among scientists that the SCT makes sense and that concepts are logically connected (Baranowski, Perry, & Parcel, 1997). Numerous hypotheses have been derived from the theory and tested. The concepts have been logically applied in a variety of studies conducted by scientists concerning academic behaviors (Rudolph, Lambert, Clark, & Kurlakowsky, 2001) and health behaviors (Strecher, DeVellis, Becker, & Rosenstock, 1986).

Examined in more detail, however, SCT contains numerous constructs that are at times difficult to categorize as belonging to the person, the environment, or the behavior components of the theory. For example, self-regulatory capability is conceptualized as an aspect of the person, but self-regulation can be observed as the person's behavior. Similarly, symbols are derived from the environment but are internalized as an abstract representation within the person. How one constructs a matrix to determine the logical adequacy of the theory thus becomes perplexing.

Usefulness

Social cognitive theory is useful in explaining many behaviors and has been found especially useful in understanding health behavior and changes in health behaviors. SCT has been useful as a framework to describe a large variety of behaviors across a wide range of ages. For example, it has been used to study adolescent sexual offenders (Burton, Miller, & Shill, 2002), gender role development and functioning (Bussey & Bandura, 1999), unhealthy eating patterns of adolescents (Cusatis & Shannon, 1996), development of attitudes toward smoking (Sargent et al., 2002), and physical activity in early adolescents (Strauss, Rodzilsky, Burack, & Colin, 2001).

It has also been used successfully as the framework for a health promotion intervention to prevent substance use in high-risk adolescents (Tencati, Kole, Feighery, Winkleby, & Altman, 2002), an intervention to develop problem-solving skills among middle school students (Sharma, Petosa, & Heaney, 1999), and an intervention for HIV prevention education (Evans, Edmundson-Drane, & Harris, 2000). SCT has also been used as a framework for interventions to promote healthy behaviors across the life span (Hardin et al., 2002; Lytle & Perry, 2001).

Testability

Social cognitive theory is complex and comprehensive. These attributes make it difficult to operationalize and test directly (Brown, 1999). Bandura and Jourden (1991) noted that "ongoing interaction between behavioral, cognitive, and environmental factors cannot be sufficiently controlled to elucidate causal processes" (p. 941). Thus, many of the postulates of the theory have been tested by simulation rather than in vivo.

Winters, Petosa, and Charlton (2003) tested selected concepts from the theory to predict leisure-time physical exercise in a convenience sample of 248 students. The sample consisted of 150 females and 98 males who were an average of 15 years old. Concepts of SCT selected for the study were social situation, self-efficacy, outcome expectation values, and self-regulation. These researchers controlled for gender and found that the selected variables accounted for 29% of the variance in the frequency of vigorous exercise. Three of the variables (i.e., social situation, outcome expectation values, and self-regulation) accounted for 11% of the variance in the frequency of leisure-time moderate physical exercise. Although these findings give some support to the relationships among selected constructs, they do not support the predictive capability of the theory.

Empirical Referents

Social Cognitive Theory contains many constructs that have not been well defined in operational terms. However, a few samples of valid measures are described briefly below.

Generalized Expectancy for Success Scale. Self-regulation has been measured by the Generalized Expectancy for Success Scale (Fibel & Hale, 1978). The scale contains 30 items with a five-point, Likert-type response format. Reported internal consistency reliability was .92 in a sample of 174 undergraduate university students (Kocovski & Endler, 2000).

Self-Regulation for Physical Activity. The Self-Regulation for Physical Activity Scale measures five dimensions of self-regulation: goal-setting, self-monitoring, social support, plans to overcome barriers, and reinforcement. The scale contains 38 items and has internal reliability coefficients of .78 to .94 for the subscales (Winters et al., 2003).

Perceived Control Scale. The Perceived Control Scale for Children contains 24 items with a 4-point, Likert-type response format. The scale was designed to assess a person's beliefs about his or her ability to control the outcomes of events in social, academic, and behavioral domains (Weisz, Southam-Gerow, & Sweeney, 1998). In a sample of 360 youth between 8 and 17 years old ($M = 11.8 \pm 2.3$), the alpha coefficient of internal consistency was .88, and the 6-month test-retest reliability coefficient was .57.

Application to Practice

Condom Use Among College Students. DiIorio, Dudley, Soet, Watkins, and Maibach (2000) collected data from college students and universities (n = 6) to test the relationship among social cognitive theory variables related to condom use behaviors. Participants included a total of 1380 students (63% females) between 18 and 25 years old (mean age 20.6 years ± 1.76). Most participants were either White (50%) or African American (42.5%), with only a few Hispanic (2.9%) and Asian Americans (3.9%). These researchers used structural equation modeling to test a model that illustrates relationships among anxiety, self-efficacy, outcome expectancies, alcohol use, and condom use. Results from this study showed that self-efficacy was related directly to condom use and indirectly through outcome expectancies. Although self-efficacy was directly and negatively related to anxiety, anxiety was not related to condom use. Use of alcohol during sexual encounters was related directly and negatively to outcome expectancies but not to condom use. DiIorio and colleagues (2000) concluded that the findings supported the model based on SCT and could be used for developing interventions to increase condom use in this population. Moreover, they suggested that based on their findings, interventions that focused on reducing anxiety related to obtaining condoms and negotiating with a partner for condom use might not be useful strategies.

School-Based Nutrition Education Program. Social cognitive theory was identified as the theoretical framework for a school-based nutrition education program. The aim of the study, titled Teens Eating for Energy at School, was to assist young adolescents in middle or junior high schools to increase their daily consumption of fruits and vegetables and lower their daily consumption of fat foods. Citing Bandura's (1986) model of triadic determinism (i.e., person, environment, behavior), Lytle and Perry (2001) assert that this model explains the health-risk behavior of adolescents who have unhealthy diets. For example, the environment in which most adolescent behavior takes place provides adolescents with unhealthy choices of food, such as fast foods with high fat content, rather than fruits and vegetables. Adolescents may have insufficient or inaccurate knowledge about the benefits of eating more fruits and vegetables and fewer fats. Moreover, they may lack motivation and self-efficacy to alter their behavior in the face of increasing knowledge and motivation. Behavioral factors include reinforcement of past eating behaviors that affects current choices. In a study using a group-randomized design (Lytle & Perry, 2001), eight schools received the 2-year intervention for students in seventh and eighth grades, and eight control schools received the intervention at the end of the 2-year trial. The outcome measure was the comparison of fruit and vegetables consumed and energy from fat assessed through 24-hour recall. Steps taken to develop the intervention are shown in Table 9.1 (Chapter 9) and focus on changing health-risk behavior. Personal, environmental, and behavioral factors from the SCT model are identified as predictive factors, and sample intervention objectives are outlined to address each of these. After objectives are outlined, curriculum is developed to address individual factors and behavior by targeting the school and the family environments.

Intervention to Prevent Violence in Early Adolescents. A 13-module intervention to prevent violence, based on social cognitive theory, was delivered to 292 sixth grade students. These students, along with 412 students from control schools, completed pre- and post-test measures at intervals of 2 weeks before and 2 weeks after the intervention, respectively. The two groups were not significantly different at the time of the pretest on measures of age, gender, depression, or exposure to violence. At the post-test, there was a decrease in violence by participants in the intervention group and an increase among the students in the control group (DuRant, Barkin, & Krowchuk, 2001).

Self-Efficacy Theory

Origins

Bandura (1997) referred to his conceptualizations of self-efficacy both as a theory and as "the *self-efficacy component* of the theory [SCT]" (p. 34). He distinguished between the two by saying that "Social cognitive theory posits a multifaceted causal structure that addresses both the development of competencies and the regulation of action" (p. 34).

Purpose

The purpose of self-efficacy as a theory is to provide a framework that explains the origin, structure, function, and processes of how a person's beliefs influence his or her actions. Moreover, as a theory, it purports to offer guidelines for people to learn how to have more control in their lives and thus effect desired change (Bandura, 1997).

Meaning of the Theory

Bandura (1977) identified self-efficacy as the critical element operating in human agency or the ability of one to take action on one's own behalf. He asserted that individuals who judge their capacity to perform a specific action as high are more likely to be motivated to perform and actually accomplish the specified action. The corollary to this is that individuals who believe they are not capable of performing a particular action will avoid that activity. Bandura further asserted that the self-referent aspect of efficacy was a perception of one's judgment that one could perform a particular task rather than that one possessed a global trait of capacity. Self-efficacy also refers to the amount of effort individuals will put into performing a particular behavior and how much time they will spend in this endeavor.

Individuals' belief in their ability to exhibit some control over what happens in their lives provides a framework for their actions. "Perceived self-efficacy refers to beliefs in one's capabilities to organize and execute the courses of action required to produce given attainments" (Bandura, 1997, p. 3). Although much of human behavior is determined by multiple factors, people contribute their beliefs to this dynamic mixture. Behavior that is volitional (done freely with some intention) is affected by the beliefs held by the actor.

Bandura (1997) is quick to point out that perceived self-efficacy is not the same concept as locus of control. Whereas locus of control is a general belief about whether or not actions can affect outcomes, perceived self-efficacy is beliefs about one's ability to perform a specific behavior. He illustrates the difference by stating that a person who lacks the skill to perform a particular behavior (e.g., correctly apply a condom) may still believe that the outcome of the activity is under his or her control. Thus, the person may demonstrate an internal locus of control but have a low sense of self-efficacy for performance of the requisite skill. Bandura distinguishes between performance and outcome in that the former refers to an accomplishment and the latter refers to something that comes after the accomplishment. To extend the example, adolescents may believe they are in control of preventing an unplanned pregnancy (outcome) but may not be able to apply a condom correctly (performance).

Self-efficacy has a critical position within SCT because of its interaction with other determinants of behavior. Beliefs of self-efficacy influence a person's motivation to acquire a knowledge base on which performance skills are based. These beliefs also contribute to self-regulation and motivation by "shaping aspirations and the outcomes expected for one's efforts" (Bandura, 1997, p. 35).

Beliefs in personal efficacy are developed most effectively through mastery experiences. Self-efficacy beliefs can also be developed vicariously by watching other people who are successful at the targeted behavior. A third way to enhance self-efficacy is through social persuasion. Through encouragement, people are able to mobilize and sustain the efforts needed to master the behavior. Finally, people relate their self-efficacy to internal awareness of stress and tension. Thus, self-efficacy can be enhanced through stress reduction and positive emotional states (Bandura, 2000).

Beliefs about self-efficacy have been shown to regulate human behavior and emotions through four processes: cognitive, affective, motivational, and selective (Bandura, 1997). In addition to having an impact on behaviors, then, self-efficacy, or rather the lack of it, can contribute to a person's feelings of sadness and despair. For example, individuals who lack confidence in their ability to perform a skill or to develop satisfying social relationships may be unable to attain desired goals and may, consequently, experience feelings of disappointment and depression. At the cognitive level, such people may also be unable to control negative or depressing thoughts, thus compounding their feelings of disappointment and despair. Bandura, Pastorelli, Barbaranelli, and Caprara (1999) conducted a longitudinal study of 282 young adolescents (mean age = 11.5 years). What they found was that children who had high self-efficacy to regulate learning and master academic work showed very few problem behaviors. Those children who had low social self-efficacy and low academic self-efficacy also showed signs of high levels of depression at baseline testing and again 1 year later. Using path analysis, this research team further showed that the effect of low academic self-efficacy on depression was mediated by prior depression, academic achievement, and problem behaviors. Low social self-efficacy had a stronger impact on the outcome of depression in females than in males.

In a prospective study of 464 adolescents 14 to 19 years old, researchers (Bandura, Caprara, Barbaranelli, Gerbino, & Pastorelli, 2003) examined the influence of perceived self-efficacy for affect regulation on various aspects of psychosocial functioning. The purpose of the study was to examine how adolescents manage transitional stressors associated with development. Specifically, the theory of self-efficacy for affect regulation was purported to influence three psychosocial outcomes: prosocial behavior, delinquent behavior, and depression. The hypothesized causal structure through which perceived self-efficacy for affect regulation works together with action-oriented efficacy beliefs to influence these three outcomes is depicted in Figure 8.3.

The model indicates that "perceived self-efficacy to regulate positive and negative affect influences depression, delinquent conduct, and prosocial behavior both directly and mediationally by their impact on perceived academic self-efficacy, resistive self-regulatory efficacy, and empathic self-efficacy" (Bandura et al., 2003, p. 771). Five sets of self-efficacy predictors and the three psychosocial domains of functioning were measured at time 1 and psychosocial functions at time 2, which was two years later. At time 1, the average age of the participants was 16 years, and at time 2, their average age was 18 years. Eighty-eight percent of the original sample participated in time 2 data collection.

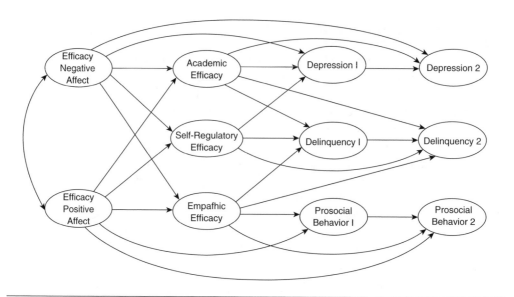

Figure 8.3   Affective Self-Regulatory Efficacy and Psychosocial Functioning in Older
Adolescents

SOURCE: Bandura et al. (2003, p. 773). © Society for Research in Child Development. Reprinted with
permission.

The data provided a good fit with the model [X^2 (90, 459) = 233.61, $p < .001$;
CFI = .93]. The only paths in the proposed model that were not significant
were (a) the direct path from self-efficacy to regulate positive affect to prosocial behavior, time 2; (b) the direct path from empathic efficacy to delinquency,
time 1; (c) the direct path from academic efficacy to delinquency, time 2;
and (d) the direct path from academic efficacy to depression, time 2. A
significant direct path not specified in Figure 8.3 was the direct path from
empathic efficacy to depression, time 2. Bandura and colleagues concluded
that the findings from this study support the theoretical utility of SCT.

Scope, Parsimony, and Generalizability

Self-efficacy theory purports to apply to all kinds of behaviors. Concepts
of the theory are difficult to isolate, and thus parsimony cannot be determined at this time. The central components of the theory, however, may
apply to persons across the life span, among various ethnic and cultural
groups, and to those in other countries.

Logical Adequacy

Scientists from various disciplines agree that the self-efficacy construct
and theory and their relationship to health-related behaviors make sense.
Hypotheses can be derived from the theory and tested.

Usefulness

Self-efficacy theory has been useful in the study of eating disorders, alcohol use and abuse, depression, and athletic performance (Bandura, 1997). The theory has also been useful in the study of safer sex behaviors (Crosby et al., 2001; DiIorio et al., 2000) and alcohol use in adolescents (Petraitis, Flay, & Miller, 1995). Similarly, it has been identified as a significant motivator to engage in physical exercise, control weight, and modify addictive behaviors (Schwarzer & Fuchs, 1996). The concept of self-efficacy has also been useful in the development of interventions based on social cognitive theory, the theory of planned behavior, and on models of health promotion (Pender, Bar-Or, Wilk, & Mitchell, 2002; Pender, Murdaugh, & Parsons, 2002).

Testability

Because of the lack of clarity about whether self-efficacy is a component of social cognitive theory or a theory in its own right, testability is unclear. There is no doubt that self-efficacy has been a useful construct in exploring health-related behaviors, and the concept itself is measurable.

Empirical Referents

Because self-efficacy refers to one's confidence in performing a specific behavior, measures of self-efficacy must be behavior specific. Thus, many scales have been developed to measure a person's confidence in performing a variety of behaviors. For example, DiIorio and colleagues (2000) report the use of self-efficacy scales to measure "self-efficacy for resisting pressures to have sex," "self-efficacy to put on a condom," and "self-efficacy to discuss the partner's sexual history" (p. 210). These scales used a 10-point response format from 1 (unsure of ability to engage in the behavior) to 10 (complete confidence).

Smith, McGraw, Costa, and McKinlay (1996) reported on the validity of a self-efficacy scale to measure HIV risk behaviors among Latino youth between 14 and 22 years old. The scale contained nine items that asked about the respondent's confidence in talking about safe sex with a partner, buying condoms, using condoms correctly, and refusing to share needles. Factor analysis yielded two factors: refusal and neutral actions. Alpha coefficients ranged from .75 to .78. A major limitation of the scale is the variety of behaviors addressed in a single scale.

Related Theories and Research

Expanded Health Belief Model. The Health Belief Model, which will be presented as a model for health promotion in Chapter 9, was expanded to include the concept of self-efficacy and to therefore enhance its explanatory power. The expanded health belief model (EHBM) is widely used in research on health behaviors. The six major constructs in the model are (a) perceived susceptibility, (b) perceived severity of condition and its sequelae, (c) perceived benefits of action, (d) perceived barriers to taking action, (e) cues to action, and (f) self-efficacy. Other demographic variables, such as education, may also influence a person's perception and have indirect effects on health behaviors. Lack of self-efficacy is conceptualized as a barrier to taking a health-promoting or -protecting action. The original health belief model hypothesized that health behavior or action depended on three interacting factors: concern about health; belief in vulnerability or susceptibility; and belief that engaging in the health behavior would benefit the person, would reduce the risk of disease, and could be done at a reasonable cost (Rosenstock, Strecher, & Becker, 1988; Strecher et al., 1986; Strecher & Rosenstock 1997).

In a study in Thailand of 391 vocational school students between 18 and 22 years old, Thato, Charron-Prochownik, Dorn, Albrecht, and Stone (2003) used the EHBM to study predictors of condom use. There were significant bivariate correlations between actual condom use and (a) perceived benefits, (b) perceived barriers, (c) condom self-efficacy, and (d) intention to use condoms. The modifying variables of age, gender, alcohol use, knowledge of STDs, and duration of sexual relationship were not significantly related to use of condoms. Using multiple linear regression, including interaction terms, the researchers found that the research participants were more likely to use condoms when they (a) believed in the benefits, (b) were male, (c) were females with high intentions to use condoms, (d) had high knowledge of STDs, (e) believed that friends also engaged in health behaviors, (f) had lower levels of alcohol use, and (g) were younger. These factors explained 27% of the variance in condom use. Condom self-efficacy, however, was significantly related to condom use ($r = .22$, $p < .01$) but was not a significant explanatory factor in multivariate analysis. In addition, two other variables of the EHBM were not significant in predicting condom use: perceived susceptibility to STDs and perceived barriers. Thus the study provides only partial support for the EHBM.

In a similar study of the EHBM (Mahoney, Thombs, & Ford, 1995), 366 college students from 18 to 24 years old participated. Only the constructs of perceived susceptibility, perceived benefits, perceived barriers, and condom use self-efficacy were measured. The measure for condom use self-efficacy was multidimensional and consisted of four subscales: mechanics; partner's disapproval; assertiveness; and being under the influence of intoxicants such as alcohol, other drugs, or strong emotions. The measure of perceived susceptibility had two dimensions: self and partner. Only perceived susceptibility and self-efficacy differentiated among nonusers ($n = 70$), sporadic users ($n = 157$), and consistent users ($n = 107$). Perceived susceptibility of both partner and self were significant [$F(2, 331) = 7.16$, $p < .001$] and

$[F(2, 331) = 8.36, p < .001]$ respectively. Three of the four dimensions of condom use self-efficacy were significant. These were assertiveness $[F (2, 331) = 9.78, p < .001]$, partner's disapproval $[F (2, 331) = 4.81, p < .05]$, and influence of intoxicants $[F (2, 331) = 3.17, p < .05]$. Again, these findings lend some support to the EHBM (Mahoney et al., 1995). Bear in mind that this was not a test of the full model.

Protection-Motivation Theory. Protection-motivation theory is an integration of concepts from social learning theory and the health belief model. The focus of the theory is on the person's perception of threat or vulnerability and the severity of that threat. Other variables in the model include self-efficacy, beliefs about costs, and beliefs about rewards. A person's response to stimuli results in an appraisal of threat and vulnerability and recognition of the severity of the threat. Individuals produce an adaptive response when they increase their coping appraisal and self-efficacy and decrease the rewards for producing a maladaptive response (Rippetoe & Rogers, 1987; Rogers, 1983).

Theories of Reasoned Action and Planned Behavior

Origins

Ajzen and Fishbein's (1980) theory of reasoned action (TRA) was developed within the discipline of social psychology. These theorists were influenced by the work of L. L. Thurston, who developed a method for measuring attitudes with an interval scale, and by Louis Guttman, who developed a method for measuring beliefs. They were also influenced by the work of Gordon W. Allport, who suggested that there was a complex relationship between attitudes and behavior. The theory of planned behavior (TPB) was developed by Ajzen (1985, 1991) when he added a third major construct to the theory of reasoned action. The theories are based on the assumption that people are rational and use information to inform their actions (Ajzen & Fishbein, 1980). Other assumptions are that to change a behavior, one must change beliefs about that behavior, and if beliefs change, intentions toward enacting the behavior will also change (Ajzen & Fishbein, 1980).

Purpose

The purpose of the theories is twofold: (a) to explain and predict human behavior in terms of motivational influences (e.g., attitudes and beliefs) that are not under the person's complete volitional control and (b) to describe strategies for changing behavior. "The theory of planned behavior is an extension of the theory of reasoned action (Ajzen & Fishbein, 1980; Fishbein & Ajzen, 1975) made necessary by the original model's limitations in dealing with behaviors over which people have incomplete volitional control" (Ajzen, 1991, p. 181).

Meaning of the Theory

The theory of planned behavior is depicted in Figure 8.4. The theory explains how attitudes and beliefs affect behaviors, and it is best applied to those behaviors that are, at least to some extent, under the volitional control of a person. Intention is the major construct of the TRA and TPB models, conceptualized as the immediate determinant of a person's action. *Behavioral intent* is a person's attitude toward performing a specific behavior, combined with that person's perception that important other people view the performance of this behavior as desirable. Intention reflects a person's motivation to enact a particular behavior. This intention is determined by the person's attitude toward the behavior and her or his perception of social pressures to engage or not engage in that behavior (Ajzen & Fishbein, 1980). For example, intention to eat a balanced diet indicates how hard a person is willing to work to engage in this activity and how much the person believes that other important people want him or her to engage in it. A proposition of the theory is that the stronger a person's intention to enact a particular behavior, the more likely it is that the person will actually enact it. Intention can be translated into actual behavior only when the particular behavior is under the volitional control of the person. Many behaviors cannot be performed under complete volitional control of the person because enactment may also depend on the availability of resources and opportunities (Ajzen, 1991).

A person's perception of the importance of the behavior to other people is known as a *subjective norm*. A person's attitude includes beliefs about a particular behavior, possible outcomes of the behavior, beliefs about the normative behavior of peers, and a motivation to comply with the behavior. Attitude is the primary element and the subjective norm is the secondary element in determining a person's behavioral intent. The subjective norm is a predictor of intention to perform a behavior and reflects perceived social pressure to do so (Beck & Ajzen, 1991).

A final construct, *perceived behavioral control*, is not found in the TRA but is in the TPB model. Perceived behavioral control includes individuals' beliefs about how much control they have over the behavior (control beliefs) and how much they believe they can perform the behavior successfully (perceived power). Individuals may have a positive attitude toward performing a particular behavior, but if they believe they do not have the power to perform that behavior successfully, it is not likely that they will display

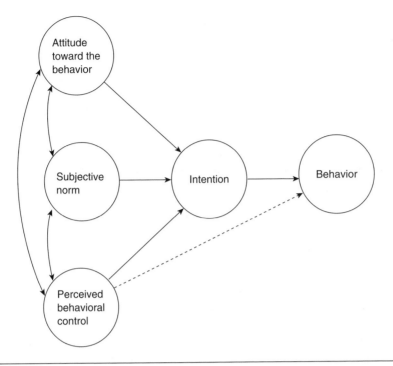

Figure 8.4   The Theory of Planned Behavior

SOURCE: Beck and Ajzen (1991, p. 287). © 1991 Elsevier Science. Reprinted with permission.

the behavioral intent to perform it. It is important to note that the TPB emphasizes perceived control rather than actual control. Unlike the concept of generalized locus of control (Rotter, 1966), perceived behavioral control varies across circumstances and refers to how easy or difficult the person perceives the behavior to be (Ajzen, 1991).

The major hypotheses of the TPB are that attitude toward the behavior, subjective norms, and perceived behavioral control independently determine a person's intention to perform a particular behavior, as depicted in Figure 8.4 (Ajzen, 1991). The relative influence of each of these independent predictors varies across circumstances and behaviors. Because intentions change over time, it is imperative that the time between intention and behavior be short. Put another way, intention can predict behavior "only if the intention does not change before the behavior is observed" (Ajzen & Fishbein, 1980, p. 52).

Scope, Parsimony, and Generalizability

The TRA and TPB are broad in scope because they are applicable to many behaviors. The two theories are parsimonious because they explain many different behavioral phenomena with just a few concepts. The theories can be generalized to many different ages and ethnic groups of people.

Logical Adequacy

The relationships among the major constructs in the TPB model are depicted in Figure 8.5. These reflect logical adequacy of the theory. There is agreement among scientists (see "Usefulness" section) that the theory makes sense and hypotheses can be derived from the theory (Ajzen, 1991).

Usefulness

The theory of reasoned action has been used to understand and predict a variety of health behaviors, including physical activity (Motl et al., 2002), substance use (Carvajal, Evans, Nash, & Getz, 2002), smoking, tobacco chewing (Gerber, Newman, & Martin, 1988), performing testicular self-examination (Brubaker & Wickersham, 1990), weight loss, and sexual activity (Conner & Flesch, 2001). The theory of planned behavior has been used to predict behavioral intentions regarding adolescents' consumption of fruits and vegetables (Lien, Lytle, & Komro, 2002) and organic foods (Monaco Bissonnette & Contento, 2001), intentions to engage in physical activity (Hagger, Chatzisarantis, & Biddle, 2001), intentions to practice testicular self-examination (Murphy & Brubaker, 1990), and adherence to training in competitive swimming (Mummery & Wankel, 1999), as well as pedestrians' road crossing decisions (Evans & Norman, 1998). The TPB has also been found useful in understanding binge drinking in college students (Norman, Bennett, & Lewis, 1998). Both theories have been applied in numerous studies of condom use (Albarracin, Johnson, Fishbein, & Muellerleile, 2001; Bennett & Bozionelos, 2000; Bryan, Fisher, & Fisher, 2002; Lugoe & Rise, 1999).

Construct	A	B	C	D	E
A	=	±	±	±	±
B		=	±	±	±
C			=	±	±
D				=	±
E					=

Legend: A = attitude toward the behavior; B = subjective norm; C = perceived behavioral control; D = intention; E = behavior. The symbol = refers to the same concept; ± means that the relationship may be either positive or negative.

Figure 8.5   Relationships Among Constructs in the Theory of Planned Behavior

Testability

Ajzen (1991) maintains that measures of intention and perceived behavioral control must be congruent with the behavior they are intended to predict. That is to say, they must be specific to a particular behavior and must measure the constructs within the context of a person performing that behavior. Ajzen also warns that both intention and perceived behavioral control "must remain stable in the interval between their assessment and observation of the behavior" (p. 185). Hankins, French, and Horne (2000) have offered statistical guidelines specifically for testing these theories, particularly for researchers using multiple regression and structural equation modeling techniques.

Empirical Referents

As noted earlier, there must be congruence between measures of attitudes, intention, perceived behavioral control, and the specific behavior under study. Thus empirical indicators of these major constructs must be developed specifically for the behavior of interest. For example, Beck and Ajzen (1991) sought to predict dishonest actions (i.e., cheating, shoplifting, and lying) of college students with the TPB. They obtained self-reports from participants by asking how often they had engaged in each of the behaviors. Attitudes toward each of the behaviors were measured with three semantic differential scales that evaluated the behavior as "good-bad, pleasant-unpleasant, foolish-wise, useful-useless, unattractive-attractive" (p. 292). Another scale, consisting of three items, was constructed to assess subjective norms about each of the dishonest behaviors; perceived behavioral control for each behavior was measured with four additional items. A measure of intention included three items that asked how likely participants were to engage in the behavior, whether or not they would ever engage in the behavior, and whether or not they might engage in the behavior at some time in the future. Beck and Ajzen also measured social desirability using the Marlowe-Crowne Social Desirability Scale (Crowne & Marlowe, 1964).

Other researchers have clearly shown how they have constructed scales specifically for the types of behavior under investigation (Evans & Norman, 1998), and occasionally, single items are used to measure one of the constructs in the theory (Lien et al., 2002). For example, several scales exist to measure intentions to use condoms. One such Likert-type scale contains eight items that assess one's intentions to use condoms with a casual sex partner (four items) and with a steady partner (four items). Internal consistency coefficients of reliability were .93 for a steady partner and .90 for a casual partner (Rosengard et al., 2001).

Related Research

The theory of reasoned action has been refined through research to include the variables of self-efficacy and past behavior (Hagger et al., 2001) for use in predicting physical activity intention in young people. Hagger and associates hypothesized that the frequency of past physical activity would attenuate the influence of attitudes, subjective norms, perceived behavioral control, and self-efficacy on the intention to engage in physical activity. Data from 1152 adolescents with a mean age of 13.5 (± 0.6) years were analyzed using confirmatory factory analyses and structural equation modeling. The confirmatory factor analysis supported the measures used for constructs in the theory of planned behavior.

Structural equation modeling showed that the intention to engage in physical activity was strongly predicted by attitudes and self-efficacy but that subjective norms and perceived behavioral control were not. Past behavior predicted all variables in the model. Past behavior was most strongly associated with attitude (standard coefficient = .50, $p < .01$) and self-efficacy (standardized coefficient = .63, $p < .01$) (Hagger et al., 2001, p. 720). Moreoever, the structural equation modeling analysis showed that the relationship between intention and perceived behavioral control was attenuated by self-efficacy. The hypothesis that past behavior would attenuate the influence of attitude, subjective norm, perceived behavioral control, and self-efficacy on intention to engage in physical activity was not supported. Hagger and colleagues (2001) concluded that the variables of past behavior and self-efficacy should be included in the theory of planned behavior. They also noted that past behavior in adolescents played a different role than it did with adults.

Prototype/Willingness Model

Origins

The prototype/willingness (P/W) model is based on theories of social cognition. In particular, it draws heavily on the theory of reasoned action.

Purpose

The purpose of the P/W model is to explain and predict complex health-risk behaviors in adolescent and young adult populations (Gibbons & Gerrard, 1995; Gibbons, Gerrard, Blanton, & Russell, 1998).

Meaning of the Model

The P/W model is based on the following assumptions:

1. Among adolescents, health-risk behaviors are volitional but may not be either intentional or rational.

2. Among adolescents, health-risk behaviors are social events and are not pursued in isolation.

3. Social images associated with health-risk behaviors have an impact on adolescents' decision to engage in them (Gibbons, Gerrard, Blanton, et al., 1998).

The primary focus of the P/W model is the concept of behavioral willingness. Behavioral willingness is different from behavioral intention because it reflects a lack of planning. Willingness is a reaction to the opportunity to engage in risky behaviors. It involves the perception that peers are engaging in the behavior and would not be disapproving (subjective norms). Behavioral willingness is associated with positive attitudes toward the behavior in question. A favorable attitude toward the behavior is associated with having enacted the behavior in the past. A final antecedent to the behavior is the prototype or social image the person has about the type of person who would engage in the particular behavior. According to this theory, the influence of prototypes on behavior is mediated by the behavioral willingness of the person (Gibbons, Gerrard, Ouelette, & Burzette, 1998).

With respect to a particular health-risk behavior, an adolescent has a prototypical image of the kind of person who engages in that behavior (e.g., a driving daredevil). Adolescents understand that if they engage in the behavior around their peers, they will acquire this image themselves (i.e., they will be seen as driving daredevils). The more acceptable the behavior and image are to a person, the more she or he is willing to engage in it. Engaging in such behavior is not planned or necessarily intended. Thus the perception of prototype is related to health-risk behaviors and to behavior changes (Gibbons & Gerrard, 1995).

Scope, Parsimony, and Generalizability

The P/W model applies broadly to health-risk behaviors and contains few variables; thus it is parsimonious. It may be generalized to adolescents across various cultures and at various stages of development.

Logical Adequacy

The logical adequacy of the P/W model is depicted in Figure 8.6. There are no logical inconsistencies, and it is possible to derive testable hypotheses.

Usefulness

The P/W model has been used to predict smoking and drinking behaviors in adolescents and pregnancy-risk behaviors in college students (Blanton,

Concept	A	B	C	D	E	F
A	=	+	+	+	+	+
B		=	±	±	+	+
C			=	+	+	+
D				=	+	+
E					=	+
F						=

Legend: A = health-risk behavior; B = subjective norms; C = positive attitude toward behavior; D = past engagement in behavior; E = behavioral willingness (expectation); F = prototype. The symbol = refers to the same concept; ± means that the relationship may be either positive or negative.

Figure 8.6   Logical Adequacy of the Prototype/Willingness Model of Health-Risk Behavior

Gibbons, Gerrard, Conger, & Smith, 1997; Gibbons, Gerrard, Blanton, et al., 1998).

Testability

The P/W model has been tested primarily by Gibbons and colleagues, who developed the model. A longitudinal study of 679 college students provided support for the relationship between prototype and four health-risk behaviors: reckless driving, inconsistent contraceptive use, smoking, and drinking (Gibbons & Gerrard, 1995). Three additional tests of the model provide evidence of support for it. In particular, findings support the hypotheses "(a) that much adolescent health-risk behavior is not planned and (b) that willingness and intention are related but independent constructs, each of which can be an antecedent to risk behavior" (Gibbons, Gerrard, Blanton, et al., 1998, p. 1164).

Empirical Referents

No standardized tests have been developed to measure the various constructs in the model. Because the model is specific for individual health-risk behaviors, specialized scales must be developed to match the targeted health-risk behavior. Previous studies have described the measurement of subjective norms, willingness, and prototype (Blanton et al., 1997; Gibbons, Gerrard, Blanton, et al., 1998).

Peer Cluster Theory

Peer cluster theory focuses on the influences of family and peers on the social learning of adolescents. Propositions of the theory are that within close-knit groups of peer clusters (e.g., best-friend dyads, girlfriend-boyfriend dyads) ideas and information are exchanged (Swaim, Bates, & Chavez, 1998). Attitudes and beliefs about how to act are formed and altered through this exchange of ideas and information. Individuals who comprise the peer clusters contribute to group norms and thus to behaviors that are considered appropriate or normal to the group. The theory has been tested to determine the relationship between association with deviant peers and the development of deviant behaviors in adolescents. Results of a study of 910 Mexican American and White non-Hispanic school dropouts partially supported the theory. That is, an adolescent's association with drug-using peers was the strongest predictor of the adolescent's drug use.

Decision-Making Models

Adolescents make decisions every day about a variety of things, including what to wear and eat, where and when to go places, what friends to "hang with" and what other people to avoid, and what to do in a multitude of settings. Learning to make decisions is a cognitive developmental process that consists of four steps: (a) setting a goal (e.g., going somewhere with friends), (b) identifying alternative ways to meet the goal (e.g., go to the movie, go to someone's home, go to the bowling alley), (c) listing the alternatives in rank order (e.g., going to the movie is better than going to the bowling alley, but not better than going to someone's home), (d) selecting the alternative with the highest ranking (e.g., going to someone's home) (Byrnes, 2003). Decision-making models have been constructed to explain and predict how adolescents make decisions about many behaviors that have short- and long-term consequences for their health. These models are presented in more detail in Chapter 10.

Self-Regulation Theory

Origins

Theories of self-regulation originated in the work of Rotter (1966) that focused on a person's beliefs about control over behaviors and on Bandura's (1986) social cognitive theory.

Purpose

The purpose of self-regulation theories is to describe and predict how people think about their actions. The main idea is that through self-observation, reflection, and evaluation, individuals alter their behavior to be consistent with personal goals.

Meaning of the Theory

There are several models or theories of self-regulation. In general, "Self-regulation refers to the process by which people initiate, adjust, interrupt, terminate or otherwise alter actions to promote attainment of personal goals, plans or standards" (Heatherton & Baumeister, 1996). Self-regulation is a synthesis of beliefs, cognitions, evaluations, and behaviors that influence goal-directed action and emotion (Rudolph et al., 2001). Self-regulatory beliefs include perceptions of control over the outcomes of events (Rotter, 1966). Self-regulatory beliefs may be adaptive, leading to health, or maladaptive, contributing to a lack of health.

A model of self-regulation that has implications for understanding health and health-risk behavior in adolescence is the Self-Regulation Model of Decision-Making (SRM) proposed by Byrnes (1998). The SRM is considered a developmental explanation because of three attributes: It describes an earlier state of some system, it describes a later state of the same system, and it contains a developmental mechanism that explains how the earlier state can be changed into the later state (Byrnes, Miller, & Reynolds, 1999). The model is based on the assumption that people have a tendency to regulate themselves and is presented in detail in Chapter 10.

Testability

In a longitudinal study of 187 adolescents in transition from elementary to middle schools, Rudolph and colleagues (2001) used self-regulation theory to test hypotheses about differences between youth who experienced a school transition and those who did not. They hypothesized that students' self-regulatory beliefs would be more strongly related to perceived school stress and depression among those youth who experienced a transition in schools than among those who did not. They also hypothesized that students who had high perceptions of academic control and high investment in success would exhibit greater effort and persistence in spite of challenge and better performance in school than students with low perceptions and low investment.

Self-Regulation and Substance Use

Data from two samples of adolescents ($n = 1699$, $n = 1225$) with mean ages of 15.4 and 15.5 years, respectively, were analyzed to test predictions about factors that moderate the relationship between levels of alcohol, tobacco, and marijuana use and problems associated with such use. For those participants who exhibited good self-control, protective moderation effects were found that reduced the relationship between level of substance use and problems associated with that use. In contrast, for those participants who exhibited poor self-control, risk-enhancing moderation effects were found. These findings provide support for the self-regulation model tested in this study (Wills, Sandy, & Yaeger, 2002).

Research Applications

Hardin et al. (2002) tested the effects of a long-term psychosocial nursing intervention to decrease distress in youth who had experienced a catastrophic event. Based on an integration of concepts from social learning theories (i.e., cognitive understanding, self-efficacy, and social support), they randomly assigned 545 adolescents to the intervention and 550 to the control group. This was a multiethnic sample (44% White, 54% African American) that ranged in age from 13 to 18 years. The intervention was designed for youth who had experienced Hurricane Hugo in the South Carolina area. The intervention consisted of three sessions, each 3.5 to 4 hours long, each year for three years. Didactic and problem-solving methods were used to improve cognitive understanding and increase healthy coping. Other strategies were used to increase social support and self-efficacy.

A study of 471 adolescent males was conducted to test hypotheses of a social cognitive theory that addressed the etiology of adolescent sexual offending (Burton et al., 2002). The researchers described a social learning framework in which some children who were sexually victimized became sexual offenders in adolescence and others did not. Specifically, the framework suggested that if the sexual perpetrator is closely related to the child who is victimized, the child is more likely to learn from this and model this behavior later, thus becoming a sexual perpetrator. Children who are victimized by a male perpetrator are more likely to learn to model this behavior in adolescence because male perpetrators use more force and therefore reinforce learning. The use of force is also likely to contribute to feelings of powerlessness and fear in the victim, leading to acting-out behavior by the victim to gain control of the situation.

Using a cross-sectional survey design, Burton and colleagues (2002) tested the following six hypotheses to compare sexually victimized, nonsexually offending delinquents with sexually victimized, sexually offending delinquents:

1. Participants who were sexual offenders were more closely related to their own perpetrators than participants who were not sexual offenders.

2. Participants who were sexual offenders were more likely to have been victimized by a male perpetrator than participants who were not sexual offenders.

3. Participants who were sexual offenders were subjected to more forceful victimization than participants who were not sexual offenders.

4. Participants who were sexual offenders were more likely to have experienced penetration in their own victimization than participants who were not sexual offenders.

5. Participants who were sexual offenders were more likely to have experienced longer duration of sexual victimization than participants who were not sexual offenders.

6. Participants who were sexual offenders were younger at the time they were sexually victimized than participants who were not sexual offenders.

Findings supported four of the hypotheses. The researchers found that the adolescents who were sexual offenders were more closely related to their perpetrators, were more likely to have been abused by a male, and experienced longer duration of victimization and more forceful victimization than those who were not sexual offenders.

Related Research

Citing the increasing incidence of obesity and overweight in preadolescent and adolescent girls, Pender, Bar-Or, and associates (2002) conducted a study to determine relationships between exercise self-efficacy and various aspects of exercise. A convenience sample of 103 girls between 8 and 17 years old was recruited from several social institutions in Canada. Exercise self-efficacy was measured prior to and after engaging in exercise (pedaling for 20 minutes on a cycle ergometer). Participants who scored high on perceived self-efficacy for exercise reported lower perceptions of exertion during exercise than participants who initially scored lower on the measure of exercise self-efficacy. Pre-exercise self-efficacy and perceived exertion during exercise were associated with postexercise self-efficacy. The researchers concluded that the brief exercise task increased the participants' self-efficacy for exercise and that this finding could be potentially valuable for developing interventions to increase physical activity among preadolescent and adolescent girls.

Applications to Practice

Health-risk behaviors among adolescents are the focus for a variety of programs intended to change those behaviors. One highly successful process for developing a communitywide program of behavior change is manifested in the research of Cheryl Perry and her colleagues from the University of Minnesota. The findings of this research team indicate that programs targeting parents, teachers, the school, and community environments, as well as the adolescents themselves, have led to greater changes in behaviors such as smoking and alcohol use than those programs that targeted only the classroom setting (Luepker et al., 1996; Perry et al., 1996; Perry et al., 1998).

Increasing Dietary Intake of Fruits and Vegetables. In a study of 53 African American adolescents, Wilson et al. (2002) found significant differences between participants randomized to one of three intervention groups. The groups included (a) a motivational intervention of strategic self-presentation plus social cognitive theory, (b) an intervention using social cognitive theory only, and (c) education only. Each intervention lasted 12 weeks and focused on increasing dietary intake of fruits and vegetables and increasing physical activity. The group with the motivational intervention received a self-representation videotape session. Measures of a 3-day food record, 4-day activity monitor, and self-reports of self-concept and self-efficacy were completed pre- and postintervention. Both groups that included the social cognitive theory–based intervention showed significant increases in dietary intake of fruits and vegetables compared to the education-only group ($p < .05$), but there were no significant differences among groups for physical activity. Only the group that received the motivational intervention along with social cognitive theory showed significant correlations between dietary self-efficacy and intake of fruits and vegetables at postintervention ($r = .65$, $p < .05$) and dietary self-efficacy and change in intake of fruits and vegetables from pre- to postintervention ($r = .85$, $p < .05$). This group also showed significant correlations between dietary self-concept and fruit and vegetable intake at postintervention ($r = .58$, $p < .05$) and change in intake of fruits and vegetables from pre- to postintervention ($r = .67$, $p < .05$). Although the study was small, it was strengthened by the experimental design and suggests that the addition of the motivational intervention that focused on self-presentation shows promise.

Chapter Summary

In this chapter, theories that focus on social cognitions have been highlighted. Specifically, social cognitive theory and its special emphasis on self-efficacy were presented, along with evidence of the usefulness of the theory in planning health-promoting interventions. The theory of reasoned action and its extension, the theory of planned behavior, were described. Both have been deemed useful in understanding and predicting several health behaviors among adolescents, including physical activity and testicular examination, as well as in predicting intentions to improve nutritional practices and adhere to training for competitive sports. The prototype/willingness model and peer cluster theory were explored briefly. Self-efficacy and self-regulation, which are both constructs in social cognitive theory, were presented as theories with testable hypotheses having relevance for adolescent health-risk behaviors.

Suggestions for Further Study

Theories of social cognition have provided valuable frameworks for the study of health-risk behaviors in adolescence. Further study is warranted to determine how adolescents develop their beliefs about health and about health-risk behaviors. We need to learn not only how these beliefs are developed but how they change over time during adolescence. Longitudinal studies using concepts from SCT or TPB could be performed to examine developmental changes in perceived behavioral control, self-efficacy for specific health-risk behaviors, and intentions to engage in behaviors that are more health promoting. Based on findings from such longitudinal studies, interventions could then be developed and tested for critical times to deliver such interventions to improve the short- and long-term health outcomes of adolescents.

It is also important to focus not only on cognitions and cognitive development but on emotions that affect health-risk behaviors. For example, the prototype/willingness model is fairly new but may be useful for further study of the emotional aspects of decision making. We need to know more about the central constructs of behavioral willingness and how people develop prototypes. Qualitative studies could provide important elaborations of these concepts and what they mean to adolescents. Further, valid measures of these concepts need to be developed and tested. To date, the P/W model has been used with a limited number of health-risk behaviors, and this research needs to be extended to other similar behaviors. The assumption that much of adolescent health-risk behavior is unplanned is an intriguing one, suggesting that emotion and immediate gratification may play a big part in these behaviors. This assumption is also in direct contrast to the theory of planned behavior. Changing this assumption into a testable hypothesis could be very helpful.

Health-risk behaviors are learned and enacted in social settings. Therefore, we need more information about what these behaviors mean to adolescents at various stages of development and how much they perceive themselves as at risk for short- and long-term health consequences. Answers to these questions could be sought through qualitative methods, such as focus groups and phenomenology. These methods will be discussed in detail in Chapter 11.

More work needs to be done with the protection-motivation theory. Specifically, this theory could frame studies about adolescents' perception of vulnerability, as well as beliefs about costs and rewards associated with specific health-risk behaviors. For example, we need to know more about how adolescents think about the major threats to their health and well-being. We also need to understand more about how social environments reward those behaviors that increase rather than decrease their vulnerability to these threats. Only then will we be able to craft interventions that minimize threats and maximize rewards for behaviors that protect and promote health and well-being.

Others have suggested adding variables to the theory of planned behavior and to consider making the theory "a dual-process model of attitude-behavior relationships" (Conner & Armitage, 1998). The additional concepts that might be added to the TPB include self-identity, past behaviors and habits, moral norms, affective beliefs, perceived behavioral control versus self-efficacy, and belief salience. Advantages of adding these concepts and variables to the theory are as follows: (a) interventions could be designed that target the salient beliefs of the target population, (b) habits have been shown to influence intentions and behavior in previous studies, (c) conceptual clarity could be established concerning differences between self-efficacy and perceived behavioral control, (d) including moral norms would address the affective and spiritual dimensions of development and their influence on behavior, (e) inclusion of self-identity and affective beliefs might clarify the role of intentions in regard to behaviors, and (f) more causal relationships might be identified. Again, longitudinal studies are needed to make claims about causality regardless of the theory or model used.

Related Web Sites

Information-Motivation-Behavioral Skills Model:

http://socialpsych. uconn.edu/Fisher_et_al_2002_psych.pdf

Self-Efficacy:(Albert Banduras and Self-Efficacy)

http://www.emory.edu/ EDUCATION/mfp/efficacy.html

(A measure of self-efficacy)

http://www.ivey.uwo.ca/faculty/Compeau_Self%20Efficacy_Measure.PDF

Self-Regulation:

(Self-regulation through visualization and imagery)

http://www.cjnetworks.com/~lifesci/

(Self-monitoring and self-regulation)

http://www.athleticinsight.com/ Vol4Iss1/SelfRegulation.htm

Theories of reasoned action and planned behavior:

(Summary and application to advertising)

http://www.ciadvertising.org/ studies/student/97_fall/practitioner/belding/theory.html

(Explanation and useful information)

http://www-unix.oit.umass.edu/ ~aizen/tpb.html

(Overview)

http://www.med.usf.edu/~kmbrown/TRA_TPB.htm

Suggestions for Further Reading

Akers, R. L. (1996). A longitudinal test of social learning theory: Adolescent smoking. *Journal of Drug Issues, 26*(2), 317-343.

Bandura, A., Pastorelli, C., Barbaranelli, C., & Caprara, G. V. (1999). Self-efficacy pathways to childhood depression. *Journal of Personality and Social Psychology, 76,* 258-269.

Guthrie, B. J., Young, A. M., Williams, D. R., Boyd, C. J., & Kintner, E. K. (2002). African American girls' smoking habits and day-to-day experiences with racial discrimination. *Nursing Research, 51,* 183-190.

Jemmott, J. B., III, Jemmott, L. S., Hines, P. M., & Fong, G. T. (2001). The theory of planned behavior as a model of intentions for fighting among African American and Latino adolescents. *Maternal and Child Health Journal, 5,* 253-263.

Kocovski, N. L., & Endler, N. S. (2000). Self-regulation: Social anxiety and depression. *Journal of Applied Biobehavioral Research, 5*(1), 80-91.

Lavoie, F., Hébert, M., Tremblay, R., Vitaro, F., Vézina, L., & McDugg, P. (2002). History of family dysfunction and perpetration of dating violence by adolescent boys: A longitudinal study. *Journal of Adolescent Health, 30,* 375-383.

9

Health Belief and Health-Promotion Models

I n the mid-1970s, the focus of public health in the United States and other industrialized countries such as Canada shifted from a biological model concerned with controlling microscopic, disease-causing organisms through technology to a model of greater self-responsibility for a healthy lifestyle. This new model was that of health promotion and was reflected in the Health Information and Health Promotion Act passed by Congress through PL 94–317. This law resulted in the establishment of the Office of Disease Prevention and Health Promotion and in the first Surgeon General's Report on Health Promotion and Disease Prevention in 1979.

National Objectives to Promote Public Health

The Surgeon General's report, *Healthy People,* was a prelude to *Healthy People 2000* (U.S. Department of Health and Human Services [USDHHS], 1992a), which was the first published document based on research evidence that set forth a national agenda to promote the public health and prevent disease (Green, 1999). This guide was accompanied by a compendium of numerous health promotion and disease prevention objectives directed at mothers, children, and adolescents titled *Healthy Children 2000* (USDHHS, 1992a). Among the objectives directed at health-risk behaviors of adolescents set forth in this document were the following:

- Reduce cigarette smoking
- Reduce smokeless tobacco use by males between 12 and 24 years old
- Enforce laws that prohibit the sale of tobacco products to those younger than 19 years old
- Increase the age of first use of alcohol, marijuana, and cigarettes
- Reduce pregnancies among girls younger than 17 years old
- Increase the proportion of sexually active youth younger than 19 years old who use contraception
- Reduce the incidence of suicide attempts among youth 14 to 17 years old

- Reduce the incidence of weapon carrying among adolescents 14 to 17 years old
- Reduce deaths caused by motor vehicle crashes

The goals and objectives identified in these documents were ambitious, and not all were met. However, having such an agenda was instrumental in directing the nation's attention to the needs for health promotion across the life span.

In 2000, the next set of goals and objectives was published, again by the USDHHS, and was titled *Healthy People 2010*. The two overarching goals of this document were to increase the quality and years of healthy life of Americans and to eliminate health disparities. In addition to establishing measurable objectives related to many of the same health risk-behaviors of adolescents identified in *Healthy People 2000*, the goal of eliminating health disparities has particular salience for adolescents. Among the groups with documented inequalities in health status and health-care access are females; members of minority racial and ethnic groups; and people who are gay, lesbian, bisexual, or transgendered.

A growing interest in self-responsibility and empowerment for health and a consumer orientation to health care were responses to a number of social changes that occurred in the decade of the 1960s. These included the women's movement and the proliferation of self-help programs (Green, 1999). Related to this sharper focus on health promotion was an interest in understanding how beliefs about health influenced people's healthy and unhealthy behaviors. Thus the Health Belief Model became an important step toward further development of public health programs that were population based rather than resource based.

Health Belief Model

Origins

The Health Belief Model (HBM) has served as a conceptual map for understanding health behavior for nearly 50 years. It was developed by social scientists and psychologists working with the U.S. Public Health Service to explain why people were not participating in screening programs designed to detect or prevent disease. In the early 1950s, the public health agenda focused on prevention rather than on treatment of disease, but it was evident that people failed to accept free or low-cost measures such as Pap smear screening for cervical cancer or x-ray screening for tuberculosis. This context set the stage for social psychologists to develop theory that would address the behavior of people who were not experiencing a disabling disease (Becker, 1974; Rosenstock, 1974c).

At that time, social psychology was dominated by two major types of learning theories: stimulus-response theory, set forth by Skinner, Watson, and Hull, and the cognitive theory of Kurt Lewin. Stimulus-response theory focused on the temporal association between a behavior and reinforcements or rewards for that behavior. Cognitive theory, on the other hand, advanced the idea that a person's behavior was related to the subjective value that the person placed on the outcomes of the behavior. This concept was labeled *value expectancy.* Cognitive theories were characterized by their focus on cognitive processes, including reasoning, thinking, and expecting (Strecher & Rosenstock, 1997).

Purpose

The purpose of the HBM was to identify a model that could explain a particular health problem in terms amenable to programs for changing health behaviors. The model was to focus on dynamics present in a person's immediate environment that motivated behavior. The development of the theory was deliberately intended to build a body of scientific knowledge rather than simply solve a particular problem (Rosenstock, 1960, 1974c).

Meaning of the Theory

The HBM is based on the assumption that a person's perception of the world determines what that person will do. The major concepts may be categorized as individual perceptions, modifying factors, and likelihood of action (Figure 9.1). Individual perceptions vary widely and include one's beliefs about susceptibility to some health condition (*perceived susceptibility*) and one's convictions about how serious that health condition is (*perceived seriousness*). Modifying factors include demographic variables of age, sex, race, and ethnicity, psychosocial variables of personality, social class status, and reference group pressure, as well as structural variables such as knowledge about and prior experience with the health condition or disease. Also included in modifying factors are the individual's *perceived threat of disease,* as well as *cues to action* (i.e., internal or external pressures that trigger a response in the individual). These cues include mass media campaigns, advice or encouragement from other people, or the illness of a peer or family member. The likelihood of action results from the individual's *perceived benefits* minus the *perceived barriers* to taking action. Perceived benefits reflect knowledge and beliefs about how a particular behavior may modify the susceptibility or seriousness of a health condition or disease. Perceived barriers, often experienced simultaneously with perceived benefits, include perceptions that the behavior or action will be inconvenient, unpleasant, or expensive (Rosenstock, 1974c).

Scope, Parsimony, and Generalizability

The HBM is fairly broad in scope because it may apply to nearly all health-related behaviors. Its relatively few concepts explain a wide variety of

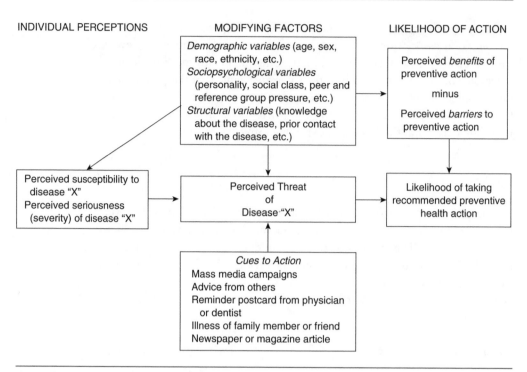

Figure 9.1   The Health Belief Model
SOURCE: Rosenstock, I. M. (1974b, p. 334).

behaviors and it is thus deemed parsimonious. There is nothing in the model that would suggest that it is limited to any particular age or cultural group. However, because it is a cognitive model, it is not generalizable to infants, very young children, or cognitively impaired persons.

Logical Adequacy

The logical adequacy of the HBM is illustrated in Figure 9.2. Based on the concepts and statements that comprise the theory, it is clear that there are no logical inconsistencies and that relationships are clearly identified. Hypotheses can be drawn from the stated relationships among concepts, and there has been agreement among scientists that the model makes sense.

Usefulness

The HBM has been used primarily for public health protection or prevention. The emphasis of the model on avoiding negative outcomes limits its usefulness to primary prevention strategies, such as immunization for

	1	2	3	4	5	6	7	8	9
1	=	+	+	+	+	+	±	+	±
2		=	+	+	+	+	±	+	±
3			=	+	+	+	+	+	±
4				=	+	+	±	· +	±
5					=	±	±	±	±
6						=	±	+	±
7							=	+	±
8								=	+
9									=

Legend: 1 = perceived susceptibility; 2 = perceived seriousness; 3 = demographics; 4 = knowledge and prior experience; 5 = perceived threat; 6 = cues to action; 7 = likelihood of action (benefits minus barriers); 8 = human being; 9 = behavior

Symbols: = refers to the same concept, + refers to positive relationship between concepts, − refers to negative relationship between concepts, ± refers to either a positive or negative relationship between concepts.

Figure 9.2   Logical Adequacy of the Health Belief Model

specific diseases; secondary prevention through screening so that individuals may access treatment early in a disease process; and tertiary prevention through efforts directed at minimizing long-term disabling conditions associated with a disease (Pender, Murdaugh, & Parsons, 2002). The HBM has also been useful in providing a framework for other scientists to develop more complex models of health promotion (see the section titled "Pender's Health-Promotion Model") and has been adapted for use with children and adolescents (see the section titled "Health Belief Model for Children and Adolescents").

Testability

Hochbaum (1958) provided preliminary support for the model in his study about why people did or did not participate in public x-ray screening for tuberculosis. He found that the decision to get x-rayed depended on a psychological state of readiness that included individuals' belief that they might contract tuberculosis, that they could have the disease and not be aware of symptoms, and that they might benefit from early diagnosis. He also found that outside influences, such as posters and radio announcements, provided cues to action for many people, particularly those who displayed all three components of the state of readiness. Moreover, he found that some people who were not in such a state of readiness also responded to external influences and showed up for the x-ray screening, whereas others who had a high state of readiness plus a fear of finding out they had the disease did not participate in the screening.

Rosenstock (1974a) reported moderate support for the model based on a review of studies in which particular action was found to be a function of the interaction of one's perceived susceptibility and perceived benefits. In addition to Hochbaum's work on the prevention of tuberculosis (cited earlier), Rosenstock discussed findings from a study of screening for dental problems; another on screening for Tay-Sachs syndrome, a genetic disorder; and others that focused on participation in a physical activity program and in obtaining annual physical examinations.

Janz and Becker (1984) conducted a critical review of 46 studies based on the HBM. They computed a significance ratio by dividing the number of statistically significant findings by the number of studies reporting significance for that dimension of the HBM. Their findings provided considerable empirical support for the model with findings from both prospective and retrospective studies with similar findings.

Health Belief Model
for Children and Adolescents

The Health Belief Model (Rosenstock, 1974b, 1974c) was adapted by Bush and Iannotti (1990) for use with school-aged children and early adolescents. Borrowing concepts from the HBM, social cognitive theory (Bandura, 1986), cognitive development theory (Piaget & Inhelder, 1958), and behavioral intention theory (Fishbein & Ajzen, 1975), they developed a model (shown in Figure 9.3) with three sets of factors: modifying, readiness, and behavior. The model specified the cognitive and affective variables and enabling and environmental variables that modified the relationship between the child or adolescent's demographics and the behavioral outcome of taking prescribed medicines. Bush and Iannotti hypothesized that demographics, modifying factors, and readiness factors would predict a child's expectations to take medicines and that the health beliefs and expectations of the child's caretakers would increase the child's readiness and expectations to use these medicines.

Bush and Iannotti (1990) tested the model with 300 children in grades 3 through 7 (ages 8-14.7 years, mean age 10.7 years) and 270 of their primary caretakers, 93% of whom were mothers. Path analysis resulted in explaining 63% of the variance in expected medicine use. Highest path coefficients were for two of the readiness factors: perceived severity of illness and perceived benefits of taking the medicine. Perceived vulnerability and illness concern were also significantly related to the outcome. Although this model is not directly related to

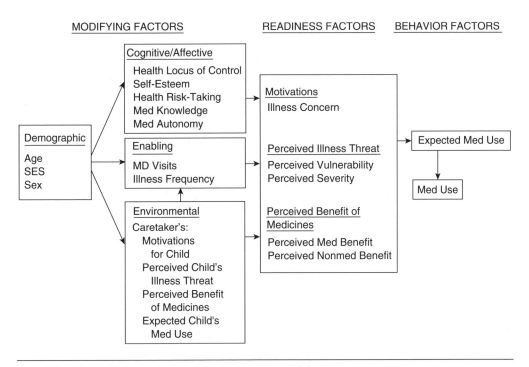

Figure 9.3   Health Belief Model for Children and Adolescents

SOURCE: Bush and Iannotti (1990, p. 71). © 1990 Lippincott, Williams and Wilkins. Reprinted with permission.

lifestyle patterns associated with health promotion, it is an interesting illustration of the way concepts from several theoretical bases can be combined to create new ways of looking at behaviors.

Pender's Health-Promotion Model

Origins

The original version of the Health-Promotion Model (HPM) was published by Nola J. Pender in 1982 primarily for the discipline of nursing. The HPM was based on constructs from expectancy-value theory, including the Health Belief Model, and social cognitive theory (see Chapter 10). Pender provided a positive framework for health behavior based on a holistic view of persons across the life span.

Purpose

The purpose of the Health-Promotion Model was to guide the exploration of complex biological, psychological, and social processes that motivate people to engage in behaviors to enhance their health.

Meaning of the Model

Assumptions of the HPM include the following:

1. Human beings live in such a way as to express a unique potential for health.

2. Human beings are reflective and can assess their own capabilities.

3. Human beings seek to achieve a balance between stability and change.

4. Human beings desire to regulate their personal behavior.

5. Human beings interact with the environment in ways that transform both.

6. Health professionals who are part of a human being's environment influence that person throughout the life span.

7. For behavior change to occur, a person must initiate a rearrangement of her or his pattern of interaction with the environment (Pender, Murdaugh, & Parsons, 2002, p. 63).

The HPM focuses on competence rather than fear as the major motivation for engaging in health behaviors. It is applicable "to any health behavior in which threat is not proposed as a major source of motivation for the behavior" (Pender, Murdaugh, & Parsons, 2002, p. 61) and is applicable across the life span. Major concepts of the theory are grouped as individual characteristics and experiences, behavior-specific cognitions and affect, and behavioral outcomes. These concepts and their relationships are depicted in Figure 9.4. Individual characteristics and experiences include two major constructs: prior related behavior and personal factors such as biological, psychological, and sociocultural characteristics. Behavior-specific cognitions and affect include (a) perceived benefits of action; (b) perceived barriers to action; (c) perceived self-efficacy; (d) activity-related affect; (e) interpersonal influences, such as family, peers, care providers, subjective norms, social support, and models; and (f) situational influences, such as options, aesthetics, and demand characteristics. Mediators of behavior include commitment to a plan of action and immediate competing demands and preferences. Behavioral outcomes are health-promoting behaviors.

The Health-Promotion Model consists of 14 theoretical propositions:

1. An individual's characteristics, including prior related behaviors plus acquired and inherited attributes, influence beliefs, feelings, and health-promoting behaviors.

2. Individuals will commit to a behavior if they perceive a valued benefit.

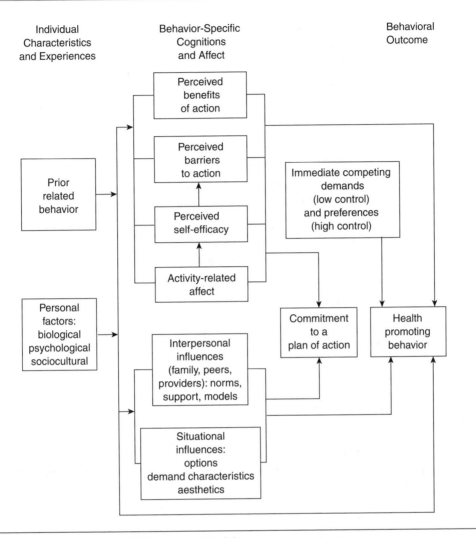

Figure 9.4   Pender's Health-Promotion Model

SOURCE: Pender, Murdaugh, & Parsons, 2002, p. 60. © 2002 Pearson Education, Inc. Reprinted by permission.

3. Perceived barriers to enacting a behavior can stifle a person's commitment to action as well as the actual health-promoting behavior.

4. Self-efficacy to enact a behavior increases the likelihood of a person's commitment to take action as well as actual enactment of that behavior.

5. As self-efficacy increases, perceived barriers to action decrease.

6. An individual's positive feelings toward a specific health behavior lead to an increase in perception of self-efficacy, which then leads to increased positive affect.

7. The probability of commitment to a behavior and actual enactment of the behavior is increased when there is an associated positive affect.

8. Commitment to and enactment of a specific health behavior are increased when significant others in a person's life model, expect, and support the behavior.

9. Commitment to and enactment of a specific health behavior are positively or negatively related to interpersonal influences from family, peer, and professionals.

10. Commitment to and enactment of a specific health behavior are positively or negatively related to situational influences.

11. Greater commitment to a plan of action is related to increased likelihood that a person will maintain a health behavior over time.

12. Competing demands that require immediate attention and over which a person has little or no control interfere with the person's commitment to the health behavior.

13. When other behaviors are preferred or perceived as more attractive, commitment to a plan of action and subsequent enactment of behavior are less likely to occur.

14. Individuals create incentives for health actions by modifying cognitions, affect, and environments (both physical and interpersonal).

Scope, Parsimony, and Generalizability

The HPM applies to a variety of health behaviors across the life span and across a variety of cultures. For example, the HPM has been used to predict health-promoting lifestyles among blue-collar workers (Weitzel, 1989), as well as among adolescent females (Gillis, 1997). Although it has several constructs, it is moderately parsimonious. The model is generalizable across the life span and across cultural backgrounds. However, it has the same limitations as other cognitive models because it cannot be applied to infants, very young children, or those with cognitive impairments.

Logical Adequacy

The logical adequacy of Pender's Health-Promotion Model is depicted in Figure 9.5. The figure depicts both positive and negative relationships between concepts. Nursing scientists have agreed that the theory makes sense (Gillis, 1993; Weitzel, 1989).

Usefulness

The HPM has been useful in developing programs to enhance the health and well-being of individuals across the life span and for predicting an

	1	2	3	4	5	6	7	8	9	10	11
1	=	+	+	+	+	+	±	±	+	+	+
2		=	+	+	+	+	+	+	+	+	+
3			=	−	?	+	±	±	+	±	+
4				=	−	−	±	±	−	±	−
5					=	+	±	±	+	±	+
6						=	±	±	+	±	+
7							=	±	±	±	±
8								=	±	±	±
9									=	−	+
10										=	−
11											=

Legend: 1 = person (personal factors); 2 = prior related behavior; 3 = perceived benefits; 4 = perceived barriers; 5 = perceived self-efficacy; 6 = activity-related affect; 7 = interpersonal influences; 8 = situational influences; 9 = commitment to plan of action; 10 = immediate competing demands; 11 = health-promoting behavior

Symbol: = refers to the same concept, + refers to positive relationship between concepts, − refers to negative relationship between concepts, ± refers to either a positive or negative relationship between concepts.

Figure 9.5 Logical Adequacy of Pender's Health-Promotion Model

overall health-promoting lifestyle. It is applicable to a wide variety of health behaviors in multiethnic populations.

Testability

Wu and Pender (2002) examined the relationships among interpersonal influences, behavior-specific cognitions, competing demands, and physical activity in a convenience sample of 832 Taiwanese adolescents. Using structural equation modeling, they found that the best predictor of physical activity was perceived self-efficacy. The interpersonal influences of social support, norms, and modeling (i.e., total from parents and from peers) had no direct effects on physical activity but had indirect effects through perceived self-efficacy and perceived benefits. When considered separately, peer influence had a direct and significant effect (see Figure 9.6) on physical activity as well as indirect effects through (a) perceived self-efficacy and (b) perceived barriers and perceived self-efficacy. The total model explained 30% of the variance in physical activity. Wu and Pender concluded that the findings indicated that peers had a stronger influence on the physical activity of adolescents in the study than did parents.

Empirical Referents

Adolescent Health Promotion Scale. The Adolescent Health Promotion Scale contains 40 self-report items with a 5-point Likert-type response format that measures frequency of behaviors (i.e., range is from *never* to *always*). There is evidence of construct validity and reliability of the instrument, based on responses from 1128 Taiwanese adolescents (54.7% females) with a mean age of 16.8 years. A six-factor structure explained 51.4% of the variance. The six factors were social support, life appreciation, health responsibility, nutritional behaviors, exercise behaviors, and stress management. The Cronbach alpha coefficient of reliability was .93 for the total scale and .75 to .88 for the subscales (Chen, Wang, Yang, & Liou, 2003).

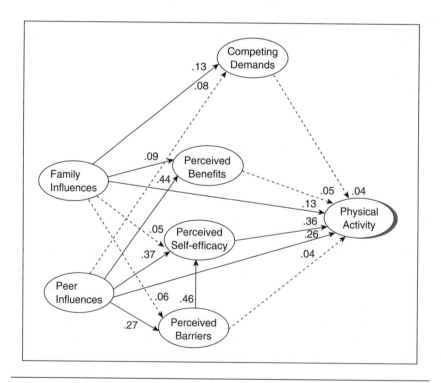

Figure 9.6   Path Model to Predict Physical Activity Among Taiwanese Adolescents

SOURCE: Wu and Pender (2002, p. 31). © 2002 John Wiley and Sons. Reprinted with permission.

Revised Personal Lifestyle Questionnaire. The Personal Lifestyle Questionnaire was developed originally to measure positive health practices of older adolescents and adults. It has recently been revised for use with younger adolescents. The questionnaire contains 24 items with six subscales: exercise, nutrition, health promotion, relaxation, substance use, and safety. Validity of the scale for older adolescents (15 to 21 years old) was achieved through factor analysis and correlation with perceived health status (Mahon, Yarcheski, & Yarcheski, 2002). The revised scale was submitted to a panel of experts in adolescent health to establish content validity. Using propositions from Pender's Health-Promotion Model, evidence of construct validity was determined in a sample of 224 students in seventh and eighth grades (average age 12.9 ± 0.63 years). The majority of the sample (76%) was European American, and 24% were Asian American, American Indian, African American, or Latino. Construct validity was supported through significant correlations between the questionnaire and measures of perceived health status ($r = .46$, $p < .001$), symptom patterns ($r = -.47$, $p < .001$), and well-being ($r = .60$, $p < .001$). Overall scale reliability was .84 (Mahon, Yarcheski, & Yarcheski, 2003).

Health Promotion Among Latino Adolescents. Researchers recruited Latino adolescents from two public health clinics ($N = 609$) to participate in a prevention program for adherence to tuberculosis treatment. Participants were an average of 15 years old (age range: 11-19 years) and most were females (51.2%). All participants had received a positive diagnosis of nonactive tuberculosis. They completed a face-to-face interview in which they were asked about demographics, acculturation, problem behaviors (e.g., cigarette, alcohol, marijuana, and other drug use), and health-promoting behaviors. Higher levels of acculturation were significantly related to increased problem behaviors and decreased health-promoting behaviors. All problem behaviors were found to co-occur, but this pattern of co-occurrence was not found among all of the health-promoting behaviors. The only significant correlations between health-promoting behaviors were between hours of sleep, which correlated with vitamin use ($p < .05$) and eating breakfast ($p < .05$), between eating breakfast and seat belt use ($p < .001$), and between dental visits and vitamin use ($p < .001$). The researchers concluded that less acculturated Latino adolescents exhibited a more healthy lifestyle than those who were more acculturated (Ebin et al., 2001).

PRECEDE-PROCEED Model

Origins

The PRECEDE-PROCEED Model was developed as a framework for planning health-promotion programs. Although it is not a theory in the sense used in this text, it has become an important model for many successful programs used to promote the public's health and therefore has implications for adolescent health. The model has its roots in the discipline of epidemiology, which is the study of the etiology of diseases and other health problems and how these conditions are distributed within various populations. Revolutionary changes in public health in the 19th century were attributed not only to the germ theory of disease but to dramatic changes in social reform and subsequent lifestyle, particularly among people living in North America and Europe. From the mid-1900s until the present, a number of significant changes in how health-care services were provided and paid for paved the way for the development of health-promotion policy and programs. An increased emphasis on personal responsibility for knowledge about health and reliance on oneself for engaging in daily activities that promoted health resulted from both federal and private efforts to educate populations about the relationship between lifestyle and health. Aspects of the model have also been derived from anthropology, developmental psychology, health-care administration, and sociology (Green & Kreuter, 1980, 1999).

Purpose

The purpose of the PRECEDE-PROCEED model was to provide a systematic framework for developing health-promotion interventions within health-care agencies and institutions.

Meaning of the Model

The PRECEDE-PROCEED model is based on a belief that organized activities or programs mediate or intervene in the process of development or change. The purpose of a health-promotion intervention is "to maintain, enhance, or interrupt a behavior pattern or condition of living that is linked to improved health or to increased risks for illness, injury, disability, or death" (Green & Kreuter, 1999, p. 32). PRECEDE and PROCEED are acronyms for nine stages of planning and evaluating health-promotion programs. PRECEDE refers to the first five phases in assessment: "predisposing, reinforcing, and enabling constructs in educational/environmental diagnosis and evaluation"; PROCEED refers to four stages of implementation and evaluation: policy, regulatory, and organizational constructs in educational and environmental development (p. 508).

The nine phases of the PRECEDE-PROCEED model are depicted in Figure 9.7. The process begins at the end (depicted at the far right of the figure) with a social assessment phase. The model emphasizes *outputs* (health changes or outcomes) over *inputs* (processes of intervention); thus the person or group planning a health-promotion intervention or program begins at the end to identify the desired outcome. Phases 2 through 5 focus on the assessment activities that necessarily precede the outcome and, in fact, also precede the development of an intervention. The initial phase of social assessment begins with the concept of *quality of life,* which refers to the perception that a person or group's basic needs for maintaining health and a sense of well-being are being met. The source of information in this phase is the target population itself, whose subjective definition of a problem or priority for change is paramount. In Phase 2, the work of assessment shifts from the target population to that of professionals who must consider the scope of the problem or behavioral change desired by the target community. This epidemiological assessment considers a variety of indicators of a problem, such as risk factors, morbidity, and mortality, and describes the parameters in terms such as prevalence, intensity, or duration. Phase 3 is characterized by assessment of both behavioral and environmental indicators and dimensions of the problem. In Phase 4, three sets of factors are assessed: predisposing factors, such as knowledge and beliefs; reinforcing factors, such as behaviors of health professionals and parents; and enabling factors, such as availability of and access to resources. Phase 5 culminates the assessment phases by addressing the administrative support and resources available to initiate the desired program (Green & Kreuter, 1999).

Phases 6 through 9 focus on implementation and evaluation of the health-promotion intervention. As depicted in Figure 9.7, the implementation flows directly from the assessment of predisposing, reinforcing, and enabling factors identified in Phase 4 as well as the assessment of administration and policy support and resources identified in Phase 5. Implementation is defined as "the act of converting program objectives into actions through policy changes, regulation, and organization" (Green & Kreuter, 1999, p. 190). Evaluation flows directly from the program objectives and is based on standards of acceptable outcomes that are clearly defined during the assessment phases.

The PRECEDE-PROCEED model leads to two propositions (Green & Kreuter, 1999): "(1) health and health risks have multiple determinants and (2) because health and health risks are determined by multiple causes, efforts to effect behavioral, environmental, and social change must be multidimensional or multisectoral" (p. 43).

The construct of lifestyle is central to this health-promotion model and is a general reference to a pattern of behavior related to culture, geographic location, socioeconomic conditions, and social relationships. More specifically, lifestyle is "The culturally, socially, economically, and environmentally conditioned complex of actions characteristic of an individual, group, or community as a pattern of habituated behavior over time that is health related but not necessarily health directed" (Green & Kreuter, 1999, p. 507).

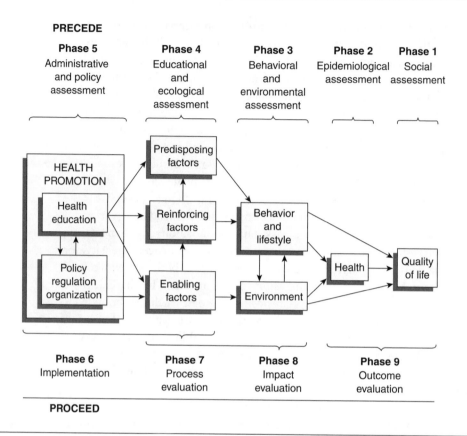

Figure 9.7   The PRECEDE-PROCEED Model for Health Promotion

SOURCE: Green and Kreuter (1999, p. 35). © 1999 McGraw-Hill Companies. Reprinted with permission.

Scope, Parsimony, and Generalizability

The scope of the model is wide, it contains a finite number of steps, and it can be generalized to many behaviors and to various populations. It is limited, however, to use in developed countries that actually have public policies related to health and health-related behaviors.

Logical Adequacy

There is considerable agreement among scientists that the PRECEDE-PROCEED model for health promotion makes sense as a framework for developing community-based health-promotion programs in schools (Alteneder, Price, Telljohann, Didion, & Locher, 1992), communities (Becker, Hendrickson, & Shaver, 1998; Fawcett, 1995; Taylor, 1994), and health-care and educational institutions (Bartholomew, Parcel, & Kok, 1998; Bartholomew et al., 2001).

Usefulness

The PRECEDE-PROCEED model of health promotion is a robust framework that has been applied to literally thousands of programs in the United States and abroad. It provides a general framework for interventions that may themselves include other theories, such as ecological theories of development or social learning theory. The model has applications ranging from framing a master's thesis on health-screening behavior (Allen, 1992) to guiding the development of a health communication campaign designed by the Centers for Disease Control and Prevention (Donovan, 1995).

Testability

Because it is a model for program planning, the criterion of testability does not apply.

Health-Promotion and Health-Risk Behaviors

A number of researchers have examined the relationship between health-promoting and health-risk behaviors. A national survey of 2787 high-risk inner city youth 14 to 19 years old, 76% of whom were female, was conducted to examine the association between health-risk and health-promoting behaviors (Kulbok, Earls, & Montgomery, 1988). The sample was primarily African American (84%). Using principal components analysis of behavior variables, the researchers identified three factors that described the types of behaviors exhibited by participants:

- Problem behaviors, including activities such as drug, alcohol, and tobacco use; sexual activity; skipping school; infrequent use of contraception; carrying a weapon; engaging in physical fights; and lying to get out of trouble
- Health-promoting behavior, including attention to grades in school, getting physical examinations, brushing teeth, having a dental or eye examination, participating in extracurricular activities and hobbies, using a seat belt, reading, and participating in religious activities
- Group activity, including spending more time in sports than in chores, more time with friends than in watching television, lying to get out of trouble (Kulbock et al., 1988), physical fighting, and sexual activity

The researchers concluded that the clustering of behaviors along dimensions of health risk versus health promotion was an important factor in understanding the lifestyle patterns of adolescents and in developing interventions to protect them from harm (Kulbok et al., 1988).

Settings for Health-Promotion Interventions and Programs

The setting in which health-promotion interventions and programs are developed and implemented is a fundamental concept for theory development and practice. The setting portrays the boundaries of time and space that form the context in which such interventions and programs are needed and advanced. Health-promotion interventions and programs respond to the health needs of particular audiences or target populations. Empowerment of individuals and communities is a hallmark of health promotion. Other characteristics of health-promotion activities are that they are holistic, addressing the physical, social, psychological, and spiritual dimensions of persons and that they emphasize social justice and equity among persons (Green, Poland, & Rootman, 2000).

Settings for health promotion refer to those specific arenas bounded by space and time where people gather to engage in particular goal-directed activities such as work, as well as other areas with long-standing policies or institutions where people have sustained interactions with one another—such as the family. The boundaries between settings are permeable, and people move in and out of various settings during their daily activities (Green et al., 2000).

The family is the primary setting in which health promotion may operate and one that is important to recognize as an ecological environment wherein health values and beliefs are taught and health behaviors are modeled and performed. Family processes that encourage direct communication and reinforce the autonomy of individual members are congruent with health promotion. The family is also embedded in a larger community or ethnic culture and is thus influenced by the values, beliefs, and behaviors of these settings. The family may be the setting in which specific health-promotion interventions or programs are delivered because it provides a natural learning environment, particularly for children (Soubhi & Potvin, 2000). The family also provides a filter for interpreting messages coming in from the larger community or ethnic culture. In addition to the social interactions of its members, families live in homes, which are physical environments with variable resources to promote health (Kalnins, 2000).

The school is another major setting in which health-promotion activities occur. The next section, on program planning and evaluation, will address this setting in more detail. The workplace also is a setting conducive to health-promotion activities. In addition to concerns about workplace and occupational safety, workplace health-promotion functions can provide information and opportunities for skill building in various aspects of health promotion. These settings, like the home, may contribute resources to facilitate engagement in health-promoting behaviors, such as providing physical spaces for exercise and stress reduction.

Health-care institutions are yet another setting in which health-promotion programs are provided. The health-care institution is organized not only to provide specific services for persons who are ill or who are interested in learning about health-promoting lifestyles; they are also the workplace for health-care providers. Thus they may serve as dual settings for health-promotion activities. Some barriers to the development of health-promotion programs within health-care institutions include the bureaucratic nature of the system, the cultural values, and the personnel hierarchies inherent in them (Johnson, 2000).

Health-Promotion Program Planning and Evaluation

Since the mid-1970s, increasing numbers of health-promotion programs have been developed for adolescents as well as for children and adults. In general, these programs are based on the premise that health promotion is a desirable process that "enables individuals to acquire a greater degree of autonomy and responsibility for their own health" (Maggs, Schulenberg, & Hurrelmann, 1997, p. 522). Health-promotion programs for adolescents should be based on the concept of enhancing the well-being of the person rather than only preventing infirmity and should have explicit, targeted behaviors. The approach is generally comprehensive, involving an entire community rather than focusing on just a few youth who are at highest risk.

School-Based Health Promotion

Schools are a common arena for offering health-promotion programs that focus on modifiable risk factors for future health and quality of life. There are both advantages and disadvantages in conducting interventions for youth within schools. According to Parcel, Kelder, and Basen-Engquist (2000), the advantages are as follows:

- The majority of U.S. adolescents attend school.
- School is the major social environment for adolescents.
- School is the major physical environment for adolescents.
- Organization of students by development and skills facilitates program development that is congruent with these characteristics.
- Health promotion is congruent with the school's mission to promote academic achievement.

The disadvantages of basing such programs in schools (Parcel et al., 2000) are as follows:

- Teachers are already burdened with numerous responsibilities.
- There is a lack of support and resources with which to address social problems.
- There is disagreement among administrators, parents, and teachers about the importance of certain health topics (e.g., sex education).

School-based health-promotion programs reflect a number of different models: knowledge based, affective, behavioral, and youth empowerment. Knowledge-based programs were among the first developed to address the health-risk behaviors of smoking and alcohol use. This approach of providing information only has been shown to be less effective than later programs with multiple components. Similarly, programs that focused primarily on affective education were developed to address health-risk behaviors by emphasizing interpersonal skills and enhancing self-esteem. These affective education models were also found to make no significant change in behaviors such as substance use (Parcel et al., 2000).

Behavioral programs, often based on social cognitive theory (SCT), were more successful than programs emphasizing knowledge or affect only. They incorporated multiple domains, such as knowledge of the consequences of health-risk behaviors, skill in resisting peer pressure, recognizing the truth in mass media campaigns, including peer leaders as role models, establishing new norms for behavior, and encouraging individuals to make commitments to specific behavior changes. Youth empowerment models based on individual responsibility for problem identification and action have shown great promise for health-promotion programs. In contrast to many of the other school-based models, youth empowerment models involve adolescents in defining the health-risk problem area and what meaning it has in their lives. Such programs include taking some kind of social action, such as changing the smoking policy at a school, and affective objectives that address the adolescents' attitudes and fears about the health-risk problem (Parcel et al., 2000).

Community-Based Health Promotion

Still other health-promotion programs have been successful by addressing not only the school arena in the adolescent's life but the family and larger community as well. These programs are based on the assumption that parents and communities have control over the resources and reinforcements inherent in establishing health-promoting behaviors. For example, parents purchase food to be consumed at home. They may also model drug or alcohol use and physical activity (Parcel et al., 2000). Similarly, the neighborhood or community may be dominated by fast-food restaurants and covertly enable adolescents to consume alcohol. Moreover, the community may not have resources to stimulate youth to engage in prosocial activities after school hours or on weekends.

Community Capacity

The concept of *community capacity* as a way to improve the public health of communities is currently gaining attention from members of several disciplines. The idea of the community as the unit of analysis or intervention stands in sharp contrast to the notion of the individual as the unit of concern. *Community* may refer to a real entity, such as a housing development with distinct parameters, or to a more abstract notion of a social grouping of people with common values, identity, and a shared history and vision for the future. Community capacity is described by Norton, McLeroy, Burdine, Felix, and Dorsey (2002) as "an evolving construct" (p. 198) with multiple definitions. Various dimensions of community capacity are identified and include (a) the nature of social relationships within the community, (b) communication networks and associations among members of the community, (c) community members' access to resources and the skills to manage them, (d) participation of both leaders and followers within the community, (e) shared values and vision among members of the community, and (f) a culture for learning about the community (Norton et al., 2002).

The concept of community capacity is appealing to public health researchers whose focus is on the health of the community rather than the individual. At the present time, however, there is no reliable and valid measure of the concept for theory development and intervention testing. Norton and colleagues (2002) suggest that such measurement and theory development are possible, but they also suggest that qualitative methods of grounded theory and case studies (see Chapter 11) may be equally likely to provide important knowledge about how communities can facilitate health and health-promoting behaviors.

Social Capital

Social capital is another concept emerging in frameworks for community-based health-promotion interventions and programs. According to Kreuter and Lezin (2002), the term has multiple meanings but in general has these aspects: (a) defined by function, social capital allows social groups to attain mutual goals; (b) social capital is manifested through trust and cooperation among persons; and (c) social capital has the capacity to access scarce resources through multiple social networks. This concept, like that of community capacity, is difficult to measure at present but does hold promise for further theory development that could guide community interventions to deal effectively with health-promotion issues.

Multicomponent Health-Promotion Programs

Project Northland is an excellent example of a health-promotion program with multiple components. The purpose of Project Northland was to reduce the use of alcohol and problems associated with its use among adolescents in Minnesota. The intervention program was implemented in 24 school districts and their surrounding communities. It was divided into two phases: early adolescence (sixth to eighth grades) and older adolescence (11th and

12th grades). The first phase focused on decreasing the demand for alcohol use, and the second phase focused on decreasing the supply of alcohol to older adolescents. Project Northland was a unique synthesis of school curricula, parental involvement, mass media campaigns, opportunities for youth to develop leadership skills, and community task forces committed to taking action. Outcome data for Phase I were promising: There were significant decreases in alcohol consumption, smoking cigarettes, and smoking marijuana (Perry, 1999). The Phase II intervention with older adolescents had a positive effect on their tendency to obtain and use alcohol and on binge drinking. The fact that there was no intervention when the students were in 9th and 10th grades had a significant and negative effect on their use of alcohol (Perry & Williams, 2003).

In developing Project Northland, Perry and her research team followed the 10 steps outlined in Table 9.1. Although the steps are presented in linear fashion, "the process may be more of a spiral, with some of the steps repeated as necessary" (Perry, 1999, p. 14).

The first step in developing a multicomponent health-promotion program is to select the target health behavior. Because health-risk behaviors may involve multiple motivations or predictive factors, it is best to restrict the scope to only one or two related behaviors in a single program. The target behavior should be one that (a) is prevalent throughout the community, (b) compromises adolescents' health or well-being, (c) is in the public domain or visible in public interactions, and (d) the community will support. In the second step of program development, a thorough review of the literature is imperative to establish the rationale for the targeted behavior. That is, the program designer should be able to demonstrate that (a) the behavior compromises adolescents' health or well-being; (b) there are both short- and long-term consequences to youth for engaging in the behavior; (c) the behavior is prevalent and is or is not related to age, gender, socioeconomic status, and race or ethnicity; and (d) there are modifiable causes of the behavior.

Table 9.1   Developing Health Behavior Programs: Ten Steps

Study	*Behavioral Objectives*
Step 1:	Selecting health behaviors for a community-wide program
Step 2:	Providing a rationale for selecting a health behavior
Step 3:	Creating an intervention model of predictive factors
Step 4:	Writing the intervention objectives
Step 5:	Ensuring that the intervention objectives are applicable to the targeted population
Step 6:	Determining which types of programs are most applicable
Step 7:	Creating program components from intervention objectives
Step 8:	Constructing the health behavior program
Step 9:	Implementing community-wide health behavior programs
Step 10:	Maintaining health behavior programs

SOURCE: Perry (1999). © 1999 Sage Publications, Inc. Reprinted by permission.

The modifiable causes may be categorized as sociodemographic, social and environmental, personal, and behavioral factors (Perry, 1999).

The third step is creating the intervention model. The first component of this model is to identify the target group for whom the health behavior change is sought. The target group should be described in detail in terms of developmental stage and sociodemographic characteristics. Outcome behaviors are then identified and should be stated as attainable and measurable objectives of the program. The last step is to identify factors that are modifiable or amenable to the planned intervention. These factors should be strong or powerful predictors of the outcome behavior. Predictive factors may be identified in the social-environmental, personal, or behavioral domains (Perry, 1999).

The fourth step in designing a health-promotion program with multiple components is to write the objectives. These objectives should be closely related to the predictive factors identified in the previous step. For example, if one of the predictive factors in the social-environmental domains is "opportunity to engage in a health-promoting or health-risk behavior," then the objective should state precisely how that factor would be changed through the intervention. Closely related to writing the objectives is the fifth step, ensuring that the objectives are applicable to the targeted population. This includes writing the objectives in the language used and understood by this population. These two steps require intensive involvement of the targeted population through individual interviews, observations, and focus groups (Perry, 1999).

Step six is to determine the types of programs that are most applicable to the desired behavioral outcomes. As noted earlier, there are advantages and disadvantages to different types of programs. These should be examined carefully, including consideration of the costs involved in the various types. After determining whether to use a school-based type of program or a community-based program, for example, the seventh step is to create the program components. This step may include modifying an existing successful program or creating an altogether new one. A team that includes representatives of the various stakeholders, including adolescents themselves and their parents, should be assembled to determine how the objectives can best be met. In step eight, the program is actually created and a plan for it documented. Resources of personnel, time, money, and potential settings must be considered. Possible barriers and supports for implementation of the program should be clearly identified (Perry, 1999).

The last two steps of the process are implementing and maintaining the health-promotion program. The implementation begins by ensuring that all key personnel who need to approve and support the program have been contacted. This step also includes training to ensure that the program is carried out as planned and ongoing evaluation to report progress to the community and make revisions as needed. The ongoing evaluation done in step nine will contribute to the decision about whether to continue the program.

A program that facilitates the desired behavioral outcome should be maintained and updated regularly. A program that has equivocal outcomes should be reevaluated and modified as concern and resources allow (Perry, 1999).

Multicultural Aspects of Health Promotion

The population of the United States is characterized by racial, ethnic, and cultural diversity. In recent years, much greater attention has been paid to the role that culture plays in influencing behavior. As seen in Chapter 4, ethnic identity is a salient component in adolescent development and associated health and health-risk behaviors. The concept of culture has been defined in many ways. In general, a culture may be defined by shared beliefs and values about dietary habits, shared language and pattern of communication, accepted forms of attire, and common beliefs about health and illness (Huff & Kline, 1999b). From these criteria, it can be seen that not only do diverse geographic and ethnic groups have distinct cultures, so does the developmental phase of the life span known as adolescence. Adolescents, as a culture, share beliefs and values about what they should eat. These beliefs and values may be in sharp contrast to the recommended dietary patterns suggested by the culture of health-promotion professionals who have worked long and hard to determine the nutritional intake that is most conducive to healthy growth and development. Similarly, adolescents have their own accepted styles of clothing and communication that reflect their emerging independence. Some of these seemingly innocuous aspects of the adolescent culture, however, may have an impact on health-promoting and health-risk behavior and are of concern to adults who see these things in a broader perspective. Although their beliefs about health and illness may not be too different from those of adults, many adolescents may be unable to connect current beliefs and behaviors to long-term outcomes of health. Each of these differences between the adolescent and adult cultures makes planning health-promotion activities a challenge.

Ethnicity, acculturation, and ethnocentrism are other concepts that need to be considered when planning health-promotion programs. *Ethnicity* refers to a person's sense of belonging to a particular social or ethnic group, but it is often confused or used interchangeably with race. Race has been used to categorize people on the basis of biological characteristics such as skin color, but it has been shown to be more of a social construction than an indication of genetic heredity. Ethnic groups share a history of beliefs and customs often related to a geographic area of origin. *Acculturation* refers to the way in which a person from one culture or ethnic group surrenders the attributes of the original culture to adopt the attributes of a new or dominant culture. As shown in Chapter 4, the process of acculturation is closely associated with health-risk behaviors in adolescence and therefore is an area for potential health-promotion programs. *Ethnocentrism* is the belief that one's own culture is superior and preferable to other cultures (Huff & Kline,

1999a. This type of belief can interfere with health-promotion activities on two levels. First, health-care professionals who believe that they know what is best for promoting the health of adolescents may make critical errors in planning and implementing such programs. Second, health-care professionals from a dominant ethnic group who believe that they know what is best for promoting the health of adolescents from a minority ethnic group also may make critical errors.

In recent years, there has been increased competence in developing health-promotion programs that are sensitive to multicultural groups. The burgeoning number of Mexican Americans moving into the southern states has brought attention to the differences between this culture and the cultures of Cuban Americans and Puerto Ricans. Acculturation of family members of these ethnic groups who are now second or third generation creates further challenges for developing interventions that are sensitive to ethnic and cultural differences. In addition to differences in beliefs about health and illness, certain dietary and activity habits have been implicated in the development of health disparities. For example, diabetes has become a major health problem for Hispanics, particularly those of Mexican American descent. Acculturation, however, has been identified as a protective factor through its influence on controlling obesity (Suarez & Ramirez, 1999). The numbers of overweight and obese children and adolescents have caught the attention of health providers, who must find culturally sensitive and competent ways to plan and implement programs to promote health and prevent the development of this life-threatening condition.

Huff and Kline (1999a) note that cultural assessment is an essential ingredient in the planning and development of a culturally competent health-promotion program or intervention. They suggest assessment of the following five areas:

1. Cultural or ethnic group-specific demographic characteristics

2. Cultural or ethnic group-specific epidemiological and environmental influences

3. General and specific cultural or ethnic group characteristics

4. General and specific health care beliefs and practices

5. Western health care organization and service delivery variables. (p. 483)

Huff and Kline (1999a) further emphasize that age and gender are critical demographic characteristics that vary across ethnic groups. In particular, these demographic variables are related to decision making in many cultures, a point that is well taken when planning health-promotion interventions for adolescents. Two of the cultural or ethnic group-specific variables that are also critical when planning interventions for adolescents are perceptions of self and time orientation. These two factors are strongly influenced by cultural beliefs and customs and can influence motivation to engage in a healthy lifestyle as defined by the dominant Western medical culture. Similarly, explanatory models of disease and health-care practices of a particular culture may be radically different from those of the Western health-promotion model and thus drastically affect the target population's willingness to participate in a particular program.

In providing a sociocultural model for health-promotion program planning, implementation, and evaluation for Latino populations, Castro, Cota, and Vega (1999) claim that many such programs are unable to attract and retain participants because they are not culturally relevant. They suggest the need for programs to be guided by two principles: (a) relevance, which means to begin where the people are, and (b) participation, which means to encourage ownership of the program by those who will receive it. They also differenti-ate among six levels of cultural orientation held by program planners. At the extreme negative end of the continuum is the notion of cultural destructive-ness, a concept similar to ethnocentrism. In this stage, one endows the dom-inant culture with superior attributes and labels other cultures as inferior. Only slightly better is the notion of cultural incapacity. In this stage, one asserts the value of separate but equal treatment of different groups. Cultural blindness refers to those who think that people from all cultures are equal and alike. On the positive half of the continuum are the increasingly more favor-able views of culture: cultural openness (sensitivity), cultural competence, and cultural proficiency. Cultural openness means that one at least has some understanding of the importance of cultural factors that may affect beliefs and participation in programs. Cultural competence reflects an increased capacity for understanding and appreciating more complex and subtle char-acteristics of a given culture. And finally, cultural proficiency means that one is committed to work in proactive ways with another culture to promote health in ways that are culturally relevant and appropriate.

Applying Theory to Multicultural Settings. The enterprise of developing health-promotion programs based on theory for multicultural groups may be challenging. Knowing not only the meaning and structure of the theory but acknowledging the origins and purpose of the theory as well may help the researcher or practitioner select a theory that is appropriate for the target population. The following questions may be helpful in selecting a theory base for intervention or program planning (Frankish, Lovato, & Shannon, 1999):

- What aspect of the health issue does the theory address?
- How does the theory explain or predict this aspect of the health issue?
- How congruent is the theory formulation with your understanding of the health issue?
- Are there salient aspects of the health issue that the theory does not address?
- How can the theory be translated into a health-promotion intervention or program?
- What elements of the theory would predict behavior change?

Other questions that should be answered include the following:

- Are the major concepts in the theory relevant to the target culture or population?
- Has the theory previously been tested in the population of interest?
- Have successful programs based on the theory been used previously with the target population?
- What do members of the target population think of the concepts and propositions of the theory?

Practice Applications

A health-promotion program to prevent substance use among ethnically diverse youth in a low-income community was based on social cognitive theory (see Chapter 8) and principles of empowerment. The successful program, which was called Teen Activists for Community Change and Leadership Education, involved 116 students from six different locations. The program was successful in creating a healthier environment for adolescents by involving them in the design and implementation of the program. The various components of the program are displayed in Figure 9.8.

Principles that guided this successful health-promotion program included the following:

1. Focus on environmental risk factors: Ask how to increase the awareness of adolescents and community members about a specific health-risk or health-promoting behavior.

2. Challenge adolescents through community projects: Invite them to identify their own health issues and concerns.

3. Encourage ownership of the health-promotion project: Help adolescents to establish goals and strategies for achieving the goals that are relevant to their lives.

4. Create learning opportunities that focus on participation and practicing new skills.

5. Plan interventions or programs that consist of small improvements that can serve as the foundation and motivation for a fuller involvement in meeting higher goals.

6. Foster committed relationships between adults and adolescents: Mutual respect helps to build strong teams.

7. Develop programs that are accessible to adolescents: Coordinate with other resources within the community.

8. Create safe, enjoyable, and supportive environments: Identify ground rules and incorporate activities for having fun, including the celebration of birthdays and other special occasions.

9. Provide incentives to improve accountability: Locate meetings at an attractive campsite, offer gift certificates as rewards, and so on.

10. Evaluate using a variety of methods: Obtain input from adolescents through planning and implementing the program (Tencati et al., 2002, pp. 27-28).

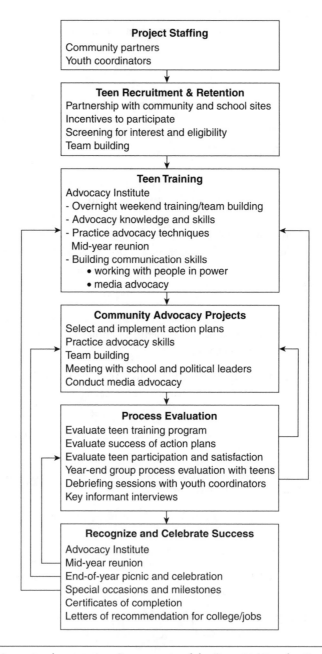

Figure 9.8   Implementation Components of the Teen Activists for Community Change and Leadership Education Program

SOURCE: Tencati et al. (2002). © 2002 Sage Publications, Inc. Reprinted by permission.

Child and Adolescent Trial
for Cardiovascular Health (CATCH)

A national health-promotion program, CATCH was developed to promote a healthy lifestyle in children and adolescents (Perry et al., 1990). This comprehensive program focused on physical activity (e.g., improving time doing moderate to vigorous physical activity) and dietary practices (decreasing fat and sodium content in meals) and included classroom instruction and family activities. Evaluation research found that time spent in physical activity increased and fat content in school lunches decreased in the CATCH schools compared to those in comparison schools (Luepker et al., 1996). Changes in diet and physical activity reported by participants 3 years after leaving the program were maintained (Nader et al., 1999). Owing to the success of the initial trials of this health-promotion initiative, program materials were provided to the public. The Paso del Norte Health Foundation in El Paso, Texas, organized a task force that soon adopted the CATCH program to address concerns about increases in diabetes mellitus (type 2) and obesity in the population. The program was well received in the primarily Hispanic neighborhoods where it was introduced and led to significant decreases in the fat content of school meals (breakfasts and lunches) and increases in moderate to vigorous physical activity during physical education classes (Heath & Coleman, 2003).

Responding to the health-promotion objectives set forth in *Healthy People 2000*, Henderson, Champlin, and Evashwick (1998) compiled a set of papers that reflected a variety of strategies for schools, health organizations, and communities to take in addressing such objectives for adolescents. In one of these papers, Scaffa (1998) addresses alcohol use among adolescents. She asserts that a comprehensive community-based health-promotion program should be based on the following factors:

- Involvement of at least three community organizations (e.g., business, education, general public, government, health-care, media, religion, and volunteer agencies)
- Community needs assessment of problems and resources
- Measurable objectives in terms of health outcomes, public awareness of health concerns, health-risk factors, and services
- Process for monitoring and evaluating the program
- Interventions that are culturally relevant and contain multiple approaches and targets for behavior change

Chapter Summary

The national objectives to promote public health include many that are directly focused on health-risk behaviors of adolescents (e.g., cigarette smoking, reducing deaths from motor vehicle accidents). Health and health-risk behaviors are closely related to the beliefs, decisions, and lifestyles of adolescents. Models presented in this chapter provide a basis for understanding a variety of factors that are antecedents, modifiers, moderators, and outcomes of the dynamic interaction of these factors. The health belief model illuminates the elements of perceived susceptibility to and threat of disease, knowledge and previous experience with that disease, perceived benefits of and barriers to taking action to prevent disease or promote health, and cues to taking action. The model has been useful in addressing a wide variety of public health problems. It has also been influential in the development of other health-promotion models, such as that of Pender.

Pender's health-promotion model focuses on competence, rather than threat or fear, as a motivation for engaging in behaviors that promote health. Fourteen theoretical propositions are clearly formulated, and the model has been applied successfully across the life span and within several different cultures, including minority adolescents in the United States and adolescents in other countries.

The PRECEDE-PROCEED model depicts a systematic framework for developing health-promotion interventions and programs. This framework, which uses a scientific reasoning and decision-making process, has been applied successfully to a great number of health-promotion programs in the United States and other countries. This model and other general principles for program planning and evaluation can be adapted for targeting the health-risk behaviors of diverse groups of adolescents. Several examples of successful community-based intervention programs are described, along with suggestions for further study.

Suggestions for Further Study

The lifestyles of adolescents provide the context in which they enact either health-promoting or health-risk behaviors. Health-care providers can plan and implement intervention programs that focus on developing lifestyle patterns that will enhance both short- and long-term health. How can theory and planning models be combined most efficaciously to facilitate positive health outcomes and contribute to the national objectives to promote the public health?

Periodic national health behavior data sets such as those established by the CDC through data collected via YRBSS provide descriptions of health-risk behaviors. These profiles, however, establish little more than a cross-sectional snapshot of the lifestyles of adolescents who attend public schools at a particular point in time. The CDC's collection of data via the YRBSS also contains only the self-reports of adolescents and tells us nothing about their development or the context of that development, including the patterns of health-promoting and health-compromising behaviors. The National

Longitudinal Data Set (Add Health), in contrast, provides data from two separate times for many of the participants and includes information about peer and family networks and geographic locations. This data set, therefore, can allow some inferences to be made about development and, to some extent, about the context of that development. Add Health also contains data from parents and school administrators that can add other perspectives to understanding health and health-risk behaviors in adolescents. Efforts among scientists from various disciplines are under way to provide integrated descriptions of factors that reflect the healthy or unhealthy lifestyle as well as quality of life of American youth. Two forms of the data are available for researchers: the public-use data set, with approximately 6500 participants, and a restricted-use contractual data set available through the Add Health Project at the Carolina Population Center, University of North Carolina. The public-use data set is available from Sociometrics Corporation in Los Altos, California. Web sites for both of these organizations are found at the end of this chapter. The Add Health data set, however, is limited to those youth who attended school.

Health-promotion interventions have targeted schools and communities because that is where most adolescents live. There is, however, a growing population of homeless adolescents in this country. Some estimates of homeless and runaway youth are as high as 2 million, some of whom are homeless with their families (Shane, 1996). This group of adolescents is at highest risk for social morbidities and mortalities related to lifestyle. These adolescents live in dangerous and unhealthy environments, often with poor nutrition, inadequate ventilation and protection from inclement weather, and limited access to health-care services (Ginsburg, Menapace, & Slap, 1997). As a group, they are at risk for developing sexually transmitted infections (STI) such as HIV and hepatitis B because they exchange sex for necessities such as food and shelter, have multiple partners, and often combine sexual activities with alcohol and other drug use. The seroprevalence rate of HIV in homeless adolescents is reported to be 2 to 10 times higher than that of other adolescent populations (Walters, 1999), and they report greater prevalence of inconsistent condom use than other adolescents (Clatts, Davis, Sotheran, & Atillasoy, 1998). These youth are also likely to be alcohol and drug users at rates that compromise their physical and mental health (Bailey, Camlin, & Ennett, 1998; Booth & Zhang, 1997; Rew, Taylor-Seehafer, & Fitzgerald, 2001).

Little research on health-promoting interventions for homeless and runaway youth has been done. Most interventions have focused on providing information about STIs, HIV, or the health risks associated with smoking, and although knowledge increased, health-promoting behaviors did not improve significantly (Booth, Zhang, & Kwiatkowski, 1999; Small, Brennan-Hunter, Best, & Solberg, 2002). Sobo, Zimet, Zimmerman, and Celcil (1997) found that almost half of the youth in shelters believed that health-care providers withheld information about HIV from them. To develop culturally relevant interventions for this underserved population, it is necessary to include them in planning. My work with homeless adolescents in Texas (Rew, Chambers, & Kulkarni, 2002) and those of others in Boston (Rosenfeld et al., 2000) included conducting focus groups to explore the adolescents' perceived needs for an intervention and to identify intervention strategies that would appeal to them. Inclusion of these underserved youth in planning health-promoting interventions is key to their success.

A consistent implication of the literature reviewed in this chapter is that the target population of youth must be given a voice in the identification of behaviors in need of change and in the design and implementation of interventions to address these behaviors. Elements of the Youth Development Model (see Chapter 3) could be incorporated into longitudinal and triangulated (e.g., combined qualitative and quantitative methods) designs to craft and test health-promotion programs for specific health-risk behaviors with particular at-risk populations of youth. These designs could also be enhanced by examining developmental trends. At present we know very little about the dosages or booster effects of interventions provided over time to promote healthy behaviors such as physical activity or adequate sleep and nutrition.

Whereas a great deal of effort has gone into understanding the health-risk behaviors of American youth, far too little effort has gone into understanding their health-promoting beliefs and behaviors. Many more lines of research need to be developed to build our knowledge base about how these behaviors are learned, valued, and enacted in young people.

Related Web Sites

Add Health: Carolina Population Center, Chapel Hill, NC, e-mail address: addhealth@unc.edu

(National Longitudinal Study of Adolescent Health home page) http://www.cpc.unc.edu/projects/addhealth/datasets.html

(Article on origins, purposes, and design) http://www.agi-usa.org/pubs/journals/gr040310.html

Sociometrics Corporation (e-mail address: socio@socio.com): http://www.socio.com/srch/summary/afda2/fam48-50.htm

PRECEDE-PROCEED Model: (Description) http://www.ulm.edu/education/hhp/PRECEDE-PROCEED. html

http://www.aahperd.org/lejhe/archive/ransdell2001.pdf

(Complete overview) http://hsc.usf.edu/~kmbrown/PRECEDE_PROCEED_Overview.htm

(Graphic depiction of model and other information) http://www.lgreen.net/ precede.htm

Project Northland:

(Summary of Project Northland II) http://www.epi.umn.edu/cyhp/r_pnII.htm

(Factsheet) http://www.epi.umn.edu/projectnorthland/Factshee.html

(Background and description) http://www.epi.umn.edu/projectnorthland/

Suggestions for Further Reading

Burkett, L. N., Rena, C. G., Jones, K., Stone, W. J., & Klein, D. A. (2002). The effects of wellness education on the body image of college students. *Health Promotion Practice, 3*(1), 76-82.

Goldman, K. D., & Schmalz, K. J. (2001). Theoretically speaking: Overview and summary of key health education theories. *Health Promotion Practice, 2,* 277-281.

Hendricks, C. S. (2001). Perceptual determinants of early adolescent health promoting behaviors: Model development. *Journal of Theory Construction & Testing, 2*(1), 13-22.

Hovell, M. F., Wahlgren, D. R., & Gehrman, C. A. (2002). The behavioral ecological model: Integrating public health and behavioral science. In R. J. DiClemente, R. A. Crosby, & M. C. Kegler (Eds.), *Emerging theories in health promotion practice and research: Strategies for improving public health* (pp. 347-385). San Francisco: Jossey-Bass.

McManus, R. P., Jr. (2002). Adolescent care: Reducing risk and promoting resilience. *Primary Care: Clinics in Office Practice, 29*(3), 557-569.

Raphael, D. (1996). Determinants of health of North-American adolescents: Evolving definitions, recent findings, and proposed research agenda. *Journal of Adolescent Health, 19*(1), 6-16.

10

Theories of Decision Making and Behavior Change

As adolescents develop increasing independence and cognitive abilities, the opportunities to engage in health-risk behaviors become more abundant. Choices about where and how to spend one's leisure time are inherent in this stage of development. Decision making reflects the power to be self-directed and autonomous in an ever-enlarging social milieu. But decision making can have either positive or negative consequences. For example, the decision to engage in sexual behavior may be accompanied by positive physical sensations and satisfactions, but it may also lead to unintended pregnancy or symptoms of sexually transmitted infections. Decision making in adolescents must address the social, affective, cognitive, and spiritual dimensions of behaviors that can either promote or threaten the adolescent's health and well-being (Elias & Kress, 1994).

Health-risk behaviors in adolescents are volitional and are therefore amenable to change. Several theories have been developed to predict who is likely to change and who is not. In this chapter, models of decision making and behavioral change are explored.

Conflict Theory of Decision Making

Origins

The conflict theory of decision making (CTDM) originated in the research on the psychology of stress, organizational decision making, and information processing within a social context (Janis & Mann, 1977). The influence of Lazarus's work on stress, principles from social learning theory and social cognitive theory, and the field theory of Kurt Lewin are evident.

Purpose

The purpose of the theory is to describe how people cope with conflicts in making decisions.

Meaning of the Theory

Janis and Mann (1977) based their theory of decision making on the assumption that conflict experienced while making a decision resulted in stress. The experience of stress was related to concern about losses that might accompany a particular decision or concern about decreases in self-esteem or personal reputation if the decision turned out to be wrong. Stress resulting from conflict in making a decision is a function of one's striving for goals. Decision-making stress is a function of a person's commitment to the present way of doing things.

Janis and Mann (1977) identified seven basic steps in high-quality decision making:

1. Examining a wide range of alternatives

2. Examining a range of goals or objectives that could be met by the decision

3. Considering the costs and risks related to consequences of each alternative

4. Searching for additional relevant information

5. Absorbing new information

6. Reconsidering the outcomes of all known alternatives

7. Planning and implementing a course of action

People have a tendency to use different styles of coping with the stress associated with difficult decisions. Five patterns may be observed: (a) unconflicted adherence, in which the decision maker ignores the possibility of risk and decides on a course of action; (b) unconflicted change, in which the decision maker simply follows a course of action without analyzing the risks, particularly if the action is highly recommended; (c) defensive avoidance, in which the decision maker procrastinates or shifts responsibility to another, thus escaping the conflict inherent in the decision-making process; (d) hypervigilance, in which the decision maker makes a hasty decision without considering all possible consequences of the alternatives; and (e) vigilance, in which the decision maker is clear about the goal, considers multiple alternatives, gathers pertinent information, and evaluates all before coming to a final decision (Janis & Mann, 1977). This last pattern, vigilance, is the only one associated with rational decision making (Mann, Burnett, Radford, & Ford, 1997).

Three conditions determine which pattern of coping with the stress that accompanies the decision-making process will be used: awareness of the risks involved in the preferred options, hope of finding a more acceptable option, and belief that one has time to search for and evaluate other options prior to making a decision. In making a decision, a person who uses vigilant coping and meets the criteria for high-quality decision making will consider all alternatives and consider both favorable and unfavorable consequences (i.e., pros and cons) associated with each alternative. This concept is known as *decisional balance*. Persons who have maladaptive coping patterns (i.e., unconflicted adherence, unconflicted change, defensive avoidance, or hyper-vigilance) will have either incomplete or unrealistic decisional balance.

In research based in CTDM, a decisional balance sheet is constructed in which individuals list all the alternatives they are considering about the decision at hand. They then specify the pros and cons for each alternative. High-quality decisions are made with complete information on both pros and cons for each alternative; poor decisions are made with incomplete or ambiguous information (Janis & Mann, 1977).

The consequences of taking action based on a decision can be categorized as one of four types: (a) utilitarian gains or losses for one's self, (b) utilitarian gains or losses for significant others, (c) self-approval or disapproval, and (d) social approval or disapproval. When the five coping strategies are compared to the seven qualities of good decision making, it becomes clear that when using the strategies of unconflicted adherence or unconflicted change, the decision maker does not thoroughly search for information, examine alternatives, or carefully evaluate the consequences. Those who use these strategies generally remain calm and experience little conflict about the decision. By using the strategy of defensive avoidance, the decision maker uses none of the seven criteria for high-quality decision making but remains calm. Using hypervigilance, the decision maker may or may not conduct a thorough search for new information, but he or she does not assimilate this information in an unbiased way and does not evaluate the consequences or plan for contingencies. Such a person experiences persistent strong anxiety and vacillates in making a decision. The person who uses vigilance meets all the criteria for quality decision making, has a moderate amount of anxiety, and vacillates moderately about the decision as new information is received (Janis & Mann, 1977).

Scope, Parsimony, and Generalizability

The CTDM has been applied in many decision-making situations; across multiple age groups (e.g., adolescents and adults); and across various cultures, including Australia, New Zealand, Taiwan, Hong Kong, Japan, and the United States (Mann et al., 1997). The theory explains decision making in these many contexts with just a few concepts, thus meeting the criterion for parsimony.

Logical Adequacy

The CTDM has logical adequacy; there are no apparent logical fallacies. A number of scientists have agreed that it makes sense, and testable hypotheses can and have been derived from it.

Usefulness

The CTDM has been used by scholars in diverse disciplines, including psychology, political science, nursing, and business management. It has been used to assess and predict smoking status (Velicer, DiClemente, Prochaska, & Brandenburg, 1985), to predict university students' decisions about writing term papers (Mann et al., 1997), and to understand the decisions of university female students to use protection against both unplanned pregnancy and STDs (Chambers & Rew, 2003).

Testability

Hypotheses derived from the concepts and statements have been tested.

Empirical Referents

Flinders and Melbourne Decision Making Questionnaires. Mann (1982) developed the Flinders Decision Making Questionnaire, which was designed to measure processes that occurred both pre- and postdecision, including attitudes and feelings. The questionnaire consisted of 31 items, with a Likert-type response format, and contained subscales to measure vigilance, hypervigilance, defensive avoidance, procrastination, buck passing, and rationalization. Through confirmatory factor analysis using LISREL, it was determined that there was not sufficient validity for the instrument. Nine items were dropped, the factor analysis yielded a model with four factors (i.e., vigilance, hypervigilance, buck passing, and procrastination), and the questionnaire was then renamed the Melbourne Decision Making Questionnaire. Cronbach alphas for the four subscales range from .74 to .87 (Mann et al., 1997).

Adolescent Decision Processes Scale. Friedman (1996) synthesized various theories and models of decision making, including that of Janis and Mann, and identified two phases of decision making: investigation-deliberation and choice implementation–resolution. Based on a matrix of the deliberation-resolution dimensions of decision making, he suggested that nine independent options could be identified. These options could further be classified into one of two groups: (a) inaction or avoidance or (b) action, with eight possible types ranging from undeliberated to thoughtful determination. Friedman developed the Adolescent Decision Processes Scale based on workshops conducted with 82 high school students in Israel. Content analysis of 150 examples of behavior identified by these adolescents resulted in six levels of decision making. An additional 652 Israeli high school students 14 to 17 years old completed questionnaires to test the fit of data to the subscales. Following factor analysis, a 17-item scale was developed and reflected three factors: undeliberated conclusion, vacillation, and thoughtful determination. These three subscales explained 41% of the variance in the scale. The 17-item scale has a 6-point Likert-type response format (1 = *never*, 6 = *always*) (Friedman, 1996, p. 889).

Related Research

Hulton (2001) conducted an integrative review of 38 research studies of adolescent decision making about becoming sexually active. Findings were that there were gender and developmental differences in making this decision. The decision to become sexually active or to abstain was related to the youth's perception of benefits (e.g., girls were supported in maintaining abstinence, but boys were encouraged to become sexually active), parental and social influences, and knowledge of human sexuality. This author also concluded that most of the research on this type of decision making was atheoretical and descriptive.

_____ A Self-Regulation Model of Decision Making

Origins

James P. Byrnes (1998), a developmental psychologist, developed the Self-Regulation Model of Decision Making (SRM) out of his concern about the limits of existing decision-making models. In particular, Byrnes thought that there was no clear and coherent picture of what decision making was or how it developed. His work was influenced by cognitive developmentalists, such as Piaget and Vygotsky; social cognitive theorists, such as Bandura; and decision-making theorists, including Janis and Mann. More directly, however, he was influenced by the work of several scholars in the area of artificial intelligence (e.g., Newell & Simon, 1972).

Purpose

The purpose of the SRM is to explain and predict a wide range of developmental differences in decision-making behavior (Byrnes, 1998).

Meaning of the Theory

The SRM is based on three assumptions about the construct of self-regulation:

1. Human behavior is goal directed. Persons adapt to their environments by setting goals related to personal survival, physical health and emotional well-being, and social or professional achievement. These are referred to as adaptive goals.

2. Successful people adapt by engaging in behaviors that increase the chances of achieving their adaptive goals.

3. Because people have innate limitations and develop attitudes and habits that prevent them from attaining adaptive goals, it is difficult for them to be successful.

Decision makers who are self-regulated tend to be successful more often than they are unsuccessful. SRM also assumes "that children are not very self regulated when they are born" (Byrnes, 1998, p. 153). Young children are incapable of coordinating a large number of goals and may be unrealistic about expected outcomes. However, children become more self-regulated as they get older and are therefore more capable of making better decisions. As children are able to experience feedback and observe capable decision makers (e.g., parents, teachers), their decision-making skills improve. Variations are related to stress and temperament.

The SRM consists of four major constructs, depicted in Figure 10.1: a generation phase, an evaluation phase, a learning phase, and moderating factors. In the generation phase, a person generates a list of options for achieving a particular goal. The person may be presented with a choice and go immediately to the evaluation phase, but most decisions begin with an environmental cue (e.g., an adolescent reads a billboard advertising a popular fast-food restaurant). The person becomes aware of hunger and sets a goal of buying lunch. A list of strategies for meeting this goal is then generated, such as remembering past experiences of eating at this fast-food restaurant or reasoning through the cost in time and money to find that particular restaurant at this time. Advice may be sought from a friend about eating at that restaurant, and the friend may suggest other alternatives. The person then moves to the evaluation phase, in which the dimensions of each option are considered (i.e., the reasons for and against selecting one of the options, which allows the options to be rank-ordered). If none of the options is acceptable, the person will then return to the generation phase to identify other alternatives (Byrnes, 1998).

Once an acceptable option has been determined, the learning phase is entered, and the person exercises the option and observes how well this option meets the original goal. Returning to the example of the hungry adolescent, she or he considers whether the meal at the fast-food restaurant met

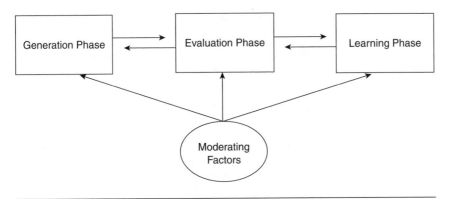

Figure 10.1   Self-Regulation Model of Decision Making

SOURCE: Byrnes (1998, p. 31). © 1998 Lawrence Erlbaum Associates, Inc. Reprinted with permission.

the original goal of reducing hunger at a price she or he was willing to pay. This is called a learning phase because what happens in this phase adds to the person's body of knowledge (e.g., memory) about the consequences of meeting a goal in a particular way. The final component is that of moderating factors, which include individual limitations, emotions, biases, and habits and affect how well the person performs in each of the three phases of decision making. Moderating factors tend to be things that prevent a person from using all available resources and include things such as the limitations of memory, stress, substance use, and personality traits (Byrnes, 1998, 2002).

Self-regulated decision makers exhibit a number of characteristics (Table 10.1) that are evident in each of the three phases and in the moderating factors. The theory further explains how these characteristics develop throughout childhood and on into adulthood. Children learn that actions lead to outcomes that help them to either meet or not meet their goals. Other people in the environment also instruct children to link their actions to outcomes and evaluate them. Adults can help children learn how to make better decisions and avoid undesirable outcomes. As children develop, those who acquire more experience in decision making and who are guided by competent adult decision makers tend to become more successful and self-regulated than those without these resources (Byrnes, 1998).

Scope, Parsimony, and Generalizability

The SRM is both broad in scope and parsimonious. It can explain and predict decision making of all types and does this with only four major constructs. However, there are additional concepts subsumed under the four general constructs of the model. The theory can be generalized to healthy people (i.e., those with intact central nervous systems) across the life span

Table 10.1   Characteristics of Self-Regulated Decision Makers

Generation phase	Pay attention to cues that are informative
	When cues are ambiguous, feel uncertain and seek additional information
	Pursue several adaptive rather than single or maladaptive goals
	Use variety of reasoning and advice-seeking strategies when uncertain how to proceed
	Seek advice such that social standing is not compromised
	Evaluate appropriateness of analogies
	Understand how causal outcomes are affected by dynamics of context, persons, and strategies
Evaluation phase	Reasonably confident of skills
	Able to evaluate strategies and rank according to importance
Learning phase	Review outcomes to incorporate accurate knowledge about self and about relationship between actions and outcomes
	Maintain high standards of success
	Have realistic knowledge of limits of decision making.
	Maintain moderate level of dogmatism, changing beliefs neither too slowly or too quickly
Moderating factors	Aware of several types of factors that affect decision making, such as emotions, memory, and personality traits
	Use various self-regulating strategies to overcome moderating factors, such as self-calming to deal with emotions

(beginning with children old enough to make decisions) and to all ethnic groups.

Logical Adequacy

The theory makes sense, and one can make a number of predictions from it. Figure 10.2 depicts the adequacy of the relationships among the constructs. Predictions can be made independent of the content of the theory. There are no questionable relationships.

Usefulness

The SRM has been used to explore differences in decision making between children and adults and between adolescents and adults. In these studies, adults learned more from feedback than adolescents did (Byrnes et al., 1999).

Concept	Generation	Evaluation	Learning	Moderating
Generation	=	+	±	−
Evaluation		=	±	−
Learning			=	−
Moderating				=

Legend: = means the same concept; + means the concepts are positively related; ± means the concepts may be positively or negatively related.

Figure 10.2   Logical Adequacy of the Self-Regulation Model of Decision Making

Testability

The SRM has been tested with children, adolescents, and adults.

Empirical Referents

Most studies to date have relied on presentation of scenarios to elicit cues, alternative strategies, and the pros and cons of the alternatives. Qualitative responses are then quantified through manifest content for further statistical analyses (Byrnes, 1998).

The Transtheoretical Model of Behavior Change

Origins

The transtheoretical model (TTM) of behavior change resulted from an analysis of competing theories of behavioral change and psychotherapy by James O. Prochaska and colleagues in the late 1970s and 1980s. These behavioral scientists were concerned about how people intentionally change addictive behaviors such as alcoholism, with and without professional treatment. They found that persons who changed their addictive behaviors moved through a series of stages. In a comparative analysis of competing systems of psychotherapy, Prochaska (1979) completed a comprehensive analysis of 18 theories of psychotherapy and identified the processes of behavior change. Because these processes were patterns that appeared in interventions based on a variety of theories, he coined the term *transtheoretical* to describe this model (Prochaska, 1979; Prochaska, DiClemente, & Norcross, 1992).

From their comparative analysis of some 300 theories, Prochaska and his research team identified 10 processes of change. They compared individuals identified as self-changers with individuals who were receiving professional treatment for smoking cessation. From this analysis, they determined that the individuals who were changing their behavior used the 10 processes at different times, leading to the discovery that change occurs in a series of stages (Prochaska, Redding, & Evers, 1997).

The theorists were strongly influenced by the decision-making model of Janis and Mann (1977), who conceptualized decision making as an approach to resolve conflict. Anticipated gains or losses in changing a behavior included the consideration of the opinion of significant others, which was translated into the concept of decisional balance in the TTM (Prochaska, Velicer, et al., 1994).

Purpose

The primary purpose of the TTM, also known as stages of change model, was to provide an integrated framework for understanding the process of intentional behavior change. Although developed primarily to assist practitioners (therapists) in guiding their clients to change behaviors in a predictable way, it has been useful in research, education, and administration. Rather than focusing on other approaches to behavior change that view people as resistant and noncompliant, this model focuses on decision making and motivation as a state of readiness to move through predictable and intentional stages of change. Behavior changes related to health may include adopting new behaviors (e.g., regular exercise), modifying a behavior (e.g., reducing carbohydrate intake), or eliminating a behavior (e.g., quitting smoking) (Velicer, Prochaska, Fava, Norman, & Redding, 1998). The TTM is a conceptualization of behavior change that delineates six stages or characteristic periods of time in which various processes of change occur. The model is applicable to changing a problem behavior or acquiring a health-promoting behavior.

Meaning of the Theory

The Transtheoretical Model consists of assumptions, clearly defined concepts, and statements or propositions. These structural components are organized around three major constructs: stages of change, processes of change, and levels of change (DiClemente & Prochaska, 1998).

Assumptions. The transtheoretical model is based on the following assumptions:

1. Behavioral change is intentional and under the volitional control of the individual.

2. No single theory can address the complex nature of behavioral change.

3. Behavioral change is a process that occurs in stages that unfold over time.

4. Stages of change and chronic behavioral risk factors are both stable and open to change.

5. People will remain stuck in early stages of change without specific planned interventions because there is no inherent motivation to progress through them when change is intentional rather than developmental.

6. Most at-risk individuals are unprepared to take action and will not respond favorably to traditional health-promotion prevention programs based solely on taking action.

7. Specific intervention principles must be matched to a person's stage of change.

8. Chronic patterns of behavior are controlled by a complex interaction of biological, social, and self-control factors (Prochaska et al., 1997).

Major Concepts. There are five basic components of the model: stages of change, processes of change, decisional balance, self-efficacy confidence, and self-efficacy temptation.

Stages of change refers to the temporal dimension of change. The six stages of change are depicted in Figure 10.3. The stages of change are depicted with relapses because most people return to a previous stage before completing the behavior change. For example, approximately 85% of smokers return to the contemplation stage after taking some action but before terminating the change.

Stages of Change

Each stage of change is associated with characteristic behaviors, goals, and tasks to be accomplished in pursuit of those goals. In precontemplation, the person may be reluctant to consider a change of behavior such as smoking cessation because it disrupts a pattern of behavior that is familiar and has possibly become a habit or an addiction. Persons in this stage of change may be rebellious and unlikely to consider change, especially if

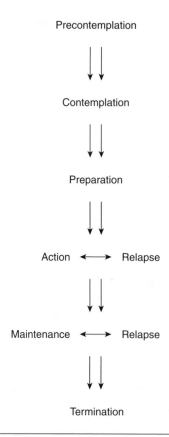

Figure 10.3   Schematic Representation of Stages of Intentional Behavior Change
as Conceptualized in the Transtheoretical Model

it is someone else's idea (e.g., court-required counseling for driving while intoxicated). Some individuals in this stage feel resigned to the behavior, believing that they are helpless to change. Others are known as *revelers* because they really enjoy engaging in the problematic behavior. The individuals most resistant to change are those who rationalize their current behavior.

Precontemplation. In the stage of precontemplation, the goal of intervention is to have the individual seriously consider a change of behavior. To that end, the interventionist works to help the person increase awareness of the need for behavior change by envisioning what life might be like if the behavioral change took place or by raising concern about what might happen to the person if the current behavior were to continue indefinitely. In this stage, a therapist avoids giving advice or confronting the individual with the undesired behavior but provides information and feedback to increase the motivation to consider the change.

Contemplation. Individuals who begin to consider a behavioral change enter the stage of contemplation, in which they reflect on the current behavior and consider their potential for change. The goal of this stage is to seriously evaluate the risks and rewards of sustaining the undesirable behavior and to make a conscious decision to change it. Tasks in this stage revolve around decision making. The therapist assists the client in completing a decisional balance exercise in which the costs and benefits of both maintaining the behavior and changing the behavior are identified.

Preparation. In the preparation stage, the person actually makes a commitment to actively participate in making and carrying out a plan to accomplish the change in behavior. The goal is a plan of action that can be enacted immediately. The tasks of the therapist are to help the client strengthen both commitment and motivation to change by providing the client with choices whenever possible. The plan must be acceptable and accessible to the client and have evidence that for other people, at least, it has been effective.

Action. This stage of change is characterized by implementation of the planned change in behavior. The goal is to establish a new pattern of behavior that can be sustained beyond the present. The therapist helps to affirm the client's commitment to change and supports the client's efforts to take the planned steps identified in the stage of preparation. At this stage, both client and therapist may discover that the client needs to develop additional skills to meet the behavioral change goal. To that end, the therapist will assist the client in identifying and rallying additional resources.

Maintenance. In the maintenance stage, people gain confidence in their ability to maintain the desired behavioral change. The focus is on preventing relapse. This stage may last from 6 months to 5 years.

Relapse. Although not identified as a stage in the transtheoretical model of change, relapse indicates that the person has reverted back to an earlier stage of change. Relapse is often followed by a second (or third, or more) experience of contemplation, preparation, and action.

Termination. Termination is the point at which a person is no longer tempted to engage in the problematic behavior. Long-term change is characterized by four criteria: (a) the lack of temptation to go back to the changed behavior under any circumstances; (b) a new self-image consistent with the new behavior pattern; (c) a solid self-efficacy or confidence that the person can engage in the new, healthier behavior; and (d) maintenance of a healthy lifestyle through changing social contacts and daily routines that influence behavior patterns (Prochaska, DiClemente, et al., 1994). This stage is particularly relevant to individuals changing addictive behaviors and may not be appropriate to those changing other behaviors such as reducing fat intake (Prochaska et al., 1997).

Although the stages of change in this model are presented linearly, Prochaska and colleagues (Prochaska, Norcross, & DiClemente, 1994) emphasize that people often have relapses and recycle through one or more of the stages. They consider this recyling as an event rather than a distinctive stage. In recycling, individuals may discover that change is more costly than first anticipated, or they may end up substituting one health-risk behavior for another. They point out that the road to behavior change is narrow but rarely straight or without obstacles. Lapses in progress are expected, but becoming distressed about the lack of progress is counterproductive. The final stage, *termination,* means that the person is leaving the cycle of change. This phase is often marked by a new self-image, a healthier lifestyle, and solid self-efficacy (Prochaska, Norcross, & DiClemente, 1994).

Processes of Change

Processes of change refers to both overt and covert activities in which people engage as they move through the six stages of change. There are 10 processes of change.

- *Consciousness raising* refers to both overt and covert actions that a person uses to progress through the stages of change. Types of interventions aimed at raising one's conscious awareness include confrontation, media campaigns, feedback, and bibliotherapy.
- *Contingency management* refers to providing consequences for taking steps toward the desired behavioral change. Examples of consequences are rewards and group recognition that tend to reinforce the desired behavior.
- *Counterconditioning* is learning about new desirable behaviors that will be followed instead of old behaviors (e.g., desensitization, positive self-talk, assertiveness, and relaxation).
- *Dramatic relief* reduces the affect that occurs when a person takes appropriate action (e.g., engaging in the desired behavior change). Types of interventions aimed at providing dramatic relief include role-playing, psychodrama, and giving personal testimonials.
- *Environmental reevaluation* refers to identifying how a particular behavior affects one's social environment and how one's behavior can serve as a model for other people. Examples of this process include family interventions and empathy training.
- *Helping relationship* is social support elicited to assist the person in changing a behavior. A helping relationship is characterized by trust,

acceptance, and openness. Examples of such relationships include therapeutic alliances and buddy systems.

- *Self-liberation* is the belief and commitment to make a change in behavior. Public testimony is an example of this process of self-liberation.
- *Self-reevaluation* is one's assessment of self-image with and without the unhealthy behavior. Examples include both affective and cognitive strategies, such as values clarification, mental imagery, and healthy role models.
- *Social liberation* refers to the opportunities one has in social settings to engage in healthy behaviors more than in health-risk behaviors. Examples of this process include institutional policies that permit access to condoms for sexually active adolescents and smoke-free zones in restaurants and other public places. Such policies promote healthy behaviors by creating a supportive environment that focuses on alternatives to the undesirable behavior.
- *Stimulus control* is removing cues for the old, unhealthy behavior and increasing the cues for alternative behaviors. Such cues can occur at individual, group, or community levels.

In TTM, *decisional balance* is a person's relative evaluation of the pros and cons of making the behavior change. This concept is based on Janis and Mann's (1977) decision-making model, which focused on the positive aspects (instrumental gains for self and others and approval for self and others) and negative aspects (instrumental costs to self and others and disapproval from self and others) of change. A two-factor model (pros and cons) of decisional balance is used in the TTM of change (Velicer et al., 1998).

Self-efficacy confidence is a person's confidence that he or she can cope with stressful or difficult situations without relapsing into the health-risk behavior. This self-efficacy is situation-specific and is based on Bandura's (1977, 1997) conceptualization of self-efficacy (see Chapter 8).

Self-efficacy temptation is the intensity of a person's urge to engage in a particular behavior (e.g., the behavior that she or he wants to change) in a stressful or difficult situation.

An integrative study headed by Prochaska, Velicer, and colleagues (1994) was done through cross-sectional comparisons of the relationship between two of the major concepts in the model: stages of change and decisional balance. Twelve problem or health-risk behaviors were examined: weight control, high-fat dieting, quitting cocaine, smoking cessation, safer sex, condom use, sunscreen use, exercise, mammography screening, physician's preventive practices, radon gas exposure, and adolescent delinquent behavior. These 12 behaviors were classified as cessation of negative (health-risk) behaviors and acquisition of positive (health-promoting or -protecting) behaviors (e.g., mammography screening and condom use).

Hypothesized relationships of the TTM that were examined across these 12 behaviors were as follows:

1. Persons in the precontemplation stage of change will judge that the positive aspects (pros) of the problem behavior outweigh the negative aspects (cons).

2. Persons in the action and maintenance stages of change will judge that the negative aspects (cons) of the problem behavior outweigh the positive aspects (pros).

Data from 12 samples with a total of 3858 participants were analyzed. Using principal-components analysis with varimax rotation, decisional balance was examined and a two-factor structure (pros and cons) was found comparable across all samples and all behaviors. This analysis provided validity for the construct of decisional balance proposed in the model. Both hypothesized relationships between stage of change and decisional balance were also supported. That is, for all of the 12 behaviors, the negative aspects of changing were rated higher than the positive aspects for those individuals in precontemplation. Similarly, for 11 of the 12 behaviors, the positive aspects of changing were rated higher than the negative aspects for individuals in the action stage. The one behavior for which this second hypothesis was not supported was quitting cocaine use (Prochaska, Velicer, et al., 1994).

The findings in support of the hypothesized relationships between these two major concepts were later restated as predictions:

1. To progress from precontemplation to contemplation, the pros of changing must increase.

2. To progress from contemplation to action, the cons of changing must decrease. (Prochaska et al., 1997, p. 67)

Two more hypotheses of the TTM were tested, using the 12 studies cited:

1. A person progressing from the precontemplation stage of change to the action stage will identify a greater increase in the positive aspects (pros) of the behavior change than decrease in the negative aspects (cons) of the change.

2. Healthy behavior change includes both cessation of unhealthy behaviors and acquisition of healthy behaviors (Prochaska, 1994, p. 47).

From these analyses, Prochaska (1994) calculated two mathematical relationships, known as the *strong and weak principles of progress* (summarized in Table 10.2). Evidence to support the first hypothesis was strong in 10 of the 12 studies (but not for mammography screening and use of sunscreen, which are health-promoting or -protecting behaviors rather than health-risk or problem behaviors). The strong principle reflects a large effect (increase of one standard deviation) and suggests that an intervention should affect 20% of the variance in the pros of change. The weak principle reflects a smaller effect size (change of 0.5 standard deviation) and suggests that an interventions should affect 5% of the variance in the cons of change. This principle was less consistent across studies. For example, for safer sex and condom use, there was little change in participants' assessments of the cons.

Levels of Change

Five levels of change are identified in the Transtheoretical Model. These levels are (a) symptom or situation, (b) maladaptive cognitions, (c) interpersonal problems, (d) systems or family problems, and (e) interpersonal conflicts. These levels are included in the model because clinicians recognized that persons with addictive behaviors often had many other problems. Changing an addictive behavior is complicated by the presence of problems that go beyond symptoms but also include negative thinking and interpersonal and intrapersonal problems (DiClemente & Prochaska, 1998).

Relationships between the stages and processes of change have been documented. This means that people in earlier stages of change (e.g., precontemplation, contemplation, and preparation) use very different strategies or processes than people who are in the stages of action and maintenance of the healthy behavior. Examples are (a) stages of precontemplation and contemplation involve the strategies of consciousness raising, dramatic relief, and environmental reevaluation; preparation involves self-liberation. (b) Stages of action and maintenance involve strategies of contingency management, counterconditioning, helping relationships, and stimulus control (Prochaska et al., 1997).

Scope, Parsimony, and Generalizability

Although this model of change was originally developed to help people overcome addictive behaviors, it has been applied to a wide variety of behaviors. Thus it is very broad in scope. The six stages reflect moderate parsimony because they can explain many different behaviors. The TTM has been applied to many kinds of people with many kinds of problem behaviors and in several countries (de Weert-Van Oene, Schippers, De Jong, & Schrijvers, 2002).

Logical Adequacy

The TTM makes sense to scientists from many different disciplines. It is possible to generate hypotheses that can be tested. There are no apparent logical fallacies.

Table 10.2 Strong and Weak Principles of Progress in the Transtheoretical Model

Principle	Mathematical Relationship	Interpretation
Strong	PC → A ≈ 1 SD ↑ Pros	To progress from contemplation to action requires increasing the pros of changing by about one standard deviation.
Weak	PC → A ≈ 0.5 SD ↓ Cons	To progress from contemplation to action requires decreasing the cons of changing by about half a standard deviation

NOTE: A indicates action; PC, to progress from contemplation; SD, standard deviation; →, to progress to the next stage; ≈, approximately; ↑, increase; ↓, decrease.

Usefulness

The Transtheoretical Model has been applied to health protective behaviors such as smoking cessation, exercise, weight control, stress management, use of sunscreen products, alcohol abuse (Velicer et al., 1998), condom use (Tigges, 2001), and screening for STDs (Banikarim, Chacko, Wiemann, & Smith, 2003). It has also been useful in planning and implementing interventions to increase exercise in adolescents (Hausenblas, Nigg, Downs, Fleming, & Connaughton, 2002) and to increase tobacco awareness and cessation among adolescents (Smith et al., 2002).

Testability

The TTM has been tested in many health-care settings. Researchers have operationalized the conceptualized stages and processes of change, self-efficacy, and decisional balance. For example, Nigg and Courneya (1998) tested the entire model for its applicability to exercise behavior among adolescents. The sample consisted of 819 students (mean age, 15 ± 1.22 years) attending five community high schools, and the data supported the model. A criterion measurement model for behavior change, which was developed to define appropriate dependent variables for testing the Transtheoretical Model, has been found useful in making predictions about the stability of each of the stages of change (Velicer, Rossi, Prochaska, & DiClemente, 1996).

Empirical Referents

Stages of Change Questionnaire. The Stages of Change Questionnaire consists of five items, one for each stage of change (Marcus, Selby, Niaura, &

Rossi, 1992). Respondents are asked to select the statement closest to their current status. Two-week test-retest reliability coefficients of .78 and .79 and evidence of validity were reported by Nigg and Courneya (1998).

Process of Change Questionnaire. The Process of Change Questionnaire consists of 39 items with a 5-point Likert-type response format (Marcus, Rossi, Selby, Niaura, & Abrams, 1992). Reliability coefficients ranging from .62 to .89 are reported in the literature (Nigg & Courneya, 1998).

Decisional Balance Questionnaire. The Decisional Balance Questionnaire consists of 10 pro items and 6 con items, with a 5-point Likert-type response format (Marcus, Rakowski, & Rossi, 1992). Coefficients of reliability are .81 for the Con subscale and .82 for the Pro subscale (Nigg & Courneya, 1998). A 24-item measure for predicting smoking status also has evidence of reliability (alpha coefficient of .87 for the Pro subscale and .90 for the Con subscale) and validity through principal component analysis, with two factors accounting for 46% of the variance (Velicer et al., 1985).

Problem Recognition Questionnaire. The Problem Recognition Questionnaire is a 24-item self-report instrument with a 4-point Likert-type response format (*strongly disagree* to *strongly agree*). It measures an adolescent's perceived seriousness of drug or alcohol use and motivation to participate in treatment (see Winters, Henly, & Stinchfield, 1987). The Cronbach alpha for the scale is .87, and the scale has established validity through factor analysis and correlations with posttreatment outcomes (Cady, Winters, Jordan, Solberg, & Stinchfield, 1996).

Theory Applied to Practice

Therapeutic Regimens Enhancing Adherence in Teens. The Transtheoretical Model served as the framework for an intervention identified by the acronym TREAT. The purpose of the program was to promote long-term adherence to highly active antiretroviral therapy (HAART) in 288 HIV-infected adolescents (Rogers, Miller, Murphy, Tanney, & Fortune, 2001). Content of the program reflected the relationships between stages and processes as outlined by Prochaska and colleagues (1997). For those in precontemplation and contemplation, information about HIV and the use of HAART were presented by way of booklets, videotapes, and audiotapes. In contemplation, self-reevaluation was employed by reframing the youth's image away from disappointment with self and toward a view of self as responsible and caring. In preparation, self-liberation processes were followed as youth gained skills and self-efficacy in taking placebo pills on the recommended schedule for HAART. These processes helped participants to believe that they could adopt the new behavior and to gain an understanding of the kind of commitment it would take to adhere to such a strict regimen. In the action and maintenance stages, contingency management, counterconditioning, and stimulus control were used to provide rewards for refraining from old habits and establishing new ones. Of the 65 participants who received the full program, 78% moved forward.

Intervention to Prevent Pregnancy and STDs. A teen-friendly intervention was developed in a community clinic among those adolescents who sought pregnancy testing and received negative results (Sadler & Daley, 2002). These nurses combined the TTM with social cognitive theory to develop the intervention, the purpose of which was to help these adolescents prevent exposure to STIs and delay pregnancy. The TTM helped the nurses determine the readiness of these adolescents to change their motivation to delay pregnancy by using preventive measures that would help the adolescents identify how much they wanted a pregnancy. Relying on SCT, the nurses also acknowledged the interrelationships among knowledge, attitudes, and behaviors in preventing pregnancy and STIs. In particular, they affirmed that self-efficacy, which had previously been shown to assist adolescents in preventing STIs, could be strengthened through modeling self-protective behavior, practicing social skills, and reinforcing both increased knowledge and demonstration of skills.

Adolescent Tobacco Use Awareness and Cessation Program. The Adolescent Tobacco Use Awareness and Cessation Program is an intervention based on the TTM that was delivered to a sample of 1601 youth in the state of Texas. The mean age of participants was 15.9 years (± 1.2 years). No ethnic or gender description of participants was provided. The intervention was implemented with small groups of 8 to 15 participants ($M = 10.9$). Most participants (95%) had smoked one or more cigarettes in their lifetime. Pre- and postintervention data were collected on tobacco use, cognitive factors, and affective factors. At the end of the study, daily tobacco use had decreased by approximately 10% ($t = 4.55$, $p < .01$), and a belief that one had the skills to quit if one chose to do so had increased ($t = 5.18$, $p < .01$). In terms of the stage of change from pre- to postintervention, there was a significant increase in the number of participants in the action stage ($n = 833$ at preintervention and $n = 1030$ at postintervention, $p < .01$). At an interval of 3 to 6 months postintervention, phone calls were made to a random sample of 100 participants and 40% of this subsample stated that they were tobacco free (Smith et al., 2002).

Intervention to Prevent Obesity and Cardiovascular Disease. An intervention based on a combined model of pender's health promotion model and the transtheoretical model of behavior change was implemented in a sample of low-income middle school students (Frenn, Malin, & Bansal, 2003). The sample included an intervention group ($n = 60$) and a control group ($n = 57$) of culturally diverse adolescents whose mean age was 13.82 years (± 1.14 years). Fifty percent of the sample was African American, 20% White, 14% Hispanic, and 15% a variety of other racial and ethnic groups.

Participants in the intervention group received four sessions of 45 minutes each that were congruent with the stage of change they were in relative to decreased dietary fat intake and increased physical activity. Participants in the control group received a general educational experience of the same length. Pretesting showed no significant differences in demographics, dietary fat intake, or physical activity between the two groups. Post-testing showed significant differences in dietary fat intake and physical activity between the two groups. From pre- to post-testing, the intervention group increased the percentage of dietary fat intake less than the control group [$t = 2.018$ (df, 99), $p = .046$] and increased exercise more than the control group [$t = 2.925$ (df, 81), $p < .004$]. Multiple analysis of variance also showed significant differences in variables by stage of change. For benefits, access, and amount of fat in food, significant differences were found between participants in precontemplation and those in the action or maintenance stages of change.

Motivational Interviewing

Origins

Motivational interviewing (MI) was originally developed to describe a method for treating people with alcohol addictions. It was based on principles of humanistic and existential psychology as expressed in the client-centered counseling theory of Carl Rogers (1951, 1957).

Purpose

The purpose of this model is to describe a method of increasing a person's intrinsic motivation to change a behavior (Miller & Rollnick, 1991). Motivational interviewing is defined as "a client-centered, directive method for enhancing intrinsic motivation to change by exploring and resolving ambivalence" (Miller & Rollnick, 2002, p. 25).

Meaning

Motivational interviewing is a method of communication that focuses on a person's intrinsic motivation to change behavior. It is not intended to impose change from outside the person. This method of communication is an adjunct to interventions that include cognitive, behavioral, and skill-building components. The focus is on collaboration between counselor and client. It is also based on the assumption that a client or person has resources and motivation within him- or herself to meet goals for change. The counselor thus affirms the client's right to change and his or her capacity to be self-directed (Miller & Rollnick, 2002).

The MI model is based on four general principles that may be viewed as theoretical constructs. These principles are to "(1) express empathy, (2) develop discrepancy, (3) roll with resistance, (4) support self-efficacy" (Miller & Rollnick, 2002, p. 36). The concept of expressing empathy is based on the notion that change may be facilitated through acceptance and reflective listening by a helping person. It is also assumed that ambivalence about change is a normal human response. Behavior change is facilitated by the realization that there is a discrepancy between one's present behavior and one's behavioral goals. Behavior change is possible only when individuals believe they have the necessary skills to make the change (i.e., self-efficacy).

Change is viewed as a normal life process, reflective of growth. The responsibility for change lies within the person, not the counselor or therapist. Expectations about one's ability to change are also an inherent assumption of this method and similar to self-efficacy in social cognitive theory. Working with supportive people such as family and friends reinforces a person's confidence in her or his ability and commitment to change. Through the process of motivational interviewing, individuals are assisted in meeting goals that are consistent with their life values (Miller, 1998).

Motivational interviewing is a way to communicate with a person who is considering a change in behavior by examining and resolving ambivalent feelings. Both interviewer and interviewee are in a collaborative relationship, within which the role of interviewer is to elicit thoughts and feelings from the interviewee. Throughout the interview, the interviewer makes every effort to clarify the client's ambivalence about changing her or his behavior through an examination of the person's values and how they relate to the decision to change at a particular point in time. Personal choice and control are integral to the process and may be experienced as resistance to change (Miller & Rollnick, 2002).

To change, a person has to have both the desire and the confidence to make the change. In the first stage of motivational interviewing, the interviewer focuses on strengthening the client's intrinsic motivation for change. This phase ends when the person exhibits a readiness for change by decreasing resistance, increasing questions about how to change, and actually experimenting with some changes. The second phase involves making a commitment to and negotiating a plan for change (Miller & Rollnick, 1991).

Scope, Parsimony, and Generalizability

MI applies to habit-forming behaviors across the life span. It relies on a few concepts and thus is parsimonious. It is valid across multiple behavioral domains, such as use of alcohol and other substances, cigarette and marijuana smoking, HIV-risk behaviors; in various age groups; and in multiple cultures (Fisher, Fisher, Williams, & Malloy, 1994; Miller, 2001; Preloran, Browner, & Lieber, 2001).

Logical Adequacy

Motivational interviewing is more of a method for intervention than a formal theory. However, its usefulness in facilitating behavior change attests to the agreement among scientists that it makes sense.

Usefulness

Motivational interviewing has been applied in medical and public health settings (Resnicow et al., 2002), criminal justice settings (Ginsburg, Mann, Rotgers, & Weekes, 2002), and in treatment of persons with dual disorders of mental illness and substance abuse (Handmaker, Packard, & Conforti, 2002). This model has been useful in understanding the motivations for adolescents' use of alcohol, cigarettes, and marijuana (Comeau, Stewart, & Loba, 2001), smoking cessation in adolescents (Dozois, Farrow, & Miser, 1995), and treatment of adolescent substance abusers (Cady et al., 1996; Friedman, Granick, & Kreisher, 1994), as well as in reducing high-risk sexual behaviors in adolescents (Brown & Lourie, 2001; Fisher, Fisher, Misovich, Kimble, & Malloy, 1996). It has also been useful in public health and other medical settings (Resnicow et al., 2002) and in conjunction with the transtheoretical model of behavior change (DiClemente & Velasquez, 2002).

Theory Application to Practice

Substance Abuse Interventions. Dunn, Deroo, and Rivara (2001) reviewed 29 randomized trials of brief interventions that had been adapted from motivational interviewing. Evidence showed that MI was effective in substance abuse interventions, but the mechanisms concerned with how it works and for whom were not explicated. Further study needs to be done to determine how effective it is with other health-risk behaviors. Murphy's research team (Murphy et al., 2001) found that a single session of feedback based on motivational interviewing was more effective than an educational intervention in reducing heavy drinking in a sample of 99 college students.

_____ Information-Motivation-Behavioral Skills Model

Origins

The information-motivation-behavioral skills (IMB) model originated in response to the need for an intervention to prevent HIV. Fisher and Fisher (2002) acknowledged the relevance of the health belief model, the theory of reasoned action, social cognitive theory, and the transtheoretical model, but they also noted that most interventions were not conceptually based and focused on general rather than on specific patterns of behavior. They also noted that extant interventions provided information, but the information was not directly related to the learner's behavior, nor did the interventions motivate people to acquire new behavioral skills.

Purpose

The purpose of the IMB model is to establish a framework for understanding how to prevent HIV infection across populations by focusing on specific informational, motivational, and behavioral skills.

Meaning of the Model

The IMB model is a linear model of information, motivation, and behavioral skills that are presumed to determine HIV-preventive behavior. The authors of the model suggest that a person who has HIV-prevention information and is motivated to prevent the disease will apply prevention behavioral skills to initiate or maintain HIV-prevention behaviors. Information about HIV is directly related to engaging in behavior. However, information is insufficient to direct behavior. A person can have adequate information but lack the motivation or skills to perform the necessary behavior. The model also acknowledges other cognitive processes whereby a person can apply simple decision-making rules to guide behavior (Fisher & Fisher, 2002).

Motivation influences behaviors and is based on beliefs about personal vulnerability and perceptions of support for engaging in prevention behaviors. Behavioral skills are specific to prevention of HIV infection, such as purchasing and using condoms and negotiating with a partner for HIV testing. Whereas HIV-prevention information and motivation have indirect influences on HIV-prevention behavior through behavioral skills, they may also have direct influences. An example of this direct effect is the pregnant woman who agrees to be tested for HIV antibodies when she learns from a health-care provider about the benefits of this behavior; no particular behavior skills are required to mediate this relationship (Fisher & Fisher, 2002).

The IMB model also includes three steps in planning and implementing an HIV-prevention intervention: elicitation, intervention, and evaluation. In the first step of elicitation, Fisher and Fisher (2002) suggest the use of focus groups (see Chapter 11) and open-ended questionnaires to determine extant levels of information, motivation, skills, and behavior in the target population. An intervention can then be designed specifically for the targeted population to address deficits in the areas of information, motivation, and skills. The evaluation process addresses all constructs of the model, using multiple sources of data.

Scope, Parsimony, and Generalizability

The IMB model was originally narrow in scope, intended to predict HIV risk behavior only, but it has also been applied to other health behaviors, including adolescent contraception and STD risk reduction, thus broadening the scope to include the understanding of other health behaviors (Fisher & Fisher, 2002). The model is parsimonious, consisting of only three major constructs. It has been generalized to diverse populations, including gay males, university and college students, and heroin addicts, and has also been tested in severely mentally ill persons and injection drug users (Fisher & Fisher, 2002).

Logical Adequacy

The relationships among the four major constructs of the IMB model are depicted in Figure 10.4. HIV-prevention information and HIV-prevention motivation are directly related to all other concepts in the model. HIV-prevention behavior skills are directly related to HIV-prevention behavior. There are no overlapping concepts and no logical fallacies.

Usefulness

The IMB model has been validated in changing HIV risk behaviors among gay men (Fisher et al., 1994), among college and university student populations (Fisher et al., 1994, 1996), and among heroin addicts (Bryan, Fisher, Fisher, & Murray, 2000). It has also been found useful in HIV prevention in minority adolescents (St. Lawrence, Brasfield, & Jefferson, 1995).

Testability

The theoretical model has been tested and supported through structural equation modeling with various populations (Bryan et al., 2000; Fisher et al., 1994).

Empirical Referents

Measures of motivation to engage in AIDS-preventive behaviors have been developed by Fisher et al. (1994). These authors also developed the Perceived Effectiveness at AIDS-Preventive Behavior Scale to measure perceptions of ability to engage in specific behaviors, such as convincing a partner to practice safer sex. Cronbach alphas ranged from .77 for gay males to .82 for university students.

Concept	1	2	3	4
1. HIV Prevention Information	=	±	±	±
2. HIV Prevention Motivation		=	±	±
3. HIV Prevention Behavioral Skills			=	+
4. HIV Prevention Behavior				=

Legend: = means the same concept; + means the concepts are positively related; ± means the concepts may be positively or negatively related.

Figure 10.4   Logical Adequacy of the Information-Motivation–Behavioral Skills Model

Chapter Summary

Decision making, motivation, and behavioral change were the focus of theories and methods described in this chapter. Adolescents are capable of advanced cognitive processes that enable them to increase self-responsibility. This means that they have increasing opportunities to decide how to act. However, some decisions to engage in behaviors that are potentially addictive increase adolescents' risk for adverse health outcomes. The conflict theory of decision making and the self-regulation model of decision making are two models for understanding how decisions are made and how they might be improved in adolescence. The transtheoretical model of behavior change and motivational interviewing may be useful in facilitating change when decision making has led to health-risk outcomes.

Suggestions for Further Study

The conflict theory of decision making has had a fairly long history but may still be used to understand more clearly how adolescents experience conflict in making decisions that affect their health. Longitudinal prospective studies that examine how decision making changes over time with respect to developmental changes could be instructive to professionals who want to facilitate healthy behaviors in adolescents.

With respect to the self-regulating model of decision making, Byrnes (1998) has suggested that further study is needed to examine developmental trends in the stages of decision making such as differences between novices and experts. For example, he suggested that developmental trends in cue detection and interpretation, goal setting, and construction of strategies should be studied in the generation phase of the process of making decisions. He also noted that more work is needed to differentiate individuals who are self-regulated decision makers and those who are "dysregulated," particularly in how they process information in the various phases of the model. Certainly more work with this model should focus on how adolescents make decisions about engaging in health-promoting versus health-risk behaviors and how these change from early to late adolescence.

The transtheoretical model and motivational interviewing have both claimed large successes in facilitating behavioral change, particularly in addictive behaviors. However, closer looks by scholars suggest that further study is warranted on both of these approaches. For example, the lack of standardized measures for the TTM limits our ability to amass a coherent body of knowledge about the stages of change. The model is not highly specified, making it difficult to derive causal hypotheses. This is important for developing interventions that closely match the stages of change. Most studies have been cross-sectional; thus it would be helpful to conduct more longitudinal studies that examine changes in cognitions across the stages and levels of change (Sutton, 2000).

While it is recognized that motivational interviewing is not a theory, its potential use in interventions to facilitate behavioral change suggests that it may be worthwhile to develop theory based on its principles and methods. Burke, Arkowitz, and Dunn (2002) have suggested that a considerable body of research has been amassed with a focus on adaptations of MI. They asserted that most studies have not tested the efficacy of a pure form of MI. These scholars further suggested that more research should be conducted to test the efficacy of pure MI in facilitating behavioral change, and they called for studies of processes. That is, more work needs to be done to understand why, how, and for whom this method of communication works to facilitate behavioral change.

Related Web Sites

Motivational interviewing:

(Resources) http://www.motivationalinterview.org/

(Explanation) http://www.motivationalinterview.org/clinical/whatismi.html

(MI and adolescent smokers) http://www.rwjf.org/reports/grr/030330.htm

Transtheoretical Model:

http://www.uri.edu/research/cprc/TTM/ detailedoverview.htm

Suggestions for Further Reading

Comeau, N., Stewart, S. H., & Loba, P. (2001). The relations of trait anxiety, anxiety sensitivity, and sensation seeking to adolescents' motivations for alcohol, cigarette, and marijuana use. *Addictive Behaviors, 26,* 803-825.

Downey, L., Rosengren, D. B., & Donovan, D. M. (2000). Sources of motivation for abstinence: A replication analysis of the Reasons for Quitting Questionnaire. *Addictive Behaviors, 26*(1), 79-89.

Fava, J. L., Velicer, W. F., & Prochaska, J. O. (1995). Applying the transtheoretical model to a representative sample of smokers. *Addictive Behaviors, 20,* 189-203.

Prochaska, J. O., & Velicer, W. F. (1997). The transtheoretical model of health behavior change. *American Journal of Health Promotion, 12,* 38-48.

Rolison, M. R., & Scheerman, A. (2002). Factors influencing adolescents' decisions to engage in risk-taking behavior. *Adolescence, 37,* 585-596.

Steinberg, L. (2003). Is decision making the right framework for research on adolescent risk taking? In D. Romer (Ed.), *Reducing adolescent risk: Toward an integrated approach* (pp. 18-24). Thousand Oaks, CA: Sage.

11

Qualitative Approaches to Knowledge Development

In addition to the empirically derived models presented in previous chapters, our understanding of health-risk behavior and interventions to promote change is increased by the findings from qualitative studies. Qualitative studies have special relevance for clinical practice because the experiences of the research participants are closer to the practice experience itself (Cohen, Kahn, & Steeves, 2002). Often these studies are important starting points for theory and instrument development. Qualitative studies are useful in providing a rich context within which to understand the lives of adolescents as they are being lived (Rich & Ginsburg, 1999). In particular, research using grounded theory and participatory action methods provides useful insights about adolescent health that are fully grounded in the experiences of the youth themselves. Qualitative researchers use these designs and methods to study phenomena in natural settings, analyzing data and interpreting their findings in terms of the meanings that people ascribe to their experiences (Denzin & Lincoln, 1998).

Qualitative Approaches to Theory Development

Strategies for conducting qualitative studies are quite varied and have evolved from multiple philosophical perspectives. Regardless of method or design, all involve collecting data in the form of words, actions, or documents (Denzin & Lincoln, 1998). Detailed information about qualitative designs and methods is beyond the scope of this text, but a general overview of the more common types that are relevant to knowledge about adolescent health and health-risk behaviors follows.

Content Analysis

One of the most basic approaches to qualitative data is that of content analysis. As the name implies, it is an analysis of the content of interviews;

focus groups; discussions; or written documents such as diaries, letters, and speeches. Two types of analysis can be done: manifest and latent. In manifest content analysis, the researcher may objectively quantify the oral or written communications, counting how many times a particular word or topic was introduced into an interview or used in a document. In latent content analysis, the researcher engages in more interpretation of the meaning of the text rather than counting the occurrences of words or phrases.

The units of analysis can be individual words, phrases, or sentences. After identifying the unit of analysis, the researcher develops a method for categorizing the data. In conducting manifest content analysis, the data may be separated into a dichotomous index (e.g., a word or phrase was used by six participants who were interviewed but not by the other seven). Content can also be ranked or rated according to criteria established prior to the analysis (Polit & Hungler, 1995).

Examples

Content analysis is useful when very little is known about a topic. The following examples illustrate how this method helps the researcher identify areas for further study.

Transition to Adulthood for Persons With Cystic Fibrosis. More and more children diagnosed with cystic fibrosis are living through the period of adolescence and maturing into young adults. These young people have typically had very close relationships with their pediatricians. Their perceptions of becoming adults and continuing to attend to their chronic disease were a topic of concern to researchers in social work. Palmer and Boisen (2002) interviewed five females and two males who were between 20 and 26 years old. They identified five themes in the participants' interviews: independence and normalization, stress, coping, new responsibilities, and resilience.

The seven participants in this study all identified their increasing independence as a normal passage from adolescence into early adulthood. Five of the seven noted that having cystic fibrosis affected their decision about where to live during college. All of the participants were nonsmokers but acknowledged that having this diagnosis did not prevent them from enjoying social drinking. The participants identified finances, health insurance, and daily therapies as sources of stress in their lives. For example, having sufficient health insurance was identified as a significant source of stress by six out of seven of the participants. All of them participated in daily chest physiotherapy but agreed that this did not stop them from having active lifestyles. Common coping strategies were keeping their disease in perspective, having a positive attitude about their disease and its treatment, and feeling support from other people. New responsibilities they encountered as young adults included the daily physiotherapy, scheduling health-care appointments, obtaining medications, and arranging for health insurance. Participants exhibited resilience through their descriptions of how the disease had made them stronger, given them confidence in their skills of management, and helped them set goals and make plans for the future. For content analysis in this study, Palmer and Boisen (2002) compared their findings to those of researchers using quantitative methods and noted that instead of the usual list of psychosocial problems delineated by other researchers, a more holistic, positive, and optimistic picture of the transition from adolescence to young adulthood emerged from the interviews.

Strategies for Coping With Loneliness. Ten homeless adolescents (three females, six males, and one who self-identified as "other") between 15 and 23 years old ($M = 19.2$) participated in individual interviews. Data from these interviews and from four focus groups, which included 32 homeless adolescents (average age 19.1 years), were analyzed using manifest and latent content analysis. Three major themes were derived from the focus group interviews: degree of loneliness, circumstances that provoked loneliness, and coping with loneliness. Using these three themes as the unit of analysis, individual interviews were analyzed. Findings from both groups indicated great variability in feelings of loneliness, from "I don't feel lonely" to "Very lonely . . . pretty much all the time" (Rew, 2000, p. 128). Circumstances that prompted feelings of loneliness included being away from family and friends, nighttime, and special events such as holidays and birthdays. Most of the participants (81%) had two critical coping strategies: friends and animal companions. Whereas friends shared information about survival, dogs provided unconditional love and motivation to keep going.

Qualitative Case Studies

Case studies may be analyzed by using either qualitative or quantitative data or some combination of both. They may include the case of an individual or a group of cases. The purpose of such study is to focus on the complexity of a particular phenomenon. Such studies generally present the uniqueness of the nature of the case, its historical development, and the various contexts and settings (e.g., legal, political, economic) of the case. The case study is often the first step in identifying a phenomenon of concern about which theory development and generalizations are then made possible. Case studies provide opportunities to study phenomena as they exist in the real world (Stake, 1998).

Example

Descriptive case studies can provide great detail about a phenomenon that may be missed when more traditional quantitative designs are used. Such studies depict more of the process inherent in phenomena, such as the two that follow. Although the subject matter is the same, the details of the population provide a richness that can lead to further hypothesizing and theory development.

Symbolism of Menarche in African American Preadolescents. The purpose of a qualitative case study conducted by Hawthorne (2002) was to describe the symbolism inherent in menarche in African American preadolescents. A purposive sample of 15 mothers and 15 daughters (between 9 and 10 years old, $M = 9.7 \pm 0.46$) was recruited through snowball sampling from a rural school district. Mothers and their daughters were interviewed together in their homes, and the mothers completed a demographic survey as well. Audiotaped interviews were transcribed verbatim, and each interview was taken back to the mother-daughter dyad for confirmation of the content. Cross-case analysis led to the identification of four symbolic themes: "(a) vaginal bleeding, (b) sexual maturation, (c) premenarcheal sexual activity, and (d) sexual payback to biological fathers" (Hawthorne, 2002, p. 491).

Various meanings were given to the vaginal bleeding theme. For some there was no special meaning attached; it was simply a concrete sign of menstruation and supported what they had learned to expect from their teachers' description. For others, it was a process of bleeding; still others thought of it as a sickness and hoped it would not return. The theme of sexual maturation was expressed by both mothers and daughters as a signal that the daughter was capable of sexual relations and getting pregnant. Both mothers and daughters gave examples that indicated that males also saw this as a signal that the girl was ready for sex. The third theme, premenarcheal sexual activity, reflected a belief of some mothers that early menarche in their daughters was evidence that the daughter or a boyfriend had been stimulating erotic parts of her body. This early menarche also meant that the mother was to be held responsible for her daughter's premenarcheal sexual activity. The final theme, sexual payback against fathers, was identified by mothers who expressed the concern that this early development in their daughters was a way to punish the girl's father for having "messed over a lot of women" (Hawthorne, 2002, p. 495). Hawthorne concluded from this study that young adolescent girls and their parents needed more information about physiological changes in puberty. She also noted that adequate information might help these families feel more confident about interactions with their daughters and equip parents to provide clear expectations about their daughter's behavior and possible consequences.

Ethnography

Ethnography is viewed as both a philosophy and a method in which qualitative data are analyzed for meanings ascribed to human behavior. Philosophically, ethnography and participant observation are interpretive as opposed to positivistic approaches (Atkinson & Hammersley, 1998). Ethnography is thus an approach to interpreting the culture of a specific social group through both participating in and observing the overt and covert behaviors of members of that group.

Focus Groups

Focus groups originated with the work of Robert K. Merton, a sociologist who introduced them as a means of asking groups of people to respond to media presentations, politicians, and marketers. The method has evolved into a legitimate form of qualitative research, one that often can reach underserved populations, such as the homeless or disenfranchised youth. This approach not only gives these populations access to the research process, it also gives them a voice in planning studies that are to their direct benefit (Litt, 2003).

Focus groups are convened with the purpose of listening to and gathering data from people to understand how they feel about a particular topic or issue. Many of the early focus groups were convened to determine what people thought about the development of various commercial products and services and to identify effective ways to market these. In the research context, however, focus groups have been useful in obtaining qualitative data to assist the investigator in planning a broader study that reflects the perspective of those being studied. They have also been useful in the early stages of development and pilot-testing of various health promotion and risk reduction interventions.

Focus groups have five general characteristics. They involve (a) people, (b) characteristic attributes of a particular group of people, (c) qualitative data generated from the people, (d) discussion within a group that is focused on a particular topic, and (e) a group that exists for a time-limited purpose. The purpose of the focus group is to help the researcher understand a specific phenomenon of concern or interest. Such groups ideally consist of 5 to 10 members who share certain characteristics (e.g., a group that is homogeneous in terms of gender, education, ethnicity) but who do not know each other. Because the objective of the focus group is to allow people to disclose truthful information about what they think and feel, it is best not to bring together a group of individuals who frequently interact in some social setting. Focus groups are not appropriate for educating a group of people or for asking them to reach consensus on an issue. They should not be used if the researcher is unable to ensure confidentiality or if the environment is emotionally charged, especially in the case of conflict between groups (Krueger, 2000).

Data generated by a focus group are often more complex than those generated by interviewing individuals because members of the group stimulate one another's thinking and responding. As a rule, data collected from three or four focus groups are sufficient to reach saturation, or that point at which the researcher has elicited a range of information and is getting no new insights. When the data are analyzed, the findings are reviewed across all groups and examined for patterns of differences and similarities (Krueger, 2000).

Four types of designs characterize focus groups: single category, multiple category, double layer, and broad involvement. The single-category or traditional focus group design has one target audience or group from which data are collected. Three or four groups of people from this target audience are interviewed in a group setting until theoretical saturation is achieved. In the multiple-category design, several target audiences may be interviewed either simultaneously or sequentially. This design permits the researcher to make within-group comparisons (i.e., one target population in two or more groups) as well as across-group comparisons (i.e., one target population compared with another target population). This more complex design may be useful when the researcher wants to plan an intervention that will include both adolescents and their parents. Analysis of the data will reflect the perspectives of both audiences. The double-layer design often addresses an issue of different target populations (layer) living in different geographic regions (layer). Thus, both adolescents and their parents living in a rural area might be compared with these same audiences living in urban and suburban areas. The broad-involvement design addresses data collected from multiple audiences: One particular audience is considered to be the target (e.g., adolescents) and other audiences, such as parents, teachers, clergy, and health-care providers, also have important perspectives (Krueger, 2000).

Qualitative data from focus groups are generated through a series of questions that are written in the language of the target audience. Such questions are posed clearly, are generally short, open ended, and one dimensional. The questions are posed through a logical sequence that has an easy beginning and that proceeds from general to specific. Types of questions that might be used in the sequence of a focus group interview are listed in Table 11.1 (Krueger, 2000).

Data from focus groups generally include verbatim transcriptions of the focus group interviews and notes recorded by one of the facilitators during the interviews. These data may be organized by using one of several computer software programs, such as NUDIST (Richards & Richards, 1998), to assist in initial coding for patterns or themes. The analysis focuses on the meaning, context, internal consistency, frequency, extent, and intensity of information provided by all groups in the study (Krueger, 1998).

Examples

Focus groups are an efficient method for giving voice to disenfranchised or marginalized populations. The advantages over case studies are that more participants can be included in the study, saving time and labor, and the group format often sparks comments from participants that would not have been elicited in a one-on-one interview.

Planning an Intervention for Homeless Adolescents. Homeless adolescents who participated in a larger study about their sexual health practices were invited to participate in one of four focus groups. Each group consisted of five or six participants, for a total of 22 in the sample (11 males and 11 females). The participants were an average of 16.18 years old and had been

Table 11.1   Sequence and Characteristics of Focus Group Questions

Sequence of Questions	*Characteristics of the Question*
Opening	Setting a conversational tone; each member asked to respond
Introductory	Introduce topic of discussion
Transition	Explore topic in more depth; connect participant to topic of discussion
Key	Focus of the study; require more time for response
Ending	Bring closure to discussion, allow participants to reflect on points made, summarize main points, determine that all has been said

homeless an average of 37.8 months. The purpose of conducting the focus groups was to explore the participants' perceived need for a brief educational intervention to promote sexual health. Following Krueger's (1998) strategies for analysis, the research team found that participants were, in general, well-informed about STDs and how to prevent them. They identified numerous barriers in the environment that interfered with their ability to apply that knowledge to protect themselves from STDs. They also described characteristics of a brief intervention that they thought would be useful to them and their peers. Such an intervention, from their perspective, should begin with respect for them as persons. They described the use of educational strategies that they considered to be applicable to them. The participants of these four groups did not come to consensus about an ideal intervention but gave the researchers a clearer picture of how to plan an intervention that was culturally relevant (Rew et al., 2002).

Pubertal Changes in African American and Latino Females. A focus-group study of African American and Latina mothers and their adolescent daughters was conducted by O'Sullivan, Meyer-Bahlburg, and Watkins (2000). The purpose of the study was to assess the meaning and cultural context that early adolescent females associated with the sexual changes of puberty. Fifty-seven pairs of mothers (51% African American between 31 and 40 years old) and daughters (10-13 years old) participated in 1 of 16 focus groups. Separate focus groups for mothers and daughters were conducted concurrently with 5 to 10 (average, 7) participants in each group. Some groups were conducted in Spanish, and the facilitators of the group were matched for ethnicity with the majority of the members of each group. Groups lasted approximately 1½ hours, and all participants received reimbursement for travel expenses and compensation for their participation.

Three major and two minor themes related to pubertal development were derived from the transcribed tapes of the focus groups. Status of major versus minor themes was determined by the number of excerpts in which the theme was identified. The first major theme was "physical maturation provides new social status of maturity" (O'Sullivan et al., 2000, p. 230). The girls ascribed high social status to peers who matured early. Some of these girls also acknowledged confusion and distress in response to unwanted attention from older males. The second major theme was "attribution of social meanings to feelings of sexual arousal" (p. 231). The research team reported that it was difficult to elicit details about feelings of arousal and that many of the girls perceived that some of their peers had "raging hormones" or had difficulty controlling their hormones. The third major theme was "strain apparent in mother-daughter relations at puberty" (p. 232). This strain was exacerbated by the girls' increasing efforts to gain autonomy and the mothers' increasing reluctance to give up control, over their daughters' relationships with boys in particular. The two minor themes were "physical development provides new social status among peers" and "menarche is a critical communication opportunity for mothers" (p. 230).

O'Sullivan and her research team (2000) noted ethnic differences between the African American and Latina participants. They noted that the African American mothers and daughters discussed the changes of puberty, sexual activity, and relationships more directly and in greater detail than the Latina participants. The African American participants were also more likely to discuss personal experiences with a sense of humor and to express positive feelings about sexuality. The Latina mothers and daughters, however, discussed the topics more vaguely, and the daughters were less knowledgeable than the African American girls of the same age. The researchers concluded that pubertal development in both African American and Latina early adolescents indicated changes in the social status and reproductive potential of these girls. They advocated early interventions to help these young women develop healthy sexual behaviors.

Grounded Theory Studies

The grounded theory approach was initially described by Glaser and Strauss (1967) as a method of generating theory through systematic data collection and analysis. Theory emerges or evolves through a constant comparative process of data collection, analysis, and interpretation. Rather than constructing theory from abstract concepts and statements, followed by model testing, those using this methodology build theory from the ground up. That is, concepts and relationships among them are grounded in the data collected for the study. Sources of data for generating this type of theory are qualitative in nature. Typical sources of qualitative data include interviews with members of the population of interest, field notes or observations recorded by the researcher, audio- and videotapes made of interviews, short answers written by research participants to questions posed by the researcher, journals or diaries, historical accounts such as autobiographies, and other printed materials.

The purpose of grounded theory methodology is to develop substantive theory. To this end, the process of verification of hypotheses or relational statements is carried out during the entire study. The method is characterized by theoretical sampling (data are derived from the population to whom the theory will apply), generating concepts through systematic coding, and integrating concepts into a coherent pattern of theory. The resulting theory consists of plausible relationships among sets of concepts that reflect the "*patterns* of action and interaction between and among various types of social units" (Strauss & Corbin, 1998, p. 169).

This methodology focuses on the processes that occur within a naturalistic environment. Theoretical concepts can be traced directly to the data, and the research theorist is an integral part of this process. The resultant theory reflects the interpretation and perspective of the researcher at a given time in history. The methodology unfolds as multiple interpretations and perspectives are considered during the collection and analysis of data from research participants (Strauss & Corbin, 1998).

Grounded theories are fluid in the sense that they are generated through the interactions of research and research participants, at a particular time in history, and through the process of constant comparison of data analysis with data collection. Grounded theories are useful in helping multiple disciplines understand the in vivo processes that pertain to the disciplinary domain of interest. Moreover, they are useful in developing policy and programs for the target population studied (Strauss & Corbin, 1998).

Examples

The following grounded theory studies of adolescent health represent valid starting points for further theory development.

Becoming a Nonsmoker. Dunn and Johnson (2001) interviewed 17 nonsmoking Canadian females who were 13 to 17 years old to discover processes used to retain their nonsmoker status. The study was based on the assumption that groups share basic social problems that they do not specifically articulate. Nonsmokers were defined as those who reported having never smoked, who had not smoked in the previous 30 days, or who had smoked less than 1 pack ($n = 20$ cigarettes) of cigarettes in their lifetime. The basic social process of remaining a nonsmoker, depicted as the three phases shown in Figure 11.1, was based on developing self-confidence. Phase I was labeled "making sense of smoking" and involved knowing the purpose of smoking, knowing the short- and long-term hazards of smoking, and trying it. Some participants who had watched their parents struggle with quitting smoking noted that this had made a lasting impression on them and they did not want this habit to control their lives. As the participants told about *making sense of smoking,* they actually decided that it was pointless or served no purpose in their lives. They had tried smoking out of curiosity or to conform to a peer group, and

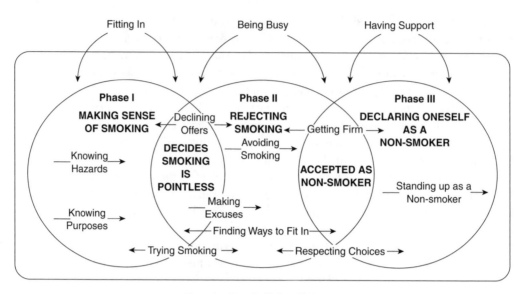

Developing Self Confidence

Figure 11.1   Making Sense of Smoking: An Example of Grounded Theory

SOURCE: Dunn and Johnson (2001, p. 291). © 2001 Society for Adolescent Medicine. Reprinted with permission.

their decision not to become a smoker meant they had to endure peer pressure. In this phase, participants reflected their self-confidence.

Phase II was labeled "rejecting smoking," which involved the application of four strategies. The adolescents declined offers to smoke, made excuses for not smoking, avoided smokers and areas where people smoked, and found other ways to fit into their peer groups. Employing these strategies increased the participants' self-confidence and helped to reinforce their decision not to become a smoker. The participants sometimes had to make excuses for not smoking and found that when they could tell others that they had tried it, their decision not to smoke seemed more credible to their peers and increased their self-confidence in deciding to be nonsmokers. Another strategy that increased their acceptance and self-confidence came from finding other ways to fit in with peers.

Phase III was labeled "declaring oneself to be a nonsmoker" and was based on the individual internalizing the belief that she was a nonsmoker and then declaring this identity publicly. Participants used three strategies in this phase: "standing up as a nonsmoker, respecting choices, and getting firm" (Dunn & Johnson, 2001, p. 294). The first strategy of "standing up" meant that they wanted their friends to respect their decision not to smoke. In turn, they respected their friends' decision to smoke and ceased commenting about the effects of secondhand smoke. In getting firm, participants had to act and speak assertively about their decision, and this in turn enhanced their self-confidence.

In this third phase, participants noted that having support increased their perceptions of self-worth and contributed to their self-confidence as well.

As with other grounded theory studies, this one is limited by the small sample size and, consequently, no claims can be made about the generalizability of the findings. However, the findings illuminate a process that may be useful in designing interventions to assist adolescents in building their self-confidence to engage in health-promoting behaviors and to resist those behaviors that may be health compromising. Of particular usefulness are the identified strategies that these participants used in the various phases of becoming a nonsmoker. As others have shown (Small et al., 2002), having factual information about the dangers of smoking is insufficient for adolescents to decide to abstain from smoking. The researchers who conducted this study noted that the process of becoming a nonsmoker took place over time within a family and social context in which social support was a critical element in the decision-making process. They suggested that there could be value in developing interventions that reflect the length of this process.

A Theory of Taking Care of Oneself. The purpose of a grounded theory study of 15 homeless adolescents between 16 and 20 years old was to describe a theory of self-care attitudes and practices displayed by adolescents living on the streets (Rew, 2003). The sample consisted of 6 females, 7 males, and 2 who self-identified as transgendered. The basic social process of "taking care of oneself in a high-risk environment" (p. 236) was identified from interview data collected in a street-outreach setting. This process, depicted in Figure 11.2, consisted of three categories: "becoming aware of oneself, staying alive with limited resources, and handling one's own health" (p. 237). As illustrated in the model (Figure 11.2), each category consisted of two processes as well as several strategies.

The first category, *taking care of oneself in a high-risk environment,* included a process of deciding to act in a way that reflected self-respect and that would enhance their sense of well-being and overall health. Participants described how this process began with developing an awareness that their lives at home were not contributing to their healthy development and that drifting to the streets represented a greater chance not only for survival but an opportunity for health. The second process described by participants was that of increasing self-reliance. This perception of self reflected their belief that trusting their own judgment was better than trusting the judgment of caretakers who had let them down. They described numerous health problems with which they had dealt successfully since leaving home and expressed confidence in their ability to handle whatever life dealt them.

The second category, *staying alive with limited resources,* meant that these participants engaged in self-preservation strategies and planned ways to protect themselves from harm. They described many things they did to preserve their sense of worth and dignity, including finding basic survival materials, such as food and water, and even finding part-time work. Participants were

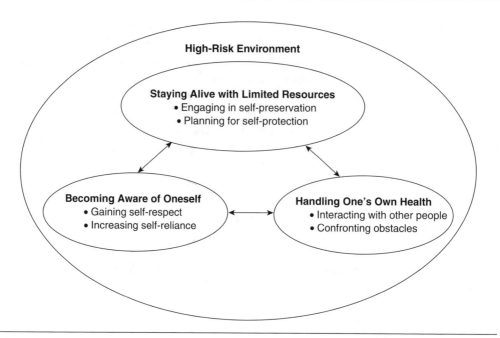

Figure 11.2 A Grounded Theory of Taking Care of Oneself in a High-Risk Environment

SOURCE: Rew (2003, p. 237). © 2003 Lippincott Williams & Wilkins. Reprinted with permission.

well aware that the environment in which they were living was hazardous. Consequently, they employed strategies to enhance their safety. Planning for self-protection meant that some carried weapons, others adopted dogs as companions, and all knew who and what to avoid to stay safe.

The third category, *handling one's own health*, came from interacting with other people and confronting the obstacles in this high-risk environment. In handling their own health, participants acknowledged that they had learned many basic facts about health promotion from other people while they were growing up and attending school. Through their experiences on the street, they also learned valuable lessons about health from other street youth and from professionals working at street outreach centers and shelters. They also acknowledged that the street environment presented numerous obstacles, such as inclement weather and staying sober when alcohol and drugs were so prevalent.

This study is limited by the small sample in one geographic location. However, findings support constructs found in theories of self-identity, self-regulation, and resilience. Many behaviors described by participants in the study are similar to the self-care requisites in Orem's (1991, 2001) theory of self-care agency. That is, participants took action on their own behalf to obtain and maintain basic health and survival necessities of air, water, food, and shelter. Youth in this study also displayed increasing independence and resilience that promoted their health and well-being in spite of having little social support or other resources.

Latinas' Definitions of Sex and Sexual Relationships. A grounded theory study was conducted with 31 late adolescents and young adults (18-36 years old, *M* = 23) to explore the meanings of sexuality among Latinas (84% Puerto Rican, 10% Dominican, and 6% Cuban) (Faulkner, 2003). The participants described three methods by which they processed the messages they received from the culture and environment about sex and sexuality. Some women rejected cultural messages and held beliefs about women's rights, that they were more than mothers and relational partners. Some of the women adjusted the messages they received to fit their own developing beliefs, incorporating some of the messages and rejecting others. The third method was to accept messages and to enact the cultural value of saving themselves for marriage (Faulkner, 2003).

Participants in this study gave various definitions of sex and pointed out that the meaning depended on the kinds of activities they had experienced and what they considered might be potentially erotic. Most defined sex as vaginal-penile intercourse. In terms of context, the definition of sex according to the church was much more rigid and included long kissing, whereas the definition of sex according to society meant sexual intercourse. *Sex* was differentiated from *making love;* sex was physical, and making love was emotional and relational. Participants defined safer sex as "smart sex" and knew how to take action to prevent pregnancy and STDs (Faulkner, 2003).

Latina participants also had strong views about men's and women's roles within a sexual relationship. Some preferred to date White men, others Latinos, but most wanted to avoid men who were "just playing" and sleeping around with several women. They differentiated the "good girl," whose relationships with men were traditional and often supervised, from the "flirt girl," whose relationships were more open and risky. These participants described the ideal relationship as reciprocal, romantic, and involving a future together. The researchers concluded that interventions to promote safer sex, especially for ethnic minority groups, should consider the group's personal and traditional definitions of sex and their levels of acculturation (Faulker, 2003).

Parents' Struggle to Understand Adolescents Who Smoke. Parents who did not smoke (N = 25) participated in a grounded theory study to describe the process parents experience when an adolescent child takes up smoking (Small et al., 2002). Participants were parents of junior high and high school students in one city in Canada. Data were collected through interviews with open-ended questions. Each interview was audiotaped and transcribed verbatim. Data analysis began with the transcript of the first interview, and a constant comparative method was used to code all data (Small et al., 2002).

Findings from the study are depicted in Figure 11.3. The basic social process was "Struggling to understand," which signified the emotional and intellectual processes that parents experienced as they discovered their child's smoking behavior and faced the problem. The figure illustrates four stages that parents went through: discovering the smoking, facing the problem,

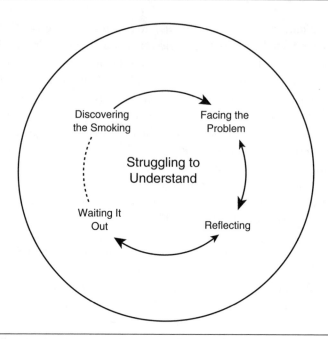

Figure 11.3   Struggling to Understand: Parents' Discovery of Adolescents'
                    Smoking Behavior

SOURCE: Small et al. (2002). © 2002 Sage Publications, Inc. Reprinted with permission.

reflecting, and waiting it out. The double-headed arrows in the figure indicate
movement between stages; larger arrowheads reflect the parent's primary
experience. The broken line shows that some parents who were waiting it out
discovered again that their child was smoking (Small et al., 2002).

In discovering the smoking, parents found evidence, such as cigarettes or
a lighter, and as the evidence was found repeatedly, the parents confronted
their children to confirm the child's behavior. Parents' responses to the
discovery were strong emotions, such as feeling shocked, disappointed, and
hurt. Many of the adolescents had worked hard to keep their behavior
a secret from their parents, and this deception increased the emotional
response of the parents (Small et al., 2002). In facing the problem, parents
acknowledged that because they were not smokers themselves, they were ill
prepared to respond to the discovery that their child had begun to smoke.
Most of the parents confronted the issue directly, some approached the
adolescent with anger, and some were passive. Most, however, finally took
a stance and indicated their displeasure with the child's behavior, established
boundaries for the behavior (e.g., not allowing the behavior in the home or
the family's car), and offered to help their children quit.

In the third phase of struggling to understand, parents reflected on their
discovery and looked for a cause, such as peer pressure. Some parents ratio-
nalized during this stage, and others questioned whether or not the behavior
could have been prevented. These parents also recognized a paradox: The

adolescents had knowledge of the risks and negative health effects but chose to initiate and continue smoking anyway. In the final stage, waiting it out, parents acknowledged that to quit smoking takes time. These parents realized they had no control over their children's behavior, but they tried to do the right thing despite their continued concern. The researchers interpreted these findings in the light of Lazarus and Folkman's (1984) theory of stress and coping (see Chapter 5). Discovery of the adolescent's smoking behavior was interpreted as a stressor and appraised as a threat. Most parents responded primarily with problem-focused coping, but some also used emotion-focused coping, particularly when they felt they had no control over the outcome. Small et al. concluded that interventions to help parents prevent and intervene in their adolescents' smoking behavior are needed. They added, "A formal theory, which explains parents' experience in the context of adolescent risk behaviors, needs to be developed" (Small et al., 2002, p. 1217).

Narrative Analysis

Narrative analysis is a qualitative method of storytelling. It is primarily for use with relatively small numbers of research participants who can provide oral, first-person descriptions of their subjective experiences. People often make sense or meaning out of traumatic experiences by putting them into a narrative or story form. The focus of analysis is on the meaning of the story to the person who experienced it (Riessman, 1993). Narrative analysis is used to explore complex social phenomena as they are experienced chronologically by individuals. It represents an initial point from which particular cases form the basis for later generalizations. The researcher is sensitized to the subjective meaning of phenomena as told in story form by research participants. In this respect, narrative analysis is very much like the case study approach to theory development.

In this context, narratives are stories about past events. They represent a person's experience, and they may or may not be told in chronological order. Narratives have a common structure: (a) an abstract or summary; (b) an orientation to time, place, person, and situation; (c) a sequence of events; (d) an evaluation or interpretations of the significance and meaning of the event or experience; (e) a resolution of events; and (f) a coda where the storyteller returns to the perspective of the present. People tell about the events of their lives in various forms, including comedy, tragedy, satire, and romance. The researcher must decide how to interpret the story for the purpose of understanding (Riessman, 1993).

Narratives are derived through personal interviews that are audiotaped. The researcher must decide how to elicit the story in a way that will facilitate the narrative outcome. Interviews may be guided by highly or loosely structured interview guides, including visual cues such as a storyboard. Audiotaped interviews are then transcribed verbatim. These transcriptions are reviewed while the reader is listening to the taped interviews, and sometimes they are revised to reflect intonation or gestures used by the research participant. Analysis may be done according to some specific structure such as the one described, or it may take a more poetic form that reflects recurrent themes or ways of expression (Riessman, 1993).

Criteria for validation of narrative analysis include persuasiveness, plausibility, correspondence, coherence, and pragmatic usefulness. Outcomes should be reasonable and convincing. Theoretical statements are supported with direct quotes from the research informants. The criterion of correspondence is met by taking the findings back to the participants and asking for validation of the researcher's interpretation. Coherence of the interpretation means that the participant's goal in telling the story is clear, the interpretation reflects the kind of effect the participant hoped to have on the listener, and the themes of the participants are unified within the text (Riessman, 1993).

Examples

Narrative analysis provides a personal glimpse of illness, the research process, and the development of resilience in the following studies of adolescents.

Children and Adolescents' Understanding of Research. One hundred and five family members were recruited for a study to describe children and adolescents' understanding of the research process (Broome, Richards, & Hall, 2001). In-depth interviews were conducted with 34 children and adolescents between 8 and 22 years old who had been diagnosed with diabetes ($n = 10$) or cancer ($n = 24$). The majority (74%, $n = 25$) were White, 9% ($n = 3$) were African American, and 9% ($n = 3$) were Hispanic or Mexican American. The other three were Japanese American, Native American, and Peruvian. All had been involved in clinical trials of new drugs to treat their medical conditions. The interviews were conducted either in the person's home, clinic, or private room at the medical facility. In addition to audio recordings of the interviews, the interviewers recorded field notes that addressed the use of space (proxemics); silences and pacing of the responses (chronemics); body language (kinesics); and changes in the tone, quality, and volume of the child or adolescent's voice (paralinguistics). Interviews were transcribed verbatim, and data were reduced through paraphrasing and summarizing the stories told by the research participants (Broome et al., 2001).

The findings included the identification of themes that reflected the structure of the clinical trials and the relationships among parents, research team members, and the child or adolescent participant. These themes were the child or adolescent's perception of disagreements between him- or herself and the parent about participation in the study, the participant's faith in the relationship between the research team and the participant's parents, concerns about the incentives for participating, treatment options if the child or adolescent decided not to participate in the clinical trial, and the participant's life outside the clinical trial situation. Three other salient themes were the child or adolescent participant's understanding of the research process and protocol, differentiation between treatment and research, and inclusion in the decision to participate in the clinical trial. These three themes were related to the age and previous research experience of the participants (Broome et al., 2001).

For the most part, adolescents were able to explain why the research was being done, and they were aware of the risks and benefits of the study. Some expressed confusion about their own participation in a clinical trial. Sometimes the decision to participate in a clinical trial was influenced by financial incentives and the opportunity to try something new or use new equipment. Those with cancer often did not participate as fully in the decision to participate as did those with diabetes because the ones with cancer were often much sicker and more fatigued. The researchers concluded from this narrative analysis that multiple factors influence the decision of children and adolescents to participate in research and that investigators should develop processes that are inclusive of these young participants throughout the informed consent process (Broome et al., 2001).

Visual Illness Narratives and Explanatory Models of Asthma. Twenty children, adolescents, and young adults (10 females and 10 males) who had moderate or severe asthma participated in a study using Video Intervention/ Prevention Assessment (Rich, Patashnick, & Chalfen, 2002). The participants, who were between 8 and 25 years old (median = 15), carried video cameras for 4 to 8 weeks, taking pictures of their daily activities and interviewing friends and relatives. The visual narratives were then analyzed to identify explanatory models, or the ways in which the participants made sense of their illness. The results were eight themes that reflected the messages the participants had received from family and health professionals and their personal experiences. The eight themes were the nature of asthma, the origin of the participant's asthma, asthma triggers, limitations of lifestyle, control of asthma, use of medications, fear of dying, and prognosis. The researchers found that their knowledge about asthma was accurate, but the understanding of the origin of the disease was less accurate. Many of them were ambivalent about taking medications and feeling that they depended on them rather than being totally in control of their own lives. As for the prognosis, many of them believed they would outgrow the asthma (Rich et al., 2002).

Resilient Development. In a study of the process of resilient development, Hauser (1999) employed narrative analysis on interviews conducted annually with adolescents who had experienced traumatic circumstances and become competent young adults. Although the methods for collecting and analyzing interview data are not made explicit in the publication of this study, Hauser identifies five content themes and a structural feature associated with this qualitative analysis of more than 35 adolescents participating in a longitudinal study. The structural feature of the findings is that the narratives are coherent. That is, the resilient individuals connected their past experiences to the present and described both success and failures throughout their transitions into adulthood. The five content themes are shown in Table 11.2.

Suicide and Prostitution Among Street Youth. Kidd and Kral (2002) analyzed the narratives of 29 street youth (19 males and 10 females) between 17 and 24 years old ($M = 21.8$). Participants were interviewed and interviews were transcribed. Kidd, the investigator, also kept a notebook with ideas and personal impressions that occurred during the interviews. The coding procedures of grounded theory methodology were followed, and interviews were analyzed by first using open coding, proceeding to theoretical coding, and finally through development of a theoretical model. Six of the interviews were not included in the final analysis because they lacked sufficient details. Results were organized in chronological order, beginning with childhood experiences, often of abuse and attempting suicide. The next phase was the life the participants encountered on the streets. For many, this involved a decrease in self-esteem and personal control as they became involved in prostitution. They related various bad experiences with prostitution and drugs that sent them down a path of thinking about or actually attempting suicide. Suicide attempts were associated with feeling alone and isolated, angry, depressed, and empty.

Street youth in this study also found help with their pain by talking to friends they had made on the streets. They acknowledged that some of the best help was to have someone listen to them. Only a few sought help from formal or professional sources. For many, this was the result of having had previous negative experiences with agencies and mental health professionals. The researchers concluded that in spite of the rather dismal picture of street life portrayed in these narratives, "There is an enormous and largely untapped potential residing in these youth, and helping them find it is a key part of the healing process" (Kidd & Kral, 2002, p. 430).

Table 11.2   Hauser's Content Themes of Resilient Outcomes

Theme	Description of Theme
Self-reflection	Increased awareness of thoughts and feelings as teenagers and further reflection as parents
Self-efficacy or agency	Beliefs and actions based on conscious choices
Self-complexity	Recognizing influences of past on present behaviors; incorporating some and rejecting others
Persistence and ambition	Taking control of one's own future
Self-esteem	Vacillating self-appraisals that became increasingly more positive over time

Participatory Action Research

Participatory action research (PAR) is based on the concept of function of social research to improve intergroup relations, originally conceptualized by Kurt Lewin (1946). Lewin believed that relationships between ethnic groups could best be studied through a process of reciprocal fact finding and planning. That is, both minority and majority groups need to study themselves and each other. The purpose of PAR is to study a social system and simultaneously collaborate with members of that system to change the system in a positive way. The members of the system under investigation become coresearchers with the scientist (O'Brien, 1998).

PAR is based on the concern that much knowledge development represents a power differential between researcher and research participant. The PAR approach challenges this tradition and promotes the production of knowledge as something that belongs to the people being studied. Specifically, this approach often begins with the everyday experiences of oppressed groups and aims to empower them to produce knowledge that they can then use. The researcher, acknowledged as an equal partner with the research participants, must be genuinely committed to dialogue and work with the target population (Reason, 1998).

The PAR methodology grew out of a concern that in the postindustrial period of this country, a knowledge society had developed. This society was based on science "as the model of truth," a claim that contributes to developing hierarchies of knowledge in which the production of knowledge belongs to an elite group of scientists or experts (Sohng, 2003, p. 2). Ordinary members of a community were deferring to experts and, consequently, silencing their own voices about what was needed to improve their daily living. Thus this methodology developed as a way to include disenfranchised citizens in answering questions about their social condition. It was a way to place research into the hands of the very people who could benefit from the findings (Sohng, 2003).

Participatory action research is a type of inquiry that informs practice. Rather than following strict scientific design, studies based on the PAR philosophy follow a method that emphasizes collaboration and dialogue between researcher and participant. The process often begins with community meetings in which groups identify issues by telling their stories. Sometimes the process begins with the collection of survey data, which are then returned to the community for interpretation. The research process is collaborative throughout. Researchers reflect on their own behavior and invite community members to do the same (Reason, 1998). The process of collaboration between researchers and research participants empowers communities by rallying isolated individuals to address a common problem or need. The process validates the experiences of ordinary citizens and provides a context for mutual reflection. As a result, knowledge of everyday life can be transformed into action (Bodner, MacIsaac, & White, 1999; Sohng, 2003).

The PAR process consists of five phases that reflect a circular, systematic, scientific reasoning process: (a) identification and diagnosis of a problem, (b) planning for action by considering alternative courses of action, (c) selecting an alternative and taking action, (d) evaluating the consequences of the action taken, and (e) identifying the general findings, which are then used to further diagnose the problem. This process is intimately connected with theory, which informs practice. Practice, in turn, refines theory (O'Brien, 1998).

Example

The purpose of a participatory action study conducted by Cargo, Grams, Ottoson, Ward, and Green (2003) in British Columbia was to "develop a theoretical framework of youth empowerment" (p. S67). Beginning with a community needs assessment initiated by a group of community health nurses, partnerships were established between a number of community-based organizations and health agencies that wanted to promote health and quality of life within the community. The needs assessment indicated that there was very little youth involvement within the community, and the research project was designed to engage youth in identifying what they needed to enhance their quality of life. This study continued for 32 months and involved 123 adolescents between 12 and 19 years old. These youth represented various ethnic groups, including East Indian, Filipino, African, and Eastern European. The youth worked with seven adult facilitators, who included community health nurses, a health promotion researcher, and a youth development worker.

Qualitative data were collected by observation of meetings and community events, six focus groups, a brainstorming session, and individual interviews with both adolescents and adults. Analysis of these data followed many of the procedures characteristic of grounded theory, including constant comparison of data as they were collected as well as open and axial coding. Data from observational notes and individual interviews were analyzed using a theoretical sampling procedure, which is also an aspect of grounded theory methodology. These analyses resulted in the formulation of a theoretical framework (see Figure 11.4) in which categories and the relationships among them were depicted (Cargo et al., 2003). The formulated theoretical framework features youth empowerment as a transactional process.

Mixed Methods Research

The mixed methods approach to research combines both quantitative and qualitative approaches to achieve the research objectives. The term *triangulation* is also used to convey the same approach. Using a combination of approaches allows the researcher to combine data from several sources, giving multiple perspectives to answer the research question. Multiple theories, multiple methods of data collection (e.g., quantitative survey data plus qualitative data from individual interviews or focus groups), and multiple investigators

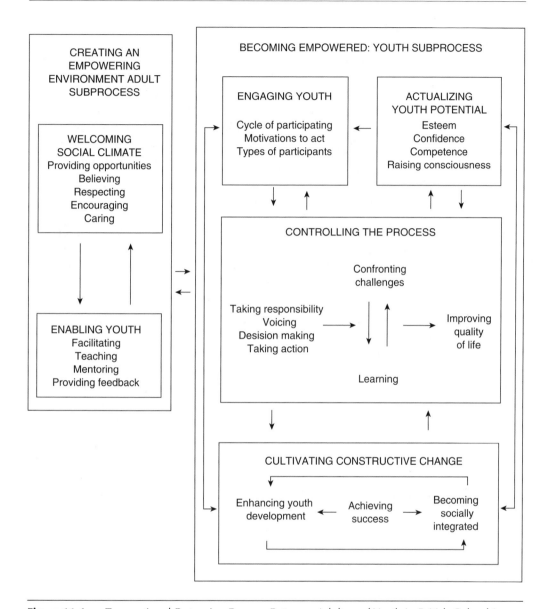

Figure 11.4 Transactional Partnering Process Between Adults and Youth in British Columbia

SOURCE: Cargo et al. (2003, p. S69). © 2003 PNG Publications. Reprinted with permission.

from diverse disciplines may be used in a single study. Using a mixture of approaches can allow the researcher to expand the breadth and scope of understanding of the problem. The use of theory to guide the collection and analysis of quantitative data plus the discovery or development of new concepts through collection and analysis of qualitative data permits the researcher to incorporate both deductive and inductive reasoning into the study (Shepard, Orsi, Mahon, & Carroll, 2002).

Example

In a study using both quantitative and qualitative data, Phinney and Devich-Navarro (1997) interviewed 52 middle class African American and 46 working class and middle class Mexican American adolescents attending schools in Southern California. The purpose of the study was to identify how the participants identified with two cultures (White American and African or Mexican American). They found three patterns of identity among the participants: blended bicultural identity, alternating bicultural identity, and separated cultural identity.

Blended Bicultural Identity. These researchers found that both African and Mexican American participants who had a blended bicultural identity felt good about being an American and felt good and proud about their individual ethnicity. Overall, they felt included in American society and valued the freedom that this status afforded them. This group of participants did not see their blended ethnic identity as a problem. However, this group did report that, unlike participants in the other two pattern groups, they experienced peer pressure to more strongly affirm their ethnic roots (Phinney & Devich-Navarro, 1997).

Alternating Bicultural Identity. Participants who reflected this pattern of identity were firmly attached to their own ethnic culture. They acknowledged being American because they were born in the United States, because they (mainly) liked the fact that being American represented a better life than they could have in some other places, and because being American meant they could enjoy freedom. For African American participants, being bicultural was more of a problem than for Mexican Americans. The African Americans acknowledged a strong unity and pride in being Black. In contrast to the participants characterized as having a blended bicultural identity, however, those with an alternating bicultural identity were aware of racial conflict. Mexican American participants in this group described an advantage in being able to speak two languages, which represented their bicultural identity (Phinney & Devich-Navarro, 1997).

Separated Cultural Identity. Participants who reflected this pattern of identity clearly asserted that they were not bicultural. In this sample, only one Mexican American displayed this pattern of identity. The other participants, who were African American, held very positive feelings about their ethnicity. They were keenly aware that America meant separation and discrimination; thus they had negative feelings associated with being an American. Moreover, they did not feel accepted by American society (Phinney & Devich-Navarro, 1997).

Although the purpose of this study was not to develop theory, it does illustrate how qualitative data can be used to generate concepts that may be useful in further research. This analysis forms a typology of ethnic identity that may be useful as a heuristic for further study and theory development.

Other Qualitative Methods

Other rigorous and complex designs for qualitative studies have been done with adolescent populations. Although detailed descriptions of these methods are beyond the scope of this text, a few are presented to illustrate the types of processes used and the types of findings that these strategies yield.

Phenomenology and Hermeneutic Interpretation

Monsen, Jackson, and Livingston (1996) were concerned about how young adolescents (12-14 years old) made decisions about becoming sexually active and using protection against disease and pregnancy. Because they were interested in understanding how these young adolescents thought in making these decisions, they used a Heideggerian hermeneutical approach to collecting and analyzing discourse data. Heidegger (1962, 1966, 1972) was a philosopher who focused on the human being's experiences of daily living and the way that humans think about this process. The qualitative approach based on this philosophy permits the researcher to identify the meaning and thinking of the research participants.

Monsen and colleagues (1996) examined extant data that had been collected from 45 adolescents attending middle school. These adolescents (25 males and 20 females with a mean age of 12.71 years; 49% African American and 51% European American) answered two open-ended questions in a health-promotion class taught by the school nurse. The questions were (a) "If you had to decide between having sex or not having sex, what factors would influence your decision?" and (b) "If you had to decide between using protection or not using protection, what would influence your decision?" (p. 184).

From the adolescents' written responses, the researchers identified an overall pattern of desiring a meaningful future that might include love and marriage as well as having children. Responses to the first question about the decision to have sex or not included comments about their relatively young age, being in a long-term relationship, and asking trusted adults for additional information. Engaging in sex at an early age was identified as something that could interrupt future plans for school, marriage, and a career, leaving the adolescent with burdensome responsibilities of child rearing or seeking treatment for infection or disease. The first theme extracted from the data was "recognizing that sexuality should be postponed until later, and for many, until marriage" (Monsen et al., 1996, p. 187).

Responses to the second question, about the decision to use protection if one had sex, included comments about abstinence, readiness to engage in sexual activity, being responsible, and using condoms. The second theme extracted from the data was "seeing sex as dangerous, involving the risks of STDs, especially AIDS as well as early pregnancy" (Monsen et al., 1996, p. 187).

Although this was a very small sample of young adolescents, from whom relatively little data were collected, the researchers concluded that these youth could express their thinking in ways that could be helpful to adults planning programs to protect their health and well-being. The findings that these young adolescents had serious concerns about their future and that they had a reasonable understanding of the risks involved in early sexual activity should be encouraging to adults working with this age group.

Chapter Summary

This chapter provided a brief overview of major qualitative designs with implications for addressing adolescent health and health-risk behaviors. Content analysis and qualitative case studies were described as introductory methods for focusing on the complexity of a particular area from which there is little extant information. The grounded theory method was presented as a systematic design for developing theory based on the experiences and language of the target population. Focus groups were another approach described as a way of giving voice to a target population and of using that voice to inform more complex research designs, including health promotion interventions. Participatory action research was portrayed as an ideal method for reducing perceived power differentials between the researcher and the research participants. Various other qualitative methods, such as narrative analysis, hermeneutic interpretation, and mixed methods (triangulation) were discussed briefly. Examples were provided of each type of qualitative design as it applied to the study of adolescent health and health-risk behavior.

Suggestions for Further Study

Theory development that begins with the experiences and words of adolescents themselves has a great deal of potential for moving the science of adolescent health forward. Here is an arena in which great creativity on the part of the investigator can be expressed. The limitations associated with measurement issues in quantitative designs are bypassed, as the researcher can go directly to the phenomenon and the person experiencing it for a rich and thick description.

A great deal of research in adolescent health has focused on an empirical deficit model. Qualitative studies have expanded our understanding of the fuller experiences of adolescence. This is clearly seen in the study of street youth by Kidd and Kral (2002) and the study of homeless adolescents by Rew (2003). Giving voice to marginalized and disadvantaged youth can and should be done more often through qualitative methods.

Further studies should also be done by aggregating qualitative findings. Aggregating results from studies that use the same methods and similar populations increases their validity and their relevance to clinical practice. This approach can lead to increasing levels of abstraction and the construction of middle-range theories (Estabrooks, Field, & Morse, 1994).

Related Web Sites

Grounded Theory Method:

(Grounded Theory Institute) http://www.groundedtheory.com/

(Article on grounded theory as scientific method) http://www.ed.uiuc.edu/EPS/PES-Yearbook/95_docs/haig.html

(Overview) http://www.scu.edu.au/schools/gcm/ar/arp/grounded.html

Narrative Analysis:

(Explanation) http://www2.chass.ncsu.edu/garson/pa765/narrativ.htm

(Update and examples) http://www.ling.upenn.edu/~wlabov/sfs.html

Participatory Action Research:

(Useful links to PAR sites) http://www.goshen.edu/soan/soan96p.htm

(Links to Action Research sites and articles and information about Kurt Lewin) http://carbon.cudenver.edu/~mryder/itc/act_res.html

Suggestions for Further Reading

Barton, W. H., Powers, G. T., Morris, E. S., & Harrison, A. (2001). Evaluating a comprehensive community initiative for children, youth, and families. *Adolescent & Family Health, 2*(1), 27-36.

Beresford, R. A., & Sloper, P. (2003). Chronically ill adolescents' experiences of communicating with doctors: A qualitative study. *Journal of Adolescent Health, 33*, 172-179.

Brackis-Cott, E., Mellins, C. A., & Block, M. (2003). Current life concerns of early adolescents and their mothers: Influence of maternal HIV. *Journal of Early Adolescence, 23*(1), 51-77.

Estabrooks, C. A., Field, P. A., & Morse, J. M. (1994). Aggregating qualitative findings: An approach to theory development. *Qualitative Health Research, 4*, 503-511.

Fielding, S. L., Edmunds, E., & Schaff, E. A. (2002). Having an abortion using mifepristone and home misoprostol: A qualitative analysis of women's experiences. *Perspectives on Sexual and Reproductive Health, 34*(1), 34-40.

Lear, D. (1996). "You're gonna be naked anyway": College students negotiating safer sex. *Qualitative Health Research, 6*(1), 112-134.

Muscari, M. E., Faherty, J., & Catalino, C. (1998). Little women: Early menarche in rural girls. *Pediatric Nursing, 24*(1), 11-15.

Parry, C. (2003). Embracing uncertainty: An exploration of the experiences of childhood cancer survivors. *Qualitative Health Research, 13*(1), 227-246.

Patton, M. Q. (2002). *Qualitative research and evaluation methods.* Thousand Oaks, CA: Sage.

Sullivan, M., Kone, A., Senturia, K. D., Chrisman, N. J., Ciske, S. J., & Krieger, J. W. (2001). Researcher and researched-community perspectives: Toward bridging the gap. *Health Education & Behavior, 28*, 130-149.

Thompson, A. M., Humbert, M. L., & Mirwald, R. L. (2003). A longitudinal study of the impact of childhood and adolescent physical activity experiences on adult physical activity perceptions and behaviors. *Qualitative Health Research, 13*, 358-377.

Wuest, J., Ford-Gilboe, M., Merritt-Gray, M., & Berman, H. (2003). Intrusion: The central problem for family health promotion among children and single mothers after leaving an abusive partner. *Qualitative Health Research, 13*, 597-622.

References _____

About Search Institute. (2004). Retrieved April 17, 2004, from http://www. search-institute.org/aboutsearch/

About the Bronfenbrenner Life Course Center. (2003, October 6). Retrieved April 17, 2004, from http://www.blcc.cornell.edu/about.html

Ackard, D. M., & Neumark-Sztainer, D. (2001). Health care information sources for adolescents: Age and gender differences on use, concerns, and needs. *Journal of Adolescent Health, 29,* 170-176.

Ajzen, I. (1985). From intentions to actions: A theory of planned behavior. In J. Kuhl & J. Beckman (Eds.), *Action-control: From cognition to behavior* (pp. 11-39). Heidelberg, Germany: Springer-Verlag.

Ajzen, I. (1991). The theory of planned behavior. *Organizational Behavior and Human Decision Processes, 50,* 179-211.

Ajzen, I., & Fishbein, M. (1980). *Understanding attitudes and predicting social behavior.* Englewood Cliffs, NJ: Prentice Hall.

Albarracin, D., Johnson, B. T., Fishbein, M., & Muellerleile, P. A. (2001). Theories of reasoned action and planned behavior as models of condom use: A meta-analysis. *Psychological Bulletin, 127,* 142-161.

Allen, K. D. (1992). *Predisposing, enabling and reinforcing factors associated with women's reported Pap smear screening behaviour.* Unpublished master's thesis. University of Toronto, Toronto, ON, Canada.

Allison, B. N., & Schultz, J. B. (2001). Interpersonal identity formation during early adolescence. *Adolescence, 36,* 509-523.

Allport, G. W. (1955). *Becoming: Basic considerations for a psychology of personality.* New Haven, CT: Yale University Press.

Allport, G. W. (1965). *Pattern and growth in personality.* New York: Holt.

Alteneder, R. R., Price, J. H., Telljohann, S. K., Didion, J., & Locher, A. (1992). Using the PRECEDE model to determine junior high school students' knowledge, attitudes, and beliefs about AIDS. *Journal of School Health, 62,* 464-470.

American Psychiatric Association. (1994). *Diagnostic and statistical manual of mental disorders* (4th ed.). Washington, DC: Author.

Archer, S. L. (1983). Identity status in early and middle adolescents: Scoring criteria. In J. E. Marcia, A. S. Waterman, D. R. Matteson, S. L. Archer, & J. L. Orlofsky (Eds.), *Ego identity: A handbook for psychosocial research* (pp. 177-204). New York: Springer.

Archer, S., & Waterman, A. (1990). Varieties of identity diffusions and foreclosures: An exploration of subcategories of the identity statuses. *Journal of Adolescent Research, 5,* 96-111.

Arias, E., & Smith, B. L. (2003). Preliminary data for 2001. *National Vital Statistics Reports, 51*(50), 1-45. Retrieved July 20, 2003, from http://www.cdc.gov/nchs/nvss.htm

Atav, S., & Spencer, G. A. (2002). Health risk behaviors among adolescents attending rural, suburban, and urban schools: A comparative study. *Family and Community Health, 17*(12), 53-64.

Aten, M. J., Siegel, D. M., Enaharo, M., & Auinger, P. (2002). Keeping middle school students abstinent: Outcomes of a primary prevention intervention. *Journal of Adolescent Health, 31,* 70-78.

Atkinson, P., & Hammersley, M. (1998). Ethnography and participant observation. In N. K. Denzin & Y. S. Lincoln (Eds.), *Strategies of qualitative inquiry* (pp. 110-136). Thousand Oaks, CA: Sage.

Backer, J. H., Bakas, T., Bennett, S. J., & Pierce, P. K. (2000). Coping with stress: Programs of nursing research. In V. H. Rice (Ed.), *Handbook of stress, coping, and health: Implications for nursing research, theory, and practice* (pp. 223-263). Thousand Oaks, CA: Sage.

Bailey, S. L., Camlin, C. S., & Ennett, S. T. (1998). Substance use and risky sexual behavior among homeless and runaway youth. *Journal of Adolescent Health, 23,* 378-388.

Bailey, S. L., Flewelling, R. L., & Rosenbaum, D. P. (1997). Characteristics of students who bring weapons to school. *Journal of Adolescent Health, 20,* 261-270.

Balistreri, E., Busch-Rossnagel, N. A., & Geisinger, K. F. (1995). Development and validation of the Ego Identity Process Questionnaire. *Journal of Adolescence, 18,* 179-192.

Bandura, A. (1977). Self-efficacy: Toward a unifying theory of behavioral change. *Psychological Review, 84,* 191-215.

Bandura, A. (1986). *Social foundations of thought and action: A social cognitive theory.* Englewood Cliffs, NJ: Prentice Hall.

Bandura, A. (1989). Social cognitive theory. *Annals of Child Development, 6,* 1-60.

Bandura, A. (1997). *Self-efficacy: The exercise of control.* New York: W. H. Freeman.

Bandura, A. (2000). Health promotion from the perspective of social cognitive theory. In P. Norman, C. Abraham, & M. Conner (Eds.), *Understanding and changing health behaviour: From health beliefs to self-regulation* (pp. 299-339). Amsterdam, The Netherlands: Harwood Academic.

Bandura, A., Caprara, G. V., Barbaranelli, C., Gerbino, M., & Pastorelli, C. (2003). Role of affective self-regulatory efficacy in diverse spheres of psychological functioning. *Child Development, 74,* 769-782.

Bandura, A., & Jourden, F. J. (1991). Self-regulatory mechanisms governing social comparison effects on complex decision making. *Journal of Personality and Social Psychology, 60,* 941-951.

Bandura, A., Pastorelli, C., Barbaranelli, C., & Caprara, G. V. (1999). Self-efficacy pathways to childhood depression. *Journal of Personality and Social Psychology, 76,* 258-269.

Banikarim, C., Chacko, M. R., Wiemann, C. M., & Smith, P. G. (2003). Gonorrhea and chlamydia screening among young women: Stage of change, decisional balance, and self-efficacy. *Journal of Adolescent Health, 32,* 288-295.

Baranowski, T., Perry, C. L., & Parcel, G. S. (1997). How individuals, environments, and health behavior interact: Social cognitive theory. In K. Glanz, F. M. Lewis, & B. K. Rimer (Eds.), *Health behavior and health education: Theory, research, and practice* (2nd ed., pp. 153-178). San Francisco: Jossey-Bass.

Barnum, B. J. (1990). *Nursing theory: Analysis, application, and evaluation* (3rd ed.). Boston: Little, Brown.

Bartholomew, L. K., Parcel, G. S., & Kok, G. (1998). Intervention mapping: A process for developing theory- and evidence-based health education programs. *Health Education and Behavior, 25*, 545-563.

Bartholomew, L. K., Parcel, G. S., Kok, G., & Gottlieb, N. H. (2001). *Intervention mapping: Designing theory- and evidence-based health promotion programs.* Mountain View, CA: Mayfield.

Bartman, B. A., Moy, E., & D'Angelo, L. J. (1997). Access to ambulatory care for adolescents: The role of a usual source of care. *Journal of Health Care for the Poor and Underserved, 8*, 214-226.

Barton, W. H., Powers, G. T., Morris, E. S., & Harrison, A. (2001). *Evaluating a comprehensive community initiative for children, youth, and families. Adolescent & Family Health, 2*(1), 27-36.

Basen-Engquist, K., Edmundson, E. W., & Parcel, G. S. (1996). Structure of health risk behavior among high school students. *Journal of Consulting and Clinical Psychology, 64*, 764-775.

Batten, M., & Oltjenbruns, K. A. (1999). Adolescent sibling bereavement as a catalyst for spiritual development: A model for understanding. *Death Studies, 23*, 529-546.

Beck, L., & Ajzen, I. (1991). Predicting dishonest actions using the theory of planned behaviour. *Journal of Research in Personality, 25*, 285-301.

Becker, H., Hendrickson, S. L., & Shaver, L. (1998). Nonurban parental beliefs about childhood injury and bicycle safety. *American Journal of Health Behavior, 22*, 218-227.

Becker, M. H. (1974). *The health belief model and personal health behavior.* Thorofare, NJ: Charles B. Slack.

Bell, C. C. (2001). Cultivating resiliency in youth. *Journal of Adolescent Health, 29*, 375-381.

Benard, B. (2000). Mentoring: New study shows the power of relationship to make a difference. In N. Henderson, B. Benard, & N. Sharp-Light (Eds.), *Mentoring for resiliency* (pp. 1-10). San Diego, CA: Resiliency in Action.

Benda, B. B. (2001). Conceptual model of assets and risks: Unlawful behavior among adolescents. *Adolescent and Family Health, 2*(3), 123-131.

Bennett, P., & Bozionelos, G. (2000). The theory of planned behaviour as predictor of condom use: A narrative review. *Psychology Health and Medicine, 5*, 307-326.

Benson, P. L., Donahue, M. S., & Erickson, J. A (1993). The Faith Maturity Scale: Conceptualization, measurement, and empirical validation. *Research in the Social Scientific Study of Religion, 5*, 1-26.

Benson, P. L., Leffert, N., Scales, P. C., & Blyth, D. A. (1998). Beyond the "village" rhetoric: Creating healthy communities for children and adolescents. *Applied Developmental Science, 2*, 138-159.

Benson, P. L., & Pittman, K. J. (2001). *Trends in youth development: Visions, realities, and challenges.* Boston: Kluwer.

Benson, P. L., & Saito, R. N. (2001). The scientific foundations of youth development. In P. L. Benson & K. J. Pittman (Eds.), *Trends in youth development: Visions, realities, and challenges* (pp. 135-154). Boston: Kluwer Academic.

Berbiglia, V. A. (1997). Orem's self-care deficit theory in nursing practice. In M. R. Alligood & A. Marriner-Tomey (Eds.), *Nursing theory: Utilization and application* (pp. 129-152). St. Louis, MO: Mosby.

Berzonsky, M. D. (1989). Identity style: Conceptualization and measurement. *Journal of Adolescent Research, 4,* 267-281.

Berzonsky, M. D. (1992). Identity style and coping strategies. *Journal of Personality, 60,* 771-788.

Berzonsky, M. D. (1993a). A constructivist view of identity formation: People as post-positivist self-theorists. In J. Kroger (Ed.), *Discussion on ego identity* (pp. 169-203). Hillsdale, NJ: Lawrence Erlbaum.

Berzonsky, M. D. (1993b). Identity style, gender, and social-cognitive reasoning. *Journal of Adolescent Research, 8,* 289-296.

Berzonsky, M. D. (1997). Identity development, control theory, and self-regulation: An individual differences perspective. *Journal of Adolescent Research, 12,* 347-353.

Berzonsky, M. D., & Adams, G. R. (1999). Reevaluating the identity status paradigm: Still useful after 35 years. *Developmental Review, 19,* 557-590.

Beyth-Marom, R., Austin, L., Fischhoff, B., Palmgren, C., & Jacobs-Quadrel, M. (1993). Perceived consequences of risky behaviors: Adults and adolescents. *Developmental Psychology, 29,* 549-563.

Blanton, H., Gibbons, F. X., Gerrard, M., Conger, K. J., & Smith, G. E. (1997). The role of family and peers in the development of prototypes associated with health risks. *Journal of Family Psychology, 11,* 271-288.

Bloom, R. (1956). *A taxonomy of educational objectives: Handbook 1 Cognitive domain.* New York: David McKay.

Blum, R. W., McNeely, C., & Nonnemaker, J. (2002). Vulnerability, risk, and protection. *Journal of Adolescent Health, 31*(1, Suppl.), 28-39.

Blyth, D. A., & Leffert, N. (1995). Communities as contexts for adolescent development: An empirical analysis. *Journal of Adolescent Research, 10*(1), 64-87.

Bodner, G., MacIsaac, D., & White, S. (1999). Action research: Overcoming the sports mentality approach to assessment/evaluation. *University Chemistry Education, 3*(1), 31-36.

Booth, R. E., & Zhang, Y. (1997). Conduct disorder and HIV risk behaviors among runaway and homeless adolescents. *Drug and Alcohol Dependence, 48*(2), 69-76.

Booth, R. E., Zhang, Y., & Kwiatkowski, C. E. (1999). The challenge of changing drug and sex risk behaviors of runaway and homeless adolescents. *Child Abuse and Neglect, 123,* 1295-1306.

Borowsky, I. W., Ireland, M., & Resnick, M. D. (2002). Violence risk and protective factors among youth held back in school. *Ambulatory Pediatrics, 2,* 475-484.

Bowlby, J. (1969). *Attachment and loss: Vol. 1 attachment.* New York: Basic Books.

Bowlby, J. (1973). *Attachment and loss: Vol. 2 separation.* New York: Basic Books.

Brener, N. D., & Collins, J. L. (1998). Co-occurrence of health-risk behaviors among adolescents in the United States. *Journal of Adolescent Health, 22,* 209-213.

Bretherton, I. (1991). Pouring new wine into old bottles: The social self as internal working model. In M. R. Gunnar & L. A. Sroufe (Eds.), *Self process and development: The Minnesota Symposia on Child Development* (Vol. 23, pp. 1-41). Hillsdale, NJ: Lawrence Erlbaum.

Brindis, C., Park, J., Ozer, E. M., & Irwin, C. E., Jr. (2002). Adolescents' access to health services and clinical preventive health care: Crossing the great divide. *Pediatric Annals, 31,* 575-581.

Broderick, P. C. (1998). Early adolescent gender differences in the use of ruminative and distracting coping strategies. *Journal of Early Adolescence, 18,* 173-191.

Bronfenbrenner, U. (1979). *The ecology of human development: Experiments by nature and design.* Cambridge, MA: Harvard University Press.

Bronfenbrenner, U. (1986a). Ecology of the family as a context for human development: Research perspectives. *Developmental Psychology, 22,* 732-744.

Bronfenbrenner, U. (1986b). Recent advances in research on the ecology of human development. In R. K. Silbereisen, K. Eyferth, & G. Rudinger (Eds.), *Development as action in context: Problem behavior and normal youth development* (pp. 287-309). New York: Springer.

Bronfenbrenner, U. (1989). Ecological systems theory. *Annals of Child Development, 6,* 187-249.

Bronfenbrenner, U., & Ceci, S. J. (1994). Nature-nurture reconceptualized in developmental perspective: A bioecological model. *Psychological Review, 20,* 568-586.

Bronfenbrenner, U., & Crouter, A. C. (1983). The evolution of environmental models in developmental research. In P. H. Mussen (Ed.), *Handbook of child psychology* (4th ed., pp. 357-414). San Francisco: Jossey-Bass.

Bronfenbrenner, U., & Evans, G. W. (2000). Developmental science in the 21st century: Emerging questions, theoretical models, research designs and empirical findings. *Social Development, 9*(1), 115-125.

Bronfenbrenner, U., McClelland, P., Wethington, E., Macu, P., & Ceci, S. J. (1996). *The state of Americans.* New York: Free Press.

Brooks, T. L., Harris, S. K., Thrall, J. S., & Woods, E. R. (2002). Association of adolescent risk behaviors with mental health symptoms in high school students. *Journal of Adolescent Health, 31,* 240-246.

Brooks-Gunn, J., Graber, J. A., Paikoff, R. L. (1994). Studying links between hormones and negative affect: Models and measures. *Journal of Research in Adolescence, 4,* 469-486.

Broome, M. E., Richards, D. J., & Hall, J. M. (2001). Children in research: The experience of ill children and adolescents. *Journal of Family Nursing, 7*(1), 32-49.

Brown, K. M. (1999). *Social cognitive theory.* Retrieved April 6, 2004, from http://www.med.usf.edu/~kmbrown/Social_Cognitive_Theory_Overview.htm

Brown, L. K., & Lourie, K. J. (2001). Motivational interviewing and the prevention of HIV among adolescents. In P. M. Monti, S. M. Colby, & T. O'Leary (Eds.), *Adolescents, alcohol, and substance abuse: Reaching teens through brief interventions* (pp. 244-274). New York: Guilford.

Brubaker, R. G., & Wickersham, D. (1990). Encouraging the practice of testicular self-examination: A field application of the theory of reasoned action. *Health Psychology, 9*(2), 154-163.

Bryan, A., Fisher, J. D., & Fisher, W. A. (2002). Tests of the mediational role of preparatory safer sexual behavior in the context of the theory of planned behavior. *Health Psychology, 21,* 71-80.

Bryan, A. D., Fisher, J. D., Fisher, W. A., & Murray, D. M. (2000). Understanding condom use among heroin addicts in methadone maintenance using the information-motivation-behavioral skills model. *Substance Use & Misuse, 35,* 451-471.

Burke, B. L., Arkowitz, H., & Dunn, C. (2002). The efficacy of motivational interviewing and its adaptations: What we know so far. In W. R. Miller & N. Heather (Eds.), *Treating addictive behaviors* (2nd ed., pp. 217-250). New York: Plenum.

Burke, P. J. (1991). Identity processes and social stress. *American Sociological Review, 56,* 836-849.

Burton, D. L., Miller, D. L., & Shill, C. T. (2002). A social learning theory comparison of the sexual victimization of adolescent sexual offenders and nonsexual offending male delinquents. *Child Abuse and Neglect, 26,* 893-907.

Bush, P. J., & Iannotti, R. J. (1990). A children's health belief model. *Medical Care, 28,* 69-86.

Bussey, K., & Bandura, A. (1999). Social cognitive theory of gender development and differentiation. *Psychological Review, 106,* 676-713.

Byrnes, J. P. (1998). *The nature and development of decision making: A self-regulation model.* Mahwah, NJ: Lawrence Erlbaum.

Byrnes, J. P. (2002). The development of decision-making. *Journal of Adolescent Health, 31,* 208-215.

Byrnes, J. P. (2003). Changing views on the nature and prevention of adolescent risk taking. In D. Romer (Ed.), *Reducing adolescent risk: Toward an integrated approach* (pp. 11-17). Thousand Oaks, CA: Sage.

Byrnes, J. P., Miller, D. C., & Reynolds, M. (1999). Learning to make good decisions: A self-regulation perspective. *Child Development, 70,* 1121-1140.

Cady, M. E., Winters, K. C., Jordan, D. A., Solberg, K. B., & Stinchfield, R. D. (1996). Motivation to change as a predictor of treatment outcome for adolescent substance abusers. *Journal of Child and Adolescent Substance Abuse, 5*(1), 73-91.

Caldwell, E. F. (2000). *Making a home for faith: Nurturing the spiritual life of your children.* Cleveland, OH: Pilgrim Press.

Caldwell, E. F. (2002). *Leaving home with faith: Nurturing the spiritual life of our youth.* Cleveland, OH: Pilgrim Press.

Call, K. T., Riedel, A. A., Hein, K., McLoyd, V., Petersen, A., & Kipke, M. (2002). Adolescent health and well-being in the twenty-first century: A global perspective. *Journal of Research on Adolescence, 12*(1), 69-88.

Calvert, W. J. (1997). Protective factors within the family, and their role in fostering resiliency in African American adolescents. *Journal of Cultural Diversity, 4,* 110-117.

Canty-Mitchell, J. (2001). Life change events, hope, and self-care agency in inner-city adolescents. *Journal of Child and Adolescent Psychiatric Nursing, 14*(1), 18-31.

Capaldi, D. M., Stoolmiller, M., Clark, S., & Owen, L. D. (2002). Heterosexual risk behaviors in at-risk young men from early adolescence to young adulthood: Prevalence, prediction, and association with STD contraction. *Developmental Psychology, 38,* 394-406.

Cargo, M., Grams, G. D., Ottoson, J. M., Ward, P., & Green, L. W. (2003). Empowerment as fostering positive youth development and citizenship. *American Journal of Health Behavior, 27*(Suppl. 1), S66-S79.

Carlson, E. A., Sroufe, L. A., Collins, W. A., Jimerson, S., Weinfield, N., Hennighausen, K., et al. (1999). Early environmental support and elementary school adjustment as predictors of school adjustment in middle adolescence. *Journal of Adolescent Research, 14*(1), 72-94.

Carvajal, S. C., Evans, R. I., Nash, S. G., & Getz, J. G. (2002). Global positive expectancies of the self and adolescents' substance use avoidance: Testing a social influence mediational model. *Journal of Personality, 70,* 421-442.

Cass, V. C. (1979). Homosexual identity formation: A theoretical model. *Journal of Homosexuality, 4,* 219-235.

Castro, F. G., Cota, M. K., & Vega, S. C. (1999). Health promotion in Latino populations: A sociocultural model for program planning, development, and evaluation. In R. M. Huff & M. V. Kline (Eds.), *Promoting health in multicultural populations: A handbook for practitioners* (pp. 137-168). Thousand Oaks, CA: Sage.

Cavendish, R., Luise, B. K., Bauer, M., Gallo, M. A., Horne, K., Medefindt, J., et al. (2001). Recognizing opportunities for spiritual enhancement in young adults. *Nursing Diagnosis, 12*(3), 77-91.

Center for Youth Development and Policy Research. (n.d.). *Mission, history, and goals.* Retrieved March 26, 2004, from http://cyd.aed.org/mission.html

Centers for Disease Control and Prevention. (2000). Youth risk behavior surveillance, 1999. *Morbidity and Mortality Weekly Report CDC Surveillance Summary, 49*(SS-5), 35-92.

Centers for Disease Control and Prevention. (2003a). *Adolescent and school health: Summary results, 2001 United States.* Retrieved June 21, 2003, from http://www.cdc.gov/nccdphp/dash/

Centers for Disease Control and Prevention. (2003b). *America's children: Key national indicators of well-being, 2002.* Retrieved June 21, 2003, from http://www.childstats.gov/ac2003/highlight.asp

Chambers, K. B., & Rew, L. (2003). Safer sexual decision making in adolescent women: Perspectives from the conflict theory of decision-making. *Issues in Comprehensive Pediatric Nursing, 26,* 129-143.

Chase, K. A., Treboux, D., & O'Leary, K. D. (2002). Characteristics of high-risk adolescents' dating violence. *Journal of Interpersonal Violence, 17*(1), 33-49.

Chassin, L., Pitts, S. C., DeLucia, C., & Todd, M. (1999). A longitudinal study of children of alcoholics: Predicting young adult substance use disorders, anxiety, and depression. *Journal of Abnormal Psychology, 108*(1), 106-119.

Chen, M., Wang, E. K., Yang, R., & Liou, Y. (2003). Adolescent Health Promotion Scale: Development and psychometric testing. *Public Health Nursing, 20,* 104-110.

Chewning, B., Douglas, J., Kokotailo, P. K., LaCourt, J., St. Clair, D., & Wilson, D. (2001). Protective factors associated with American Indian adolescents' safer sexual patterns. *Maternal and Child Health Journal, 5,* 273-280.

Christian, M. D., & Barbarin, O. A. (2001). Cultural resources and psychological adjustment of African American children: Effects of spirituality and racial attribution. *Journal of Black Psychology, 27*(1), 43-63.

Christian, B. J., D'Auria, J. P., & Fox, L. C. (1999). Gaining freedom: Self-responsibility in adolescents with diabetes. *Pediatric Nursing, 25,* 255-260.

Cicchetti, D., Rogosch, F. A., Lynch, M., & Holt, K. D. (1993). Resilience in maltreated children: Processes leading to adaptive outcome. *Development and Psychopathology, 5,* 629-647.

Clatts, M. D., Davis, W. R., Sotheran, J. L., & Atillasoy, A. (1998). Correlates and distribution of HIV risk behaviors among homeless youths in New York City: Implications for prevention and policy. *Child Welfare, 77,* 195-207.

Cohen, M. Z., Kahn, D. L., & Steeves, R. H. (2002). Making use of qualitative research. *Western Journal of Nursing Research, 24,* 454-471.

Cokkinides, V. E., Johnston-Davis, K., Weinstock, M., O'Connell, M. C., Kalsbeek, W., Thun, M. J., et al. (2001). Sun exposure and sun-protection behaviors and attitudes among U.S. youth, 11 to 18 years of age. *Preventive Medicine, 33,* 141-151.

Cokkinides, V. E., O'Connell, M. C., Thun, M. J., & Weinstock, M. A. (2002). Use of indoor tanning sunlamps by US youth, ages 11-18 years, and by their parent or guardian caregivers: Prevalence and correlates. *Pediatrics, 109,* 1124-1130.

Coles, R. (1986). *The moral life of children.* Boston: Houghton Mifflin.

Coles, R. (1990). *The spiritual life of children.* Boston: Houghton Mifflin.

Comeau, N., Stewart, S. H., & Loba, P. (2001). The relations of trait anxiety, anxiety sensitivity, and sensation seeking to adolescents' motivations for alcohol, cigarette, and marijuana use. *Addictive Behaviors, 26,* 803-825.

Conner, M., & Armitage, C. J. (1998). Extending the theory of planned behavior: A review and avenues for further research. *Journal of Applied Social Psychology, 28,* 1429-1464.

Conner, M., & Flesch, D. (2001). Having casual sex: Additive and interactive effects of alcohol and condom availability on the determinants of intentions. *Journal of Applied Social Psychology, 31,* 89-112.

Conner, M., & Norman, P. (1996). The role of social cognition in health behaviours. In M. Conner & P. Norman (Eds.), *Predicting health behavior: Research and practice with social cognition models* (pp. 1-21). Philadelphia: Open University Press.

Copeland, E. P., & Hess, R. S. (1995). Differences in young adolescents' coping strategies based on gender and ethnicity. *Journal of Early Adolescence, 15*(2), 203-219.

Coupey, S. M., Neinstein, L. S., & Zeltzer, L. K. (2002). Chronic illness in the adolescent. In L. S. Neinstein (Ed.), *Adolescent health care: A practical guide* (4th ed., pp. 1511-1536). Philadelphia: Lippincott Williams & Wilkins.

Crawford, M., & Rossiter, G. (1996). School education and the spiritual development of adolescents: An Australian perspective. In R. Best (Ed.), *Education, spirituality and the whole child* (pp. 305-318). New York: Cassell.

Crockett, L. J. (1999). Cultural, historical, and subcultural contexts of adolescence: Implications for health and development. In J. Schulenberg, J. L. Maggs, & K. Hurrelmann (Eds.), *Health risks and developmental transitions during adolescence* (pp. 23-53). Cambridge, England: Cambridge University Press.

Croll, J., Neumark-Sztainer, D., Story, M., & Ireland, M. (2002). Prevalence and risk and protective factors related to disordered eating behaviors among adolescents: Relationship to gender and ethnicity. *Journal of Adolescent Health, 31,* 166-175.

Crosby, R., DiClemente, R. J., Wingood, G. M., Sionean, C., Cobb, B. K., Harrington, K., et al. (2001). Correct condom application among African-American adolescent females: The relationship to perceived self-efficacy and the association to confirmed STDs. *Journal of Adolescent Health, 29,* 194-199.

Crowne, D., & Marlowe, D. (1964). *The approval motive.* New York: John Wiley.

Crumbaugh, J. (1968). Purpose-in-life test. *Journal of Individual Psychology, 24,* 74-81.

Cunningham, P. J., Hadley, J., & Reschovsky, J. D. (2002). The effects of SCHIP on children's health insurance coverage (Research Report No. 7). *Center for Studying Health System Change.* Retrieved April 6, 2004, from http://www.hschange.org/CONTENT/510/

Cusatis, D. C., & Shannon, B. M. (1996). Influences on adolescent eating behavior. *Journal of Adolescent Health, 18*(1), 27-34.

Dahl, R. E., & Lewin, D. S. (2002). Pathways to adolescent health: Sleep regulation and behavior. *Journal of Adolescent Health, 31*(6S), 175-184.

Deatrick, J. A., Angst, D. B., & Madden, M. (1998). Promoting self-care with adolescents. *Journal of Child and Family Nursing, 1,* 65-76.

Denyes, M. J. (1981). Development of an instrument to measure self-care agency in adolescents (Doctoral dissertation, University of Michigan, 1980). *Dissertation Abstracts International, 41,* 1716B.

Denyes, M. J. (1988). Orem's model used for health promotion: Directions from research. *Advances in Nursing Science, 11*(1), 13-21.

Denzin, N. K., & Lincoln, Y. S. (1998). *Strategies of qualitative inquiry.* Thousand Oaks, CA: Sage.

De Weert-Van Oene, G. H., Schippers, G. M., De Jong, C. A., & Schrijvers, G. A. (2002). Motivation for treatment in substance-dependent patients: Psychometric evaluation of the TCU motivation for treatment scales. *European Addiction Research, 8*(1), 2-9.

DiClemente, C. C., & Prochaska, J. O. (1998). Toward a comprehensive, transtheoretical model of change: Stages of change and addictive behaviors. In W. R. Miller & N. Heather (Eds.), *Treating addictive behaviors* (2nd ed., pp. 3-24). New York: Plenum.

DiClemente, C. C., & Velasquez, M. M. (2002). Motivational interviewing and the stages of change. In W. R. Miller & S. Rollnick (Eds.), *Motivational interviewing: Preparing people to change addictive behavior* (2nd ed., pp. 201-216). New York: Guilford.

DiClemente, R. J., Wingood, G. M., Crosby, R. A., Sionean, C., Brown, L. K., Rothbaum, B., et al. (2001). A prospective study of psychological distress and sexual risk behavior among Black adolescent females. *Pediatrics, 108,* 1-6.

DiIorio, C., Dudley, W. N., Soet, J., Watkins, J., & Maibach, E. (2000). A social cognitive-based model for condom use among college students. *Nursing Research, 49,* 208-214.

DiNapoli, P. P., & Murphy, D. (2002). The marginalization of chronically ill adolescents. *Nursing Clinics of North America, 37,* 565-572.

Donaghue, K. C., Fairchild, J. M., Craig, M. E., Chan, A. K., Hing, S., Cutler, L. R., et al. (2003). Do all prepubertal years of diabetes duration contribute equally to diabetes complications? *Diabetes Care, 26,* 1224-1229.

Donahue, M. J., & Benson, P. L. (1995). Religion and the well-being of adolescents. *Society for the Psychological Study of Social Issues, 51*(2), 145-160.

Donovan, J. E., & Jessor, R. (1985). Structure of problem behavior in adolescence and young adulthood. *Journal of Consulting and Clinical Psychology, 53,* 890-904.

Donovan, J. E., Jessor, R., & Costa, F. M. (1988). Syndrome of problem behavior in adolescence: A replication. *Journal of Consulting and Clinical Psychology, 56,* 762-765.

Donovan, R. J. (1995). Steps in planning and developing health communication campaigns: A comment on CDC's framework for health communication. *Public Health Reports, 110*(2), 215-218.

Doswell, W. M., Millor, G. K., Thompson, H., & Braxter, B. (1998). Self-image and self-esteem in African-American preteen girls: Implications for mental health. *Issues in Mental Health Nursing, 19,* 71-94.

Dowling, J. S., & Fain, J. A. (1999). A multidimensional sense of humor scale for school-aged children: Issues of reliability and validity. *Journal of Pediatric Nursing, 14*(1), 38-43.

Dozois, D. N., Farrow, J. A., & Miser, A. (1995). Smoking patterns and cessation motivations during adolescence. *International Journal of the Addictions, 30,* 1485-1498.

Dryfoos, J. G. (1992). Adolescents at risk: A summary of work in the field—programs and policies. In D. E. Rogers & E. Ginzberg (Eds.), *Adolescents at risk: Medical and social perspectives* (pp. 128-141). Boulder, CO: Westview.

Dunn, C., Deroo, L., & Rivara, F. P. (2001). The use of brief interventions adapted from motivational interviewing across behavioral domains: A systematic review. *Addiction, 96,* 1725-1742.

Dunn, D. A., & Johnson, J. L. (2001). Choosing to remain smoke-free: The experiences of adolescent girls. *Journal of Adolescent Health, 29,* 289-297.

DuRant, R. H., Barkin, S., & Krowchuk, D. P. (2001). Evaluation of a peaceful conflict resolution and violence prevention curriculum for sixth-grade students. *Journal of Adolescent Health, 28,* 386-393.

DuRant, R. H., & Smith, K. S. (2002). Vital statistics and injuries. In L. S. Neinstein (Eds.), *Adolescent health care: A practical guide* (4th ed., pp. 126-169). Philadelphia: Lippincott Williams & Wilkins.

Ebin, V. J., Sneed, C. D., Morisky, D. E., Rotheram-Borus, M. J., Magnusson, A. M., & Malotte, C. K. (2001). Acculturation and interrelationships between problem and health-promoting behaviors among Latino adolescents. *Journal of Adolescent Health, 28,* 62-72.

Eggert, L. L., Thompson, E. A., Randell, B. P., & Pike, K. C. (2002). Preliminary effects of brief school-based prevention approaches for reducing youth suicide: Risk behaviors, depression, and drug involvement. *Journal of Child and Adolescent Psychiatric Nursing, 15,* 48-64.

Eidem, B. W., Cetta, F., Webb, J. L., Graham, L. C., & Jay, S. (2001). Early detection of cardiac dysfunction: Use of the myocardial performance index in patients with anorexia nervosa. *Journal of Adolescent Health, 29,* 267-270.

Elford, K. J., & Spence, J. E. H. (2002). The forgotten female: Pediatric and adolescent gynecological concerns and their reproductive consequences. *Journal of Pediatric and Adolescent Gynecology, 15,* 65-77.

Elias, M. J., & Kress, J. S. (1994). Social decision-making and life skills development: A critical thinking approach to health promotion in the middle school. *Journal of School Health, 64,* 62-66.

Elixhauser, A., Machlin, S. R., Zoder, M. W., Chevarley, F. M., Parel, N., McCormick, M. C., et al. (2002). Health care for children and youth in the United States: 2001 annual report on access, utilization, quality, and expenditures. *Ambulatory Pediatrics, 2,* 419-437.

Ellis, N. T., & Torabi, M. R. (1994). Prevalence of adolescent health risk behaviors: School health implications. *Journal of School Nursing, 10*(4), 25-33.

Ellis, R. (1968). Characteristics of significant theories. *Nursing Research, 17*(3), 217-222.

Erikson, E. (1963). *Childhood and society.* New York: Norton.

Erikson, E. (1968). *Identity: Youth and crisis.* New York: Norton.

Erikson, E. H. (1980). *Identity and the life cycle.* New York: Norton.

Estabrooks, C. A.., Field, P. A.. & Morse, J. M. (1994). Aggregating qualitative findings: An approach to theory development. *Qualitative Health Research, 4,* 503-511.

Evans, A. E., Edmundson-Drane, E. W., & Harris, K. K. (2000). Computer-assisted instruction: An effective instructional method for HIV prevention education? *Journal of Adolescent Health, 26,* 244-251.

Evans, D., & Norman, P. (1998). Understanding pedestrians' road crossing decisions: An application of the theory of planned behaviour. *Health Education Research, Theory and Practice, 13,* 481-489.

Farmer, E. M. Z., Burns, B. J., Phillips, S. D., Angold, A., & Costello, E. J. (2003). Pathways into and through mental health services for children and adolescents. *Psychiatric Services, 54*(1), 60-66.

Farrell, M. P., Barnes, G. M., & Banerjee, S. (1995). Family cohesion as a buffer against the effects of problem-drinking fathers on psychological distress, deviant behavior, and heavy drinking in adolescents. *Journal of Health and Social Behavior, 36,* 377-385.

Faulkner, S. L. (2003). Good girl or flirt girl: Latinas' definitions of sex and sexual relationships. *Hispanic Journal of Behavioral Sciences, 25,* 174-200.

Fawcett, J., Watson, J., Neuman, B., Walker, P. H., & Fitzpatrick, J. J. (2001). On nursing theories and evidence. *Journal of Nursing Scholarship, 33,* 115-119.

Fawcett, S. B. (1995). Using empowerment theory in collaborative partnerships for community health and development. *American Journal of Community Psychology, 23,* 677-698.

Federal Interagency Forum on Child and Family Statistics. *2002 America's children: Key national indicators of well-being.* Washington, DC: U.S. Government Printing Office.

Fehring, R. J., Brennan, P. F., & Keller, M. L. (1987). Psychological and spiritual well-being in college students. *Research in Nursing and Health, 10,* 391-398.

Feldman, S. S., Fisher, L., Ransom, D. C., & Dimiceli, S. (1995). Is "what is good for the goose good for the gander"? Sex differences in relations between adolescent coping and adult adaptation. *Journal of Research on Adolescence, 5,* 333-359.

Fibel, B., & Hale, W. D. (1978). The Generalized Expectancy for Success Scale: A new measure. *Journal of Consulting and Clinical Psychology, 46,* 924-931.

Fishbein, M., & Ajzen, I. (1975). *Belief, attitude, intention, and behavior: An introduction to theory and research.* Reading, MA: Addison-Wesley.

Fisher, J. D., Fisher, W. A., Misovich, S. J., Kimble, D. L., & Malloy, T. E. (1996). Changing AIDS risk behavior: Effects of an intervention emphasizing AIDS risk reduction information, motivation, and behavioral skills in a college student population. *Health Psychology, 15,* 114-123.

Fisher, J. D., Fisher, W. A., Williams, S. S., & Malloy, T. E. (1994). Empirical tests of an information-motivation-behavioral skills model of AIDS-preventive behavior with gay men and heterosexual university students. *Health Psychology, 13,* 238-250.

Fisher, J. D., & Fisher, W. A. (2002). The information-motivation-behavioral skills model. In R. J. DiClemente, R. A. Crosby, & M. C. Kegler (Eds.), *Emerging theories in health promotion practice and research: Strategies for improving public health* (pp. 40-70). San Francisco: Jossey-Bass.

Flaskerud, J. H., & Winslow, B. J. (1998). Conceptualizing vulnerable populations' health-related research. *Nursing Research, 47,* 69-78.

Floyd, F. J., & Stein, T. S. (2002). Sexual orientation identity formation among gay, lesbian, and bisexual youths: Multiple patterns of milestone experiences. *Journal of Research on Adolescence, 12,* 167-191.

Folkman, S., Chesney, M., McKusick, L., Ironson, G., Johnson, D. S., & Coates, T. J. (1991). Translating coping theory into an intervention. In J. Eckenrode (Ed.), *The social context of coping* (pp. 239-260). New York: Plenum.

Folkman, S., Chesney, M. A., Pollack, L., & Phillips, C. (1992). Stress, coping, and high-risk sexual behavior. *Health Psychology, 11*(4), 218-222.

Folkman, S., & Lazarus, R. S. (1985). If it changes it must be a process: Study of emotion and coping during three stages of a college examination. *Journal of Personality and Social Psychology, 48,* 150-170.

Fortenberry, J. D., McFarlane, M., Bleakley, A., Bull, S., Fishbein, M., Grimley, D. M., et al. (2002). Relationships of stigma and shame to gonorrhea and HIV screening. *American Journal of Public Health, 92,* 378-381.

Fowler, J. W. (1991). Stages in faith consciousness. In F. K. Oser & W. G. Scarlett (Eds.), *New directions for child development: Religious development in child-hood and adolescence* (pp. 27-45). New York: Jossey-Bass.

Frankish, C. J., Lovato, C. Y., & Shannon, W. J. (1999). Models, theories, and principles of health promotion with multicultural populations. In R. M. Huff & M. V. Kline (Eds.), *Promoting health in multicultural populations: A handbook for practitioners* (pp. 41-72). Thousand Oaks, CA: Sage.

Frankl, V. (1978). *The unheard cry for meaning: Psychotherapy and humanism.* New York: Simon and Schuster.

French, S. A., Leffert, N., Story, M., Neumark-Sztainer, D., Hannan, P., & Benson, P. L. (2001). Adolescent binge/purge and weight loss behaviors: Associations with developmental assets. *Journal of Adolescent Health, 28,* 211-221.

Frenn, M., Malin, S., & Bansal, N. K. (2003). Stage-based interventions for low-fat diet with middle school students. *Journal of Pediatric Nursing, 18*(1), 36-45.

Frey, M. A., & Denyes, M. J. (1989). Health and illness self-care in adolescents with IDDM: A test of Orem's theory. *Advances in Nursing Science, 12*(1), 67-75.

Frey, M. A., & Fox, M. A. (1990). Assessing and teaching self-care to youths with diabetes mellitus. *Pediatric Nursing, 16,* 597-599.

Friedman, A. S., Granick, S., & Kreisher, C. (1994). Motivation of adolescent drug abusers for help and treatment. *Journal of Child and Adolescent Substance Abuse, 3*(1), 69-88.

Friedman, I. A. (1996). Deliberation and resolution in decision-making processes: A self-report scale for adolescents. *Educational and Psychological Measurement, 56,* 881-890.

Friis, R. H., & Sellers, T. A. (1996). *Epidemiology for public health practice.* Gaithersburg, MD: Aspen.

Fry, S. T. (1995). Science as problem solving. In A. Omery, C. E. Kasper, & G. G. Page (Eds.), *In search of nursing science* (pp. 72-80). Thousand Oaks, CA: Sage.

Frydenberg, E., & Lewis, R. (1991). Adolescent coping: The different ways in which boys and girls cope. *Journal of Adolescence, 14,* 119-133.

Frydenberg, E., & Lewis, R. (1993a). *Adolescent Coping Scale: Administrator's manual* (Research ed.). Melbourne: Australian Council for Educational Research.

Frydenberg, E., & Lewis, R. (1993b). Boys play sport and girls turn to others: Age, gender and ethnicity as determinants of coping. *Journal of Adolescence, 16,* 253-266.

Fulkerson, J. A., & French, S. A. (2003). Cigarette smoking for weight loss or control among adolescents: Gender and racial/ethnic differences. *Journal of Adolescent Health, 32,* 306-313.

Gagné, R. M. (1965). *The conditions of learning.* New York: Holt, Rinehart, & Winston.

Galetta, F., Franzoni, F., Prattichizzo, F., Rolla, M., Santoro, G., & Pentimone, F. (2003). Heart rate variability and left ventricular diastolic function in anorexia nervosa. *Journal of Adolescent Health, 32,* 416-421.

Garbarino, J., Bradshaw, C. P., & Vorrasi, J. A. (2002). Mitigating the effects of gun violence on children and youth. *Future of Children, 12*(2), 73-78.

Garmezy, N. (1971). Vulnerability research and the issue of primary prevention. *American Journal of Orthopsychiatry, 42,* 101-116.

Garmezy, N. (1985). Stress-resistant children: The search for protective factors. In J. E. Stevenson (Eds.), *Recent research in developmental psychopathology (Journal of Child Psychology and Psychiatry* book supplement no. 4, pp. 213-233). Oxford, England: Pergamon.

Garmezy, N. (1987). Stress, competence, and development: Continuities in the study of schizophrenic adults, children vulnerable to psychopathology, and the search for stress-resistant children. *American Journal of Orthopsychiatry, 57,* 159-174.

Garmezy, N. (1991). Resiliency and vulnerability to adverse developmental outcomes associated with poverty. *American Behavioral Scientist, 34,* 416-430.

Garmezy, N., & Masten, A. S. (1991). The protective role of competence indicators in children at risk. In E. M. Cummings, A. L. Greene, & K. H. Karrakei (Eds.), *Perspectives on stress and coping* (pp. 151-174). Hillsdale, NJ: Lawrence Erlbaum.

Garmezy, N., Masten, A. S., & Tellegen, A. (1984). The study of stress and competence in children: A building block of developmental psychopathology. *Child Development, 55,* 97-111.

Garmezy, N., & Nuechterlein, K. (1972). Invulnerable children: The fact and fiction of competence and disadvantage. *American Journal of Orthopsychiatry, 42,* 328-239.

Gavin, L. E., Black, M. M., Minor, S., Abel, Y., Papas, M. A., & Bentley, M. E. (2002). Young, disadvantaged fathers' involvement with their infants: An ecological perspective. *Journal of Adolescent Health, 31,* 266-276.

Ge, X., Conger, R. D., & Elder, G. H., Jr. (2001). The relation between puberty and psychological distress in adolescent boys. *Journal of Research on Adolescence, 11*(1), 49-70.

Gerber, R. W., Newman, I. M., & Martin, G. L. (1988). Applying the theory of reasoned action to early adolescent tobacco chewing. *Journal of School Health, 58,* 410-413.

Gibbons, F. X., & Gerrard, M. (1995). Predicting young adults' health-risk behavior. *Journal of Personality and Social Psychology, 69,* 505-517.

Gibbons, F. X., Gerrard, M., Blanton, H., & Russell, D. W. (1998). Reasoned action and social reaction: Willingness and intention as independent predictors of health risk. *Journal of Personality and Social Psychology, 74,* 1164-1180.

Gibbons, F. X., Gerrard, M., Ouelette, J., & Burzette, B. (1998). Cognitive antecedents to adolescent health risk: Discriminating between behavioral intention and behavioral willingness. *Psychology and Health, 13,* 319-340.

Gil, A. G., Vega, W. A., & Turner, R. J. (2002). Early and mid-adolescence risk factors for later substance abuse by African Americans and European Americans. *Public Health Reports, 117*(Suppl. 1), S15-S29.

Gilligan, C. (1993). *In a different voice.* Cambridge, MA: Harvard University Press.

Gillis, A. J. (1997). The Adolescent Lifestyle Questionnaire: Development and psychometric testing. *Canadian Journal of Nursing Research, 29*(1), 29-46.

Ginsburg, J. I. D., Mann, R. E., Rotgers, F., & Weekes, J. R. (2002). Motivational interviewing with criminal justice populations. In W. R. Miller & S. Rollnick (Eds.), *Motivational interviewing: Preparing people to change addictive behavior* (2nd ed., pp. 333-346). New York: Guilford.

Ginsburg, K., Menapace, A., & Slap, G. (1997). Factors affecting the decision to seek health care: The voice of adolescents. *Pediatrics, 100*, 922-930.

Glanz, K., Lewis, F. M., & Rimer, B. K. (Eds.). (1997). *Health behavior and health education: Theory, research, and practice* (2nd ed.). San Francisco: Jossey-Bass.

Glaser, B., & Strauss, A. (1967). *The discovery of grounded theory: Strategies for qualitative research.* Chicago: Aldine.

Goldberg, P. (1983). *The intuitive edge.* Los Angeles: Jeremy P. Tarcher.

Gonzales, R., & Padilla, A. M. (1997). The academic resilience of Mexican American high school students. *Hispanic Journal of Behavioral Sciences, 19*, 301-317.

Graber, J. A., Brooks-Gunn, J., & Galen, B. R. (1998). Betwixt and between: Sexuality in the context of adolescent transitions. In R. Jessor (Ed.), *New perspectives on adolescent risk behavior* (pp. 270-316). Cambridge, England: Cambridge University Press.

Graber, J. A., Lewinsohn, P. M., Seeley, J. R., & Brooks-Gunn, J. (1997). Is psychopathology associated with timing of pubertal development? *Journal of the American Academy of Child and Adolescent Psychiatry, 36*, 1768-1776.

Green, L. W. (1999). Health education's contributions to public health in the twentieth-century: A glimpse through health promotion's rear-view mirror. *Annual Review of Public Health, 20*, 67-88.

Green, L. W., & Kreuter, M. W. (1980). *Health promotion planning* (2nd ed.). Mountain View, CA: Mayfield.

Green, L. W., & Kreuter, M. W. (1999). *Health promotion planning: An educational and ecological approach* (3rd ed.). Mountain View, CA: Mayfield.

Green, L. W., Poland, B. D., & Rootman, I. (2000). The settings approach to health promotion. In B. D. Poland, L. W. Green, & I. Rootman (Eds.), *Settings for health promotion: Linking theory and practice* (pp. 1-43). Thousand Oaks, CA: Sage.

Greig, R. (2003). Ethnic identity development: Implications for mental health in African-American and Hispanic adolescents. *Issues in Mental health Nursing, 24*, 317-331.

Gross, D., & Conrad, B. (1995). Temperament in toddlerhood. *Journal of Pediatric Nursing, 10*, 146-151.

Grotevant, H. D. (1987). Toward a process model of identity formation. *Journal of Adolescent Research, 2*, 175-182.

Grotevant, H. D. (1992). Assigned and chosen identity components: A process perspective on their integration. In G. R. Adams, T. P. Gullotta, & R. Montemayor (Eds.), *Adolescent identity formation* (pp. 73-90). Newbury Park, CA: Sage.

Grotevant, H. D. (1997). Identity processes: Integrating social psychological and developmental processes. *Journal of Adolescent Research, 12*, 354-357.

Grunbaum, J. A., Lowry, R., & Kann, L. (2001). Prevalence of health-related behaviors among alternative high school students as compared with students attending regular high schools. *Journal of Adolescent Health, 29*, 337-343.

Guo, J., Chung, I. J., Hill, K. G., Hawkins, J. D., Catalano, R. F., & Abbott, R. D. (2002). Developmental relationships between adolescent substance use and risky sexual behavior in young adulthood. *Journal of Adolescent Health, 31,* 354-362.

Gurian, M. (1998). *A fine young man: What parents, mentors, and educators can do to shape adolescent boys into exceptional men.* New York: Jeremy P. Tarcher/ Putnam.

Hagger, M. S., Chatzisarantis, N., & Biddle, S. J. H. (2001). The influence of self-efficacy and past behaviour on the physical activity intentions of young people. *Journal of Sports Sciences, 19,* 711-725.

Halpern-Felsher, B. L., & Cauffman, E. (2001). Costs and benefits of a decision: Decision-making competence in adolescents and adults. *Journal of Applied Developmental Psychology, 22,* 257-273.

Hampson, S. E., Glasgow, R. E., & Toobert, D. J. (1990). Personal models of diabetes and their relations to self-care activities. *Health Psychology, 9,* 632-646.

Handmaker, N., Packard, M., & Conforti, K. (2002). Motivational interviewing in the treatment of dual disorders. In W. R. Miller & S. Rollnick (Eds.), *Motivational interviewing: Preparing people to change addictive behavior* (2nd ed., pp. 362-376). New York: Guilford.

Hankins, M., French, D., & Horne, R. (2000). Statistical guidelines for studies of the theory of reasoned action and the theory of planned behaviour. *Psychology and Health, 15,* 151-161.

Hardin, S. B., Carbaugh, L., Weinrich, S., Pesut, D., & Carbaugh, C. (1992). Stressors and coping in adolescents exposed to Hurricane Hugo. *Issues in Mental Health Nursing, 13,* 191-205.

Hardin, S. B., Weinrich, S., Weinrich, M., Garrison, C., Addy, C., & Hardin, T. (2002). Effects of a long-term psychosocial nursing intervention on adolescents exposed to catastrophic stress. *Issues in Mental Health Nursing, 23,* 537-551.

Hardy, M. E. (1997). Perspectives on nursing theory. In L. H. Nicoll (Ed.). *Perspectives on nursing theory* (3rd ed.), (pp. 89-100). Philadelphia: Lippincott.

Harrell, J. S., Bangdiwala, S. I., Deng, S., Webb, J. P., & Bradley, C. (1998). Smoking initiation in youth: The roles of gender, race, socioeconomics, and developmental status. *Journal of Adolescent Health, 23,* 271-279.

Harrison, T. W. (2003). Adolescent homosexuality and concerns regarding disclosure. *Journal of School Health, 73,* 107-112.

Harter, S. (1983). Developmental perspectives on the self-system. In P. Mussen & E. M. Hetherington (Eds.), *Handbook of child psychology: Vol. 4. Socialization personality, and social development* (4th ed., pp. 275-385). New York: John Wiley.

Harter, S. (1988). *The self-perception profile for adolescents.* Unpublished manuscript, University of Denver, Denver, CO.

Harter, S. (1999). *The construction of the self.* New York: Guilford.

Hausenblas, H. A., Nigg, C. R., Downs, D. S., Fleming, D. S., & Connaughton, D. P. (2002). Perceptions of exercise stages, barrier self-efficacy, and decisional balance for middle-level school students. *Journal of Early Adolescence, 22,* 436-454.

Hauser, S. T. (1999). Understanding resilient outcomes: Adolescent lives across time and generations. *Journal of Research on Adolescence, 9*(1), 1-24.

Hawkins, J. D., Catalano, R. F., Kosterman, R., Abbott, R., & Hill, K. G. (1999). Preventing adolescent health-risk behaviors by strengthening protection during childhood. *Archives of Pediatric and Adolescent Medicine, 153,* 226-234.

Hawthorne, D. J. (2002). Symbols of menarche identified by African American females. *Western Journal of Nursing Research, 24,* 484-501.

Heath, E. M., & Coleman, K. J. (2003). Adoption and institutionalization of the Child and Adolescent Trial for Cardiovascular Health (CATCH) in El Paso, Texas. *Health Promotion Practice, 4,* 157-164.

Heatherton, T. F., & Baumeister, R. F. (1996). Self-regulation failure: Past, present, and future. *Psychological Inquiry, 7*(1), 90-98.

Heidegger, M. (1962). *Being and time.* San Francisco: Harper & Row.

Heidegger, M. (1966). *Discourse on thinking.* New York: Harper and Row.

Heidegger, M. (1972). *On time and being.* San Francisco: Harper & Row.

Heller, S. S., Larrieu, J. A., D'Imperio, R., & Boris, N. W. (1999). Research on resilience to child maltreatment: Empirical considerations. *Child Abuse and Neglect, 23,* 321-338.

Helson, H. (1964). *Adaptation level theory: An experimental and systematic approach to behavior.* New York: Harper & Row.

Hempel, C. G. (1966). *Philosophy of natural science.* Englewood Cliffs, NJ: Prentice Hall.

Henderson, A., Champlin, S., & Evashwick, W. (1998). *Promoting teen health: Linking schools, health organizations, and community.* Thousand Oaks, CA: Sage.

Henderson, N., & Milstein, M. M. (2003). *Resiliency in schools.* Thousand Oaks, CA: Sage.

Herrenkohl, E. C., Herrenkohl, R. C., & Egolf, B. (1994). Resilient early school-age children from maltreating homes: Outcomes in late adolescence. *American Journal of Orthopsychiatry, 64,* 301-309.

Hobfoll, S. E., & Schumm, J. A. (2002). Conservation of resources theory: Application to public health promotion. In R. J. DiClemente, R. A. Crosby, & M. C. Kegler (Eds.), *Emerging theories in health promotion practice and research: Strategies for improving public health* (pp. 285-312). San Francisco: Jossey-Bass.

Hochbaum, G. M. (1958). *Public participation in a medical screening program: A socio-psychological study* (PHS Publication no. 572). Washington, DC: Government Printing Office.

Hock-Long, L., Herceg-Baron, R., Cassidy, A. M., & Whittaker, P. G. (2003). Access to adolescent reproductive health services: Financial and structural barriers to care. *Perspectives on Sexual and Reproductive Health, 35,* 144-147.

Hodge, D. R., Cardenas, P., & Montoya, H. (2001). Substance use: Spirituality and religious participation as protective factors among rural youths. *Social Work Research, 25,* 153-161.

Holahan, C. J., Valentiner, D. P., & Moos, R. H. (1995). Parental support, coping strategies, and psychological adjustment: An integrative model with late adolescents. *Journal of Youth and Adolescence, 24,* 633-648.

Huff, R. M. & Kline, M. V. (1999a). The cultural assessment framework. In R. M. Huff & M. V. Kline (Eds.), *Promoting health in multicultural populations: A handbook for practitioners* (pp. 481-499). Thousand Oaks, CA: Sage.

Huff, R. M., & Kline, M. V. (1999b). Health promotion in the context of culture. In R. M. Huff & M. V. Kline (Eds.), *Promoting health in multicultural populations: A handbook for practitioners* (pp. 3-22). Thousand Oaks, CA: Sage.

Hulton, L. J. (2001, October 3). Adolescent sexual decision-making: An integrative review. *Online Journal of Knowledge Synthesis for Nursing, 8*(4), 1-13. Retrieved April 6, 2004, from http://www.stti.iupui.edu/library/ojksn/case_study/ 080004 .htm

Humberside Partnership. (n.d.). *The Adolescent Coping Scale.* Retrieved March 29, 2004, from http://www.getting-on.co.uk/toolkit/acs.html

Hunter, A. J., & Chandler, G. E. (1999). Adolescent resilience. *Image: Journal of Nursing Scholarship, 31,* 243-247.

Institute of Medicine. (2001). *Health and behavior: The interplay of biological, behavioral, and societal influences.* Washington, DC: National Academy Press.

Jacobson, K. C., & Crockett, L. J. (2000). Parental monitoring and adolescent adjustment: An ecological perspective. *Journal of Research on Adolescence, 10*(1), 65-97.

Jalowiec, A. (2003). The Jalowiec Coping Scale. In O. L. Strickland & C. DiIorio (Eds.), *Measurement of nursing outcomes* (2nd ed., pp. 71-87). New York: Springer.

James, W. (1950). *The principles of psychology* (Vol. 1). New York: Dover.

Janis, I., & Mann, L. (1977). *Decision making.* New York: Free Press.

Janz, N. K., & Becker, M. H. (1984). The health belief model: A decade later. *Health Education Quarterly, 11*(1), 1-47.

Jelalian, E., Alday, S., Spirito, A., Rasile, D., & Nobile, C. (2000). Adolescent motor vehicle crashes: The relationship between behavioral factors and self-reported injury. *Journal of Adolescent Health, 27,* 84-93.

Jessor, R. (1982, May). Problem behavior and developmental transition in adolescence. *Journal of School Health, 56,* 295-300.

Jessor, R. (1987). Risky driving and adolescent problem behavior: An extension of problem-behavior theory. *Alcohol, Drugs, and Driving, 3*(3-4), 1-11.

Jessor, R. (1991). Risk behavior in adolescence: A psychosocial framework for understanding and action. *Journal of Adolescent Health, 12,* 597-605.

Jessor, R. (1992). Risk behavior in adolescence: A psychosocial framework for understanding and action. In D. E. Rogers & E. Ginzberg (Eds.), *Adolescents at risk: Medical and social perspectives* (pp. 19-34). Boulder, CO: Westview.

Jessor, R. (1998). *New perspectives on adolescent risk behavior.* Cambridge, England: Cambridge University Press.

Jessor, R., & Jessor, S. L. (1977). *Problem behavior and psychosocial development: A longitudinal study of youth.* New York: Academic Press.

Jessor, R., Turbin, M. S., & Costa, F. M. (1998). Protective factors in adolescent health behavior. *Journal of Personality and Social Psychology, 75,* 788-800.

Jessor, R., Van Den Bos, J., Vanderryn, J., Costa, F. M., & Turbin, M. S. (1995). Protective factors in adolescent problem behavior: Moderator effects and developmental change. *Developmental Psychology, 31,* 923-933.

Johnson, J. L. (2000). The health care institution as a setting for health promotion. In B. D. Poland, L. W. Green, & I. Rootman (Eds.), *Settings for health promotion: Linking theory and practice* (pp. 175-199). Thousand Oaks, CA: Sage.

Johnston, L. D. (2003). Alcohol and illicit drugs: The role of risk perceptions. In D. Romer (Ed.), *Reducing adolescent risk: Toward an integrated approach* (pp. 56-74). Thousand Oaks, CA: Sage.

Josselson, R. (1994). The theory of identity development and the question of intervention: An introduction. In S. L. Archer (Ed.), *Interventions for adolescent identity development* (pp. 12-25). Thousand Oaks, CA: Sage.

Kalnins, I. (2000). Commentary on homes and families as health promotion settings. In B. D. Poland, L. W. Green, & I. Rootman (Eds.), *Settings for health promotion: Linking theory and practice* (pp. 76-85). Thousand Oaks, CA: Sage.

Kann, L., Warren, C. W., Harris, W. A., Collins, J. L., Douglas, K. A., Collins, M. E., et al. (1995). Youth risk behavior surveillance: United States, 1993. *Journal of School Health, 65,* 162-171.

Kass, J. D., Friedman, R., Leserman, J., Zuttermeister, P. C., & Benson, H. (1991). Health outcomes and a new index of spiritual experience. *Journal for the Scientific Study of Religion, 30*(2), 203-211.

Kerlinger, F. N. (1973). *Foundations of behavioral research* (2nd ed.). New York: Holt, Rinehart and Winston.

Kerpelman, J. L., & Lamke, L. K. (1997). Anticipation of future identities: A control theory approach to identity development within the context of serious dating relationships. *Personal Relationships, 4,* 47-62.

Kerpelman, J. L., Pittman, J. F., & Lamke, L. K. (1997a). Revisiting the identity control theory approach: A rejoinder. *Journal of Adolescent Research, 12,* 363-371.

Kerpelman, J. L., Pittman, J. F., & Lamke, L. K. (1997b). Toward a microprocess perspective on adolescent identity development: An identity control theory approach. *Journal of Adolescent Research, 12,* 325-346.

Kerpelman, J. L., & Smith, S. L. (1999). Adjudicated adolescent girls and their mothers: Examining identity perceptions and processes. *Youth and Society, 30,* 313-347.

Kerr, M. H., Beck, K., Shattuck, T. D., Kattar, C., & Uriburu, D. (2003). Family involvement, problem and prosocial behavior outcomes of Latino youth. *American Journal of Health Behavior, 27*(Suppl. 1), S55-S65.

Kibble, D. G. (1996). Spiritual development, spiritual experience and spiritual education. In R. Best (Ed.), *Education, spirituality and the whole child* (pp. 64-74). New York: Cassell.

Kidd, S. A., & Kral, M. J. (2002). Suicide and prostitution among street youth: A qualitative analysis. *Adolescence, 37,* 411-431.

Klohnen, E. C. (1996). Conceptual analysis and measurement of the construct of ego-resiliency. *Journal of Personality and Social Psychology, 70*(5), 1067-1079.

Kobus, K., & Reyes, O. (2000). A descriptive study of urban Mexican American adolescents' perceived stress and coping. *Hispanic Journal of Behavioral Sciences, 22,* 163-178.

Kocovski, N. L., & Endler, N. S. (2000). Self-regulation: Social anxiety and depression. *Journal of Applied Biobehavioral Research, 5*(1), 80-91.

Kohlberg, L. (1963a). The development of children's orientations toward a moral order: Sequence in the development of moral thought. *Vita Humana, 6,* 11-33.

Kohlberg, L. (1963b). Moral development and identification. In H. Stevenson (Ed.), *Child psychology. 62nd yearbook of the National Society for the Study of Education* (pp. 277-332). Chicago: University of Chicago Press.

Kohlberg, L. (1978). Revisions in the theory and practice of moral development. *New Directions for Child Development, 2,* 83-88.

Krueger, R. A. (1998). Analyzing and reporting focus group results. In D. Morgan & R. A. Krueger (Eds.), *The focus group kit.* Thousand Oaks, CA: Sage.

Krueger, R. A. (2000). *Focus groups: A practical guide for applied research* (3rd ed.). Thousand Oaks, CA: Sage.

Kreuter, M. W., & Lezin, N. (2002). Social capital theory: Implications for community-based health promotion. In R. J. DiClemente, R. A. Crosby, & M. C. Kegler (Eds.), *Emerging theories in health promotion practice and research: Strategies for improving public health* (pp. 228-254). San Francisco: Jossey-Bass.

Kulbok, P. P., Earls, F. J., & Montgomery, A. C. (1988). Life style and patterns of health and social behavior in high-risk adolescents. *Advances in Nursing Science, 11*(1), 22-35.

Labre, M. P. (2002). Adolescent boys and the muscular male body ideal. *Journal of Adolescent Health, 30*, 233-242.

Lafferty, C. K., Mahoney, C. A., & Thombs, D. L. (2003). Diffusion of a developmental asset-building initiative in public schools. *American Journal of Health Behavior, 27*(Suppl. 1), S35-S44.

Lammers, C., Ireland, M., Resnick, M., & Blum, R. (2000). Influences on adolescents' decision to postpone onset of sexual intercourse: A survival analysis of virginity among youths aged 13 to 18 years. *Journal of Adolescent Health, 26*, 42-48.

Lantzouni, E., Frank, G. R., Golden, N. H., & Shenker, R. I. (2002). Reversibility of growth stunting in early onset anorexia nervosa: A prospective study. *Journal of Adolescent Health, 31*, 162-165.

Lazarus, R. S. (1966). *Psychological stress and the coping process.* New York: McGraw-Hill.

Lazarus, R. S. (1991a). *Emotion and adaptation.* New York: Oxford University Press.

Lazarus, R. S. (1991b). Progress on a cognitive-motivational-relational theory of emotion. *American Psychologist, 46*, 819-834.

Lazarus, R. S. (1993). Coping theory and research: Past, present, and future. *Psychosomatic Medicine, 55*, 234-247.

Lazarus, R. S. (1999). *Stress and emotion: A new synthesis.* New York: Springer.

Lazarus, R. S. (2000). Evolution of a model of stress, coping, and discrete emotions. In V. H. Rice (Ed.), *Handbook of stress, coping and health: Implications for nursing research, theory, and practice* (pp. 195-222). Thousand Oaks, CA: Sage.

Lazarus, R. S., & Cohen, J. B. (1977). Environmental stress. In I. Altman & J. F. Wohlwill (Eds.), *Human behavior and environment* (Vol. 2). New York: Plenum.

Lazarus, R. S., & Folkman, S. (1984). *Stress, appraisal, and coping.* New York: Springer.

Leffert, N., Benson, P.L, Scales, P. C., Sharma, A. R., Drake, D. R., & Blyth, D. A. (1998). Developmental assets: Measurement and prediction of risk behaviors among adolescents. *Applied Developmental Science, 2*, 209-230.

Lenz, E. R., Suppe, F., Gift, A. G., Pugh, L. C., & Milligan, R. A. (1995). Collaborative development of middle-range nursing theories: Toward a theory of unpleasant symptoms. *Advances in Nursing Science, 17*(3), 1-13.

Lerner, R. M. (1995a). *America's youth in crisis: Challenges and options for programs and policies.* Thousand Oaks, CA: Sage.

Lerner, R. M. (1995b, Winter). Features and principles of effective youth programs: Promoting positive youth development through the integrative vision of family and consumer sciences. *Journal of Family and Consumer Sciences*, pp. 16-21.

Lerner, R. M. (1996). Relative plasticity, integration, temporality, and diversity in human development: A developmental contextual perspective about theory, process, and method. *Developmental Psychology, 32*, 781-786.

Lerner, R. M. (1998). Theories of human development: Contemporary perspectives. In W. Damon (Ed.), *Handbook of child psychology: Vol. 1. Theoretical models of human development* (5th ed., pp. 1-24). New York: John Wiley.

Lerner, R. M. (2002). *Adolescence: Development, diversity, context, and application.* Upper Saddle River, NJ: Pearson Education.

Lerner, R. M., & Castellino, D. R. (2002). Contemporary developmental theory and adolescence: Developmental systems and applied developmental science. *Journal of Adolescent Health, 31,* 122-135.

Lerner, R. M., & Galambos, N. L. (1998). Adolescent development: Challenges and opportunities for research, programs, and policies. *Annual Review of Psychology, 49,* 413-446.

Lerner, R. M., & Hood, K. E. (1986). Plasticity in development: Concepts and issues for intervention. *Journal of Applied Developmental Psychology, 7,* 139-152.

Lerner, R. M., & Miller, J. R. (1993). Integrating human development research and intervention for America's children: The Michigan State University model. *Journal of Applied Developmental Psychology, 14,* 347-364.

Lescohier, I., & Gallagher, S. S. (1996). Unintentional injury. In R. J. DiClemente, W. B. Hansen, & L. E. Ponton (Eds.), *Handbook of adolescent health risk behavior* (pp. 225-258). New York: Plenum Press.

Leventhal, H. (1970). Findings and theory in the study of fear communications. In L. Berkowitz (Ed.), *Advances in experimental social psychology* (Vol. 5, pp. 120-186). New York: Academic Press.

Leventhal, T., Graber, J. A., & Brooks-Gunn, J. (2001). Adolescent transitions to young adulthood: Antecedents, correlates, and consequences of adolescent employment. *Journal of Research on Adolescence, 11,* 297-323.

Leventhal, H., Nerenz, D. R., & Steele, D. J. (1984). Illness representations and coping with health threats. In A. Baum, S. E. Taylor, & J. E. Singer (Eds.), *Handbook of psychology and health* (pp. 219-252). Hillsdale, NJ: Lawrence Erlbaum.

Levine, H. (1997). A further exploration of the lesbian identity development process and its measurement. *Journal of Homosexuality, 34,* 67-78.

Lewin, K. (1946). Action research and minority problems. *Journal of Social Issues, 2*(4), 34-46.

Lewin, K. (1951). *Field theory in social science: Selected theoretical papers* (D. Cartwright, Ed.). New York: Harper Torchbooks.

Lewis, C. L., & Brown, S. C. (2002). Coping strategies of female adolescents with HIV/AIDS. *ABNF Journal, 13*(4), 72-77.

Lien, N., Lytle, L. A., & Komro, K. A. (2002). Applying theory of planned behavior to fruit and vegetable consumption of young adolescents. *American Journal of Health Promotion, 16*(4),189-197.

Lieu, T. A., Newacheck, P. W., & McManus, M. A. (1993). Race, ethnicity, and access to ambulatory care among U.S. adolescents. *American Journal of Public Health, 83,* 960-965.

Limbos, M.A.P., & Peek-Asa, C. (2003). Comparing unintentional and intentional injuries in a school setting. *Journal of School Health, 73,* 101-106.

Litt, I. (2003). Focusing on focus groups. *Journal of Adolescent Health, 32,* 329-330.

Loeber, R., Farrington, D. P., Stouthamer-Loeber, M., & Van Kammen, W. B. (1998). Multiple risk factors for multiproblem boys: Co-occurrence of delinquency, substance use, attention deficit, conduct problems, physical aggression, covert behavior, depressed mood, and shy/withdrawn behavior. In R. Jessor (Ed.), *New perspectives on adolescent risk behavior* (pp. 90-149). Cambridge, England: Cambridge University Press.

Lovinger, S. L., Miller, L., & Lovinger, R. J. (1999). Some clinical applications of religious development in adolescence. *Journal of Adolescence, 22,* 269-277.

Luepker, R. V., Perry, C. L., McKinlay, S. M., Nader, P. R., Parcel, G. S., Stone, E. J., et al. (1996). Outcomes of a field trial to improve children's dietary patterns and physical activity: The Child and Adolescent Trial for Cardiovascular Health (CATCH). *Journal of the American Medical Association, 275*, 768-776.

Lugoe, W., & Rise, J. (1999). Predicting intended condom use among Tanzanian students using the theory of planned behaviour. *Journal of Health Psychology, 4*, 497-506.

Lum, C. (2002). *Scientific thinking in speech and language therapy*. Mahwah, NJ: Lawrence Erlbaum.

Luthar, S. S. (1991). Vulnerability and resilience: A study of high-risk adolescents. *Child Development, 62*, 600-616.

Luthar, S. S., & Zigler, E. (1991). Vulnerability and competence: A review of research on resilience in childhood. *American Journal of Orthopsychiatry, 61*(1), 6-22.

Lyon, B. L. (2000). Stress, coping, and health: A conceptual overview. In V. H. Rice (Ed.), *Handbook of stress, coping, and health: Implications for nursing research, theory, and practice* (pp. 3-23). Thousand Oaks, CA: Sage.

Lytle, L. A., Kelder, S. H., Perry, C. L., & Klepp, K. I. (1995). Covariance of adolescent health behaviors: The class of 1989 study. *Health Education Research, 10*, 133-146.

Lytle, L. A., & Perry, C. L. (2001). Applying research and theory in program planning: An example from a nutrition education intervention. *Health Promotion Practice, 2*(1), 68-80.

Maggs, J. L, Schulenberg, J., & Hurrelmann, K. (1997). Developmental transitions during adolescence: Health promotion implications (pp. 522-546). In J. Schulenberg, J. L. Maggs, & K. Hurrelmann (Eds.), *Health risks and developmental transitions during adolescence*. Cambridge, MA: Cambridge University Press.

Mahon, N. E., Yarcheski, A., & Yarcheski, T. J. (2002). Psychometric evaluation of the Personal Lifestyle Questionnaire for Adolescents. *Research in Nursing and Health, 25*, 68-75.

Mahon, N. E., Yarcheski, T. J., & Yarcheski, A. (2003). The revised personal lifestyle questionnaire for early adolescents. *Western Journal of Nursing Research, 25*, 533-547.

Mahoney, C. A., Thombs, D. I., & Ford, O. J. (1995). Health belief and self-efficacy models: Their utility in explaining college student condom use. *AIDS Education and Prevention, 7*, 32-49.

Mann, L. (1982). *Flinders Decision Making Questionnaire II*. Unpublished questionnaire, Flinders University of South Australia, Adelaide.

Mann, L., Burnett, P., Radford, M., & Ford, S. (1997). The Melbourne Decision Making Questionnaire: An instrument for measuring patterns for coping with decisional conflict. *Journal of Behavioral Decision Making, 10*(1), 1-19.

Marcell, A. V., Klein, J. D., Fischer, I., Allan, M. J., & Kokotailo, P. K. (2002). Male adolescent use of health care services: Where are the boys? *Journal of Adolescent Health, 30*, 35-43.

Marcia, J. E. (1966). Development and validation of ego-identity status. *Journal of Personality and Social Psychology, 3*, 551-558.

Marcia, J. E. (1980). Identity in adolescence. In J. Adelson (Ed.), *Handbook of adolescent psychology* (pp. 159-187). New York: John Wiley.

Marcia, J. E. (1989). Identity diffusion differentiated. In M. A. Luszcz & T. Nettlebeck (Eds.), *Psychological development: Perspectives across the life-span* (pp. 289-294). New York: Elsevier North-Holland.

Marcia, J. E. (1993). The ego identity status approach to ego identity. In J. E. Marcia, A. S. Waterman, D. R. Matteson, S. L. Archer, & J. L.Orlofsky (Eds.), *Ego identity: A handbook for psychosocial research* (pp. 3-21). New York: Springer.

Marcia, J. E. (1994). Identity and psychotherapy. In S. L. Archer (Ed.), *Interventions for adolescent identity development* (pp. 29-46). Thousand Oaks, CA: Sage.

Marcia, J. E., & Archer, S. L. (1993). Identity status in late adolescents: Scoring criteria. In J. E. Marcia, A. S. Waterman, D. R. Matteson, S. L. Archer, & J. L. Orlofsky (Eds.), *Ego identity: A handbook for psychosocial research* (pp. 205-240). New York: Springer.

Marcia, J. E., Waterman, A. S., Matteson, D. R., Archer, S. L., & Orlofsky, J. L. (1993). *A handbook for psychosocial research.* New York: Springer.

Marcus, B. H., Rakowski, W., & Rossi, J. S. (1992). Assessing motivational readiness and decision-making for exercise. *Health Psychology, 11,* 257-261.

Marcus, B. H., Rossi, J. S., Selby, V. C., Niaura, R. S., & Abrams, D. B. (1992). The stages and processes of exercise adoption and maintenance in a worksite sample. *Health Psychology, 11,* 386-395.

Marcus, B. H., Selby, V. C., Niaura, R. S., & Rossi, J. S. (1992). Self-efficacy and the stages of exercise behavior change. *Research Quarterly Exercise and Sports, 63,* 60-66.

Markstrom, C. A. (1999). Religious involvement and adolescent psychosocial development. *Journal of Adolescence, 22,* 205-221.

Markus, H., & Wurf, E. (1987). The dynamic self-concept: A social psychological perspective. *Annual Review of Psychology, 38,* 299-337.

Marshall, W. A., & Tanner, J. M. (1969). Variations in pattern of pubertal changes in girls. *Archives of Diseases of Children, 44,* 291-303.

Martyn, K. K., & Hutchinson, S. A. (2001). Low-income African American adolescents who avoid pregnancy: Tough girls who rewrite negative scripts. *Qualitative Health Research, 11,* 238-256.

Masten, A. S. (1986). Humor and competence in school-aged children. *Child Development, 57,* 461-473.

Masten, A. S., & Coatsworth, J. D. (1998). The development of competence in favorable and unfavorable environments: Lessons from research on successful children. *American Psychologist, 53,* 205-220.

Masten, A. S., Garmezy, N., Tellegen, A., Pellegrini, D. S., Larkin, K., & Larsen, A. (1988). Competence and stress in school children: The moderating effects of individual and family qualities. *Journal of Child Psychology and Psychiatry, 29,* 745-764.

Masters, W. H., Johnson, V. E., & Kolodny, R. C. (1995). *Human sexuality* (5th ed.). New York: HarperCollins College.

McCaleb, A., & Cull, V. V. (2000). Sociocultural influences and self-care practices of middle adolescents. *Journal of Pediatric Nursing, 15*(1), 30-35.

McClowry, S. G. (1995). The influence of temperament on development during middle childhood. *Journal of Pediatric Nursing, 10,* 160-165.

McCord, J. (1990). Problem behaviors. In S. S. Feldman & G. R. Elliott (Eds.), *At the threshold: The developing adolescent* (pp. 414-430). Cambridge, MA: Harvard University Press.

McCubbin, H. I., & Thompson, A. I. (Eds.). (1991). *Family assessment inventories for research and practice.* Madison, WI: University of Wisconsin–Madison.

McEwen, B. S., & Dhabhar, F. (2002). Stress in adolescent females: Relationship to autoimmune diseases. *Journal of Adolescent Health, 30*(4, Suppl.), 30-36.

McGuire, S., Manke, B., Saudino, K. J., Reiss, D., Hetheringon, E. M., & Plomin, R. (1999). Perceived competence and self-worth during adolescence: A longitudinal behavioral genetic study. *Child Development, 70,* 1283-1296.

McNabb, W. L., Quinn, M. T., Murphy, D. M., Thorp, F. K., & Cook, S. (1994). Increasing children's responsibility for diabetes self-care: The *In Control* study. *Diabetes Educator, 20,* 121-124.

Mead, G. H. (1934). *Mind, self and society.* Chicago: University of Chicago Press.

Medoff-Cooper, B. (1995). Infant temperament: Implications for parenting from birth through 1 year. *Journal of Pediatric Nursing, 10,* 141-145.

Meleis, A. I. (1997). *Theoretical nursing: Development and progress* (3rd ed.). Philadephia: J. B. Lippincott.

Miller, G. A. (1956). The magical number seven, plus or minus two: Some limits on our capacity for processing information. *Psychological Review, 63,* 81-97.

Miller, N. E., & Dollard, J. (1941). *Social learning and imitation.* New Haven, CT: Yale University Press.

Miller, W. R. (1998). Enhancing motivation for change. In W. R. Miller & N. Heather (Eds.), *Treating addictive behaviors* (2nd ed., pp. 121-132). New York: Plenum.

Miller, W. R. (2001). When is it motivational interviewing? *Addiction, 96,* 1770-1772.

Miller, W. R., & Rollnick, S. (1991). *Motivational interviewing: Preparing people to change addictive behavior.* New York: Guilford.

Miller, W. R., & Rollnick, S. (2002). *Motivational interviewing: Preparing people to change addictive behavior* (2nd ed.). New York: Guilford.

Millstein, S. (1993). A view of health from the adolescent's perspective. In S. G. Millstein, A. C. Petersen, & E. O. Nightingale (Eds.), *Promoting the health of adolescents* (pp. 97-118). New York: Oxford University Press.

Millstein, S. G. (2003). Risk perception: Construct development, links to theory, correlates, and manifestations. In D. Romer (Ed.), *Reducing adolescent risk: Toward an integrated approach* (pp. 35-43). Thousand Oaks, CA: Sage.

Millstein, S. G., & Halpern-Felsher, B. L. (2002). Judgments about risk and perceived invulnerability in adolescents and young adults. *Journal of Research on Adolescence, 12,* 399-422.

Millstein, S., Peterson, A. C., & Nightingale, E. O. (1993). Adolescent health promotion: Rationale, goals, and objectives. In S. G. Millstein, A. C. Petersen, & E. O. Nightingale (Eds.), *Promoting the health of adolescents* (pp. 3-10). New York: Oxford University Press.

Mithaug, D. E. (2003). Evaluating credibility and worth of self-determination theory. In M. L. Wehmeyer, B. H. Abery, D. E. Mithaug, & R. J. Stancliffe (Eds.), *Theory in self-determination: Foundations for educational practice* (pp. 154-173). Springfield, IL: Charles C Thomas.

Monaco Bissonnette, M., & Contento, I. R. (2001). Adolescents' perspectives and food choice behavior in terms of the environmental impacts of food production practices: Application of a psychosocial model. *Journal of Nutrition Education, 32,* 72.

Monsen, R. B., Jackson, C. P., & Livingston, M. (1996). Having a future: Sexual decision making in early adolescence. *Journal of Pediatric Nursing, 11,* 183-188.

Moore, J. B. (1995). Measuring the self-care practice of children and adolescents: Instrument development. *Maternal-Child Nursing Journal, 23*(3),101-108.

Moos, R. H. (2002). Life stressors, social resources, and coping skills in youth: Applications to adolescents with chronic disorders. *Journal of Adolescent Health, 30*(4, Suppl.), 22-29.

Moss, H. B., Vanyukov, M., Yao, J. K., & Kirillova, G. P. (1999). Salivary cortisol responses in prepubertal boys: The effects of parental substance abuse and association with drug use behavior during adolescence. *Biological Psychiatry, 45,* 1293-1299.

Motl, R. W., Dishman, R. K., Saunders, R. P., Dowda, M., Felton, G., Ward, D. S., et al. (2002). Examining social-cognitive determinants of intention and physical activity among Black and White adolescent girls using structural equation modeling. *Health Psychology, 21,* 459-467.

Mummery, W. K., & Wankel, L. M. (1999). Training adherence in adolescent competitive swimmers: An application of the theory of planned behavior. *Journal of Sport and Exercise Psychology, 21,* 313-328.

Munsch, J., & Wampler, R. S. (1993). Ethnic differences in early adolescents' coping with school stress. *American Journal of Orthopsychiatry, 63,* 633-646.

Murphy, D. A., Moscicki, B., Vermund, S. H., Muenz, L. R., and the Adolescent Medicine HIV/AIDS Research Network. (2000). Psychological distress among HIV+ adolescents in the REACH study: Effects of life stress, social support, and coping. *Journal of Adolescent Health, 27,* 391-398.

Murphy, J. G., Duchnick, J. J., Vuchinich, R. E., Davison, J. S., Karg, R. S., Olson, A. M., et al. (2001). Relative efficacy of a brief motivational intervention for college student drinkers. *Psychology of Addictive Behaviors, 15,* 373-379.

Murphy, W. G., & Brubaker, R. G. (1990). Effects of a brief theory-based intervention on the practice of testicular self-examination by high school males. *Journal of School Health, 60,* 459-462.

Muscari, M. E., Faherty, J., & Catalino, C. (1998). Little women: Early menarche in rural girls. *Pediatric Nursing, 24*(1), 11-15.

Myers, L. J., Speight, S. L., Highlen, P. S., Cox, C. I., Reynolds, A. L., Adams, E. M., et al. (1991). Identity development and world-view: Toward an optimal conceptualization. *Journal of Counseling and Development, 70,* 54-63.

Nader, P. R., Stone, E. J., Lytle, L. A., Perry, C. L., Osganian, S. K., Kelder, S., et al. (1999). Three-year maintenance of improved diet and physical activity: The CATCH cohort. *Archives of Pediatric and Adolescent Medicine, 153,* 695-704.

National Highway Traffic Safety Administration. (2003). *2000 annual assessment revised: Motor vehicle traffic crash fatality and injury estimates for 2000.* Retrieved April 6, 2004, from http://www-nrd.nhtsa.dot.gov/pdf/nrd-30/NCSA/Rpts/2001/Assess2K.pdf

Neinstein, L. S. (2002). *Adolescent health care: A practical guide* (3rd ed.). Baltimore: Williams & Wilkins.

Neinstein, L. S., & Kaufman, F. R. (2002). Normal physical growth and development. In L. S. Neinstein (Ed.), *Adolescent health care: A practical guide* (3rd ed., pp. 3-58). Baltimore: Williams & Wilkins.

Neinstein, L. S., & Schack, E. (2002). Nutrition. In L. S. Neinstein (Ed.), *Adolescent health care: A practical guide* (4th ed.). Philadelphia: Lippincott Williams & Wilkins.

Nelson, C. E. (2002). Reforming childish religion. *Insights, 117*(2), 3-11.

Neumark-Sztainer, D., Story, M., French, S., Cassuto, N., Jacobs, D. R., Jr., & Resnick, M. D. (1996). Patterns of health-compromising behaviors among Minnesota adolescents: Sociodemographic variations. *American Journal of Public Health, 86,* 1599-1606.

Newacheck, P. W., Wong, S. T., Galbraith, A. A., & Hung, Y. Y. (2003). Adolescent health care expenditures: A descriptive profile. *Journal of Adolescent Health, 32*(6, Suppl.), 3-11.

Newell, A., & Simon, H. A. (1972). *Human problem solving*. Englewood Cliffs, NJ: Prentice Hall.

Newman, M. A. (1994). *Health as expanding consciousness* (2nd ed.). New York: National League for Nursing Press.

Niccolai, L. M., Ethier, K. A., Kershaw, T. S., Lewis, J. G., & Ickovics, J. R. (2003). Pregnant adolescents at risk: Sexual behaviors and sexually transmitted disease prevalence. *American Journal of Obstetrics and Gynecology, 188*, 63-70.

Niemann, Y. F., Romero, A. J., Arredondo, J., & Rodriguez, V. (1999). What does it mean to be "Mexican"? Social construction of an ethnic identity. *Hispanic Journal of Behavioral Sciences, 21*(1), 47-60.

Nigg, C. R., & Courneya, K. S. (1998). Transtheoretical model: Examining adolescent exercise behavior. *Journal of Adolescent Health, 22*, 214-224.

Nightingale, F. (1946). *Notes on nursing: What it is and what it is not*. Philadelphia: J. B. Lippincott.

Norman, P., Bennett, P., & Lewis, H. (1998). Understanding binge drinking among young people: An application of the theory of planned behaviour. *Health Education Research, 13*, 163-169.

Norton, B. L., McLeroy, K. R., Burdine, J. N., Felix, M.R.J., & Dorsey, A. M. (2002). Community capacity: Concept, theory, and methods. In R. J. DiClemente, R. A. Crosby, & M. C. Kegler (Eds.), *Emerging theories in health promotion practice and research: Strategies for improving public health* (pp. 194-227). San Francisco: Jossey-Bass.

Obeidallah, D. A., Brennan, R. T., Brooks-Gunn, J., Kindlon, D., & Earls, F. (2000). Socioeconomic status, race, and girls' pubertal maturation: Results from the project on human development in Chicago neighborhoods. *Journal of Research on Adolescence, 10*, 443-464.

Oberg, C., Hogan, M., Bertrand, J., & Juve, C. (2002). Health care access, sexually transmitted diseases, and adolescents: Identifying barriers and creating solutions. *Current Problems in Pediatric Adolescent Health Care, 32*, 315-339.

O'Brien, R. (1998, April 17). *An overview of the methodological approach of action research*. Retrieved April 6, 2004, from http://www.web.net/~robrien/papers/arfinal.html

Oman, R. F., Vesely, S. K., Kegler, M., McLeroy, K., & Aspy, C. B. (2003). A youth development approach to profiling sexual abstinence. *American Journal of Health Behavior, 27*(Suppl. 1), S80-S93.

Oman, R. F., Vesely, S. K., Kegler, M., McLeroy, K. R., Harris-Wyatt, V., Aspy, C. B., et al. (2002). Reliability and validity of the Youth Asset Survey (YAS). *Journal of Adolescent Health, 31*, 247-255.

Orem, D. E. (1971). *Nursing: Concepts of practice*. New York: McGraw-Hill.

Orem, D. E. (1980). *Nursing: Concepts of practice* (2nd ed.). New York: McGraw-Hill

Orem, D. E. (1985). *Nursing: Concepts of practice* (3rd ed.). New York: McGraw-Hill.

Orem, D. E. (1991). *Nursing: Concepts of practice* (4th ed.). St. Louis: Mosby.

Orem, D. E. (2001). *Nursing: Concepts of practice* (6th ed.). St. Louis: Mosby.

O'Sullivan, L. F., Meyer-Bahlburg, H.F.L., & Watkins, B. X. (2000). Social cognitions associated with pubertal development in a sample of urban, low-income, African-American and Latina girls and mothers. *Journal of Adolescent Health, 27*, 227-235.

Ozer, E. M., Park, M. J., Paul, T., Brindis, C. D., & Irwin, C. E., Jr. (2003). *America's adolescents: Are they healthy?* San Francisco: National Adolescent Health Information Center.

Pakula, A. S., & Neinstein, L. S. (2002). Acne vulgaris. In L. S. Neinstein (Ed.), *Adolescent health care: A practical guide* (4th ed., pp. 441-482). Philadelphia: Lippincott Williams & Wilkins.

Palmer, M. K. L., & Boisen, L. S. (2002). Cystic fibrosis and the transition to adulthood. *Social Work in Health Care, 36*(1), 45-58.

Paloutzian, R. F., & Ellison, C. W. (1982). Loneliness, spiritual well-being, and the quality of life. In L. A. Peplau & D. Perlman (Eds.), *Loneliness: A source book of current theory, research and therapy* (pp. 224-237). New York: John Wiley.

Paloutzian, R. F., & Ellison, C. W. (1991). *Manual for the spiritual well-being scale.* Nyack, NY: Life Advance.

Parcel, G. S., Kelder, S. H., & Basen-Engquist, K. (2000). The school as a setting for health promotion. In B. D. Poland, L. W. Green, & I. Rootman (Eds.), *Settings for health promotion: Linking theory and practice* (pp. 86-120). Thousand Oaks, CA: Sage.

Patterson, C. J. (1995). Sexual orientation and human development: An overview. *Developmental Psychology, 31*(1), 3-11.

Pender, N. J., Bar-Or, O., Wilk, B., & Mitchell, S. (2002). Self-efficacy and perceived exertion of girls during exercise. *Nursing Research, 51,* 86-91.

Pender, N. J., Murdaugh, C. L., & Parsons, M. A. (2002). *Health promotion in nursing practice* (4th ed.). Upper Saddle River, NJ: Prentice Hall.

Perrin, E. C. (2002). *Sexual orientation in child and adolescent health care.* New York: Kluwer Academic/Plenum.

Perry, C. L. (1999). *Creating health behavior change: How to develop community-wide programs for youth.* Thousand Oaks: Sage.

Perry, C. L., Bishop, D. B., Taylor, G., Murray, D. M., Mays, R. W., Dudovitz, B. S., et al. (1998). Changing fruit and vegetable consumption among children: The 5-A-Day Power Plus program in Saint Paul, Minnesota. *American Journal of Public Health, 88,* 603-609.

Perry, C. L., Stone, E. J., Parcel, G. S., Ellison, R. C., Nader, P. R., Webber, L. S., et al. (1990). School-based cardiovascular health promotion: The Child and Adolescent Trial for Cardiovascular Health (CATCH). *Journal of School Health, 64,* 405-409.

Perry, C. L., & Williams, C. L. (2003). Project Northland II. *Center for Youth Health Promotion.* Retrieved April 6, 2004, from http://www.epi.umn.edu/cyhp/ r_pnII.htm

Perry, C. L., Williams, C. L., Veblen-Mortenson, S., Toomey, T., Komro, K. A., Anstine, P. S., et al. (1996). Project Northland: Outcomes of a community-wide alcohol use prevention program during early adolescence. *American Journal of Public Health, 86,* 956-965.

Petraitis, J., Flay, B. R., & Miller, T. Q. (1995). Reviewing theories of adolescent substance use: Organizing pieces in the puzzle. *Psychological Bulletin, 117*(1), 67-86.

Phillips, D. C. (1987). *Philosophy, science and social inquiry.* Oxford, England: Pergamon.

Phinney, J. S. (1990). Ethnic identity in adolescents and adults: A review of research. *Psychological Bulletin, 180,* 499-514.

Phinney, J. S., & Devich-Navarro, M. (1997). Variations in bicultural identification among African American and Mexican American adolescents. *Journal of Research on Adolescence, 7*(1), 3-32.

Phinney, J. S., & Kohatsu, E. L. (1997). Ethnic and racial identity development and mental health. In J. Schulenberg, J. L. Maggs, & K. Hurrelmann (Eds.), *Health risks and developmental transitions during adolescence* (pp. 395-419). Cambridge, MA: Cambridge University Press.

Phinney, J. S., & Rosenthal, D. A. (1992). Ethnic identity in adolescence: Process, context, and outcome. In G. R. Adams, T. P. Gullotta, & R. Montemayor (Eds.), *Adolescent identity formation: Advances in adolescent development* (pp. 145-172). Newbury Park, CA: Sage.

Piaget, J. (1932). *The moral judgement of the child*. New York: Harcourt, Brace.

Piaget, J., & Inhelder, B. (1958). *The growth of logical thinking from childhood to adolescence*. New York: Basic Books.

Piaget, J., & Inhelder, B. (1969). *The psychology of the child*. New York: Basic Books.

Piaget, J., & Inhelder, B. (1973). *Memory and intelligence*. New York: Basic Books.

Pickett, J. P. (Ed.). (2000). *The American heritage dictionary of the English language* (4th ed.). Boston: Houghton Mifflin.

Pickett, W., Schmid, H., Boyce, W. F., Simpson, K., Scheidt, P. C., Mazur, J., et al. (2002). Multiple risk behavior and injury: An international analysis of young people. *Archives of Pediatric and Adolescent Medicine, 156,* 786-793.

Piedmont, R. L. (1999). Does spirituality represent the sixth factor of personality? Spiritual transcendence and the five-factor model. *Journal of Personality, 67,* 985-1013.

Piedmont, R. L. (2001). Spiritual transcendence and the scientific study of spirituality. *Journal of Rehabilitation, 67*(1), 4-14.

Pipher, M. (1994). *Reviving Ophelia*. New York: G. P. Putnam.

Pittman, K., Irby, M., & Ferber, T. (2001). Unfinished business: Further reflections on a decade of promoting youth development. In P. L. Benson & K. J. Pittman (Eds.), *Trends in youth development: Visions, realities, and challenges* (pp. 3-50). Boston: Kluwer Academic.

Plant, T. M. (2002). Neurophysiology of puberty. *Journal of Adolescent Health, 31*(6, Suppl.), 185-191.

Plomin, R. (2000). Behavioural genetics in the 21st century. *International Journal of Behavioral Development, 24*(1), 30-34.

Ploof, S. (1999). *Definition: Turner's syndrome*. Retrieved March 8, 2004, from http://www.onr.com/ts-texas/turner.html

Polit, D. F., & Hungler, B. P. (1995). *Nursing research: Principles and methods* (5th ed.). Philadelphia: J. B. Lippincott.

Polk, L. V. (1997). Toward a middle-range theory of resilience. *Advances in Nursing Science, 19,* 1-13.

Porter, C. P. (2002). Female "tweens" and sexual development. *Journal of Pediatric Nursing, 17,* 402-406.

Preloran, H. M., Browner, C. H., & Lieber, E. (2001). Strategies for motivating Latino couples' participation in qualitative health research and their effects on sample construction. *American Journal of Public Health, 91,* 1832-1841.

Prinstein, M. J., Boergers, J., & Spirito, A. (2001). Adolescents' and their friends' health-risk behavior: Factors that alter or add to peer influence. *Journal of Pediatric Psychology, 26,* 287-298.

Prochaska, J. O. (1979). *Systems of psychotherapy: A transtheoretical analysis*. Homewood, IL: Dorsey.

Prochaska, J. O. (1994). Strong and weak principles for progressing from precontemplation to action on the basis of twelve problem behaviors. *Health Psychology, 13*(1), 47-51.

Prochaska, J. O., DiClemente, C. C., & Norcross, J. C. (1992). In search of how people change: Applications to addictive behaviors. *American Psychologist, 47,* 1102-1114.

Prochaska, J. O., Norcross, J. C., & DiClemente, C. C. (1994). *Changing for good.* New York: Avon Books.

Prochaska, J. O., Redding, C. A., & Evers, K. E. (1997). The transtheoretical model and stages of change. In K. Glanz, F. M. Lewis, & B. K. Rimer (Eds.), *Health behavior and health education: Theory, research, and practice* (2nd ed., pp. 60-84). San Francisco: Jossey-Bass.

Prochaska, J. O., Velicer, W. F., Rossi, J. S., Goldstein, M. G., Marcus, B. H., Rakowski, W., et al. (1994). Stages of change and decisional balance for 12 problem behaviors. *Health Psychology, 13*(1), 39-46.

Pullen, L., Modrcin-Talbott, M. A., West, W. R., & Muenchen, R. (1999). Spiritual high vs. high on spirits: Is religiosity related to adolescent alcohol and drug abuse? *Journal of Psychiatric and Mental Health Nursing, 6,* 3-8.

Rabin, B. S. (2002). Can stress participate in the pathogenesis of autoimmune disease? *Journal of Adolescent Health, 30*(4, Suppl.), 71-75.

Radzik, M., Sherer, S., & Neinstein, L. S. (2002). Psychosocial development in normal adolescents. In L. S. Neinstein (Ed.), *Adolescent health care: A practical guide* (4th ed.). Philadelphia: Lippincott Williams & Wilkins.

Rak, C. F., & Patterson, L. E. (1996). Promoting resilience in at-risk children. *Journal of Counseling and Development, 74,* 368-373.

Ratner, P. A., Johnson, J. L, & Jeffery, B. (1998). Examining emotional, physical, social, and spiritual health as determinants of self-rated health status. *American Journal of Health Promotion, 12,* 275-282.

Reason, P. (1998). Three approaches to participative inquiry. In N. K. Denzin & Y. S. Lincoln (Eds.), *Strategies of qualitative inquiry* (pp. 261-291). Thousand Oaks, CA: Sage.

Resnick, M. D., Bearman, P. S., Blum, R. W., Bauman, K. E., Harris, K. M., Jones, J., et al. (1997). Protecting adolescents from harm: Findings from the National Longitudinal Study on Adolescent Health. *Journal of the American Medical Association, 278,* 823-832.

Resnick, M. D., Harris, L. J., & Blum, R. W. (1993). The impact of caring and connectedness on adolescent health and well-being. *Journal of Paediatric and Child Health, 29*(Suppl. 1), S3-S9.

Resnicow, K., Braithwaite, R. L., & Kuo, J. A. (1997). Interpersonal interventions for minority adolescents. In D. K. Wilson, J. R. Rodrigue, & W. C. Taylor (Eds.). *Health-promoting and health-compromising behaviors among minority adolescents* (pp. 201-228). Washington, DC: American Psychological Association.

Resnicow, K., DiIorio, C., Soet, J. E., Borrelli, B., Ernst, D., Hecht, J., et al. (2002). Motivational interviewing in medical and public health settings. In W. R. Miller & S. Rollnick (Eds.), *Motivational interviewing: Preparing people to change addictive behavior* (2nd ed., pp. 251-269). New York: Guilford.

Rew, L. (1997). Health-related help-seeing behaviors in female Mexican-American adolescents. *Journal of the Society of Pediatric Nursing, 2,* 156-162.

Rew, L. (2000). Friends and pets as companions: Strategies for coping with loneliness among homeless youth. *Journal of Child and Adolescent Psychiatric Nursing, 13,* 125-132.

Rew, L. (2001). Sexual health practices of homeless youth: A model for intervention. *Issues in Comprehensive Pediatric Nursing, 24*(1), 1-18.

Rew, L. (2003). A theory of taking care of oneself grounded in experiences of homeless youth. *Nursing Research, 5,* 234-241.

Rew, L., Chambers, K. B., & Kulkarni, S. (2002). Planning a sexual health promotion intervention with homeless adolescents. *Nursing Research, 51,* 168-174.

Rew, L., Resnick, M. D., & Blum, R. W. (1997). An exploration of help-seeking behaviors in female Hispanic adolescents. *Family and Community Health, 20*(3), 1-15.

Rew, L., Taylor-Seehafer, M., & Fitzgerald, M. L. (2001). Sexual abuse, alcohol and other drug use and suicidal behaviors in homeless adolescents. *Issues in Comprehensive Pediatric Nursing, 24,* 225-240.

Rew, L., Taylor-Seehafer, M., Thomas, N. Y., & Yockey, R. D. (2001). Correlates of resilience in homeless adolescents. *Journal of Nursing Scholarship, 33*(1), 33-40.

Reynolds, N. R., & Alonzo, A. A. (2000). Self-regulation: The commonsense model of illness representation. In V. H. Rice (Ed.), *Handbook of stress, coping, and health: Implications for nursing research, theory, and practice* (pp. 483-494). Thousand Oaks, CA: Sage.

Reynolds, P. D. (1971). *A primer in theory construction.* Indianapolis, IN: ITT Bobbs-Merrill Educational.

Rich, M., & Ginsburg, K. R. (1999). The reason and rhyme of qualitative research: Why, when, and how to use qualitative methods in the study of adolescent health. *Journal of Adolescent Health, 25,* 371-378.

Rich, M., Patashnick, J., & Chalfen, R. (2002). Visual illness narratives of asthma: Explanatory models and health-related behavior. *American Journal of Health Behavior, 26,* 442-453.

Richards, T. J., & Richards, L. (1998). Using computers in qualitative research. In N. K. Denzin & Y. S. Lincoln (Eds.), *Collecting and interpreting qualitative materials.* Thousand Oaks, CA: Sage.

Riessman, C. K. (1993). *Narrative analysis.* Newbury Park, CA: Sage.

Rippetoe, P., & Rogers, R. W. (1987). Effects of components of protection-motivation theory on adaptive and maladaptive coping with a health threat. *Journal of Personality and Social Psychology, 52,* 596-604.

Rogers, A. S., Miller, S., Murphy, D. A., Tanney, M., & Fortune, T. (2001). The TREAT (Therapeutic Regimens Enhancing Adherence in Teens) program: Theory and preliminary results. *Journal of Adolescent Health, 29*(3, Suppl.), 30-38.

Rogers, C. R. (1951). *Client-centered therapy.* Boston: Houghton Mifflin.

Rogers, C. R. (1957). The necessary and sufficient conditions of therapeutic personality change. *Journal of Consulting Psychology, 21,* 95-103.

Rogers, M. E. (1970). *An introduction to the theoretical basis of nursing.* Philadelphia: F. A. Davis.

Rogers, R. W. (1983). Cognitive and physiological processes in attitudinal change: A revised theory of protection-motivation. In J. Cacioppo & R. Petty (Eds.), *Social psychophysiology* (pp. 153-176). New York: Guilford.

Rosario, M., Hunter, J., Maguen, S., Gwadz, M., & Smith, R. (2001). The coming-out process and its adaptational and health-related associations among gay, lesbian, and bisexual youths: Stipulation and exploration of a model. *American Journal of Community Psychology, 29*(1), 133-160.

Rosenfeld, S. L., Keenan, P. M., Fox, D. J., Chase, L. H., Melchiono, M. W., & Woods, E. R. (2000). Youth perceptions of comprehensive adolescent health services through the Boston HAPPENS program. *Journal of Pediatric Health Care, 14,* 60-67.

Rosengard, C., Adler, N. E., Gurvey, J. E., Dunlop, M. B. V., Tschann, J. M., Millstein, S. G., et al. (2001). Protective role of health values in adolescents' future intentions to use condoms. *Journal of Adolescent Health, 29,* 200-207.

Rosenstock, I. M. (1960). What research in motivation suggests for public health. *American Journal of Public Health, 50,* 295-301.

Rosenstock, I. M. (1974a). The health belief model and preventive health behavior. In M. H. Becker (Ed.), *The health belief model and personal health behavior* (pp. 27-59). Thorofare, NJ: Charles B. Slack.

Rosenstock, I. M. (1974b). Historical origins of the health belief model. *Health Education Monograph, 2,* 328-335.

Rosenstock, I. M. (1974c). Historical origins of the health belief model. In M. H. Becker (Ed.), *The health belief model and personal health behavior* (pp. 1-8). Thorofare, NJ: Charles B. Slack.

Rosenstock, I. M., Strecher, V. J., & Becker, M. H. (1988). Social learning theory and the health belief model. *Health Education Quarterly, 15,* 175-183.

Roth, J. L., & Brooks-Gunn, J. (2003). Youth development programs: Risk, prevention and policy. *Journal of Adolescent Health, 32,* 170-182.

Rotter, J. (1966). *Social learning and clinical psychology.* Englewood Cliffs, NJ: Prentice Hall.

Rouse, K. A. G., Ingersoll, G. M., & Orr, D. P. (1998). Longitudinal health endangering behavior risk among resilient and nonresilient early adolescents. *Journal of Adolescent Health, 23,* 297-302.

Rudolph, K. D. (2002). Gender differences in emotional responses to interpersonal stress during adolescence. *Journal of Adolescent Health, 30*(4, Suppl.), 3-13.

Rudolph, K. D., Hammen, C., Burge, D., Lindberg, N., Herzberg, D., & Daley, S. E. (2000). Toward an interpersonal life-stress model of depression: The developmental context of stress generation. *Development and Psychopathology, 12,* 215-234.

Rudolph, K. D., Lambert, S. F., Clark, A. G., & Kurlakowsky, K. D. (2001). Negotiating the transition to middle school: The role of self-regulatory processes. *Child Development, 72,* 929-946.

Runyon, M. K., & Kenny, M. C. (2002). Relationship of attributional style, depression, and posttrauma distress among children who suffered physical or sexual abuse. *Child Maltreatment, 7,* 254-264.

Rutter, M. (1980). *Changing youth in a changing society: Patterns of adolescent development and disorder.* Cambridge, MA: Harvard University Press.

Rutter, M. (1985). Resilience in the face of adversity: Protective factors and resistance to psychiatric disorder. *British Journal of Psychiatry, 147,* 598-611.

Rutter, M. (1987). Psychosocial resilience and protective mechanisms. *American Journal of Orthopsychiatry, 57,* 316-331.

Rutter, M. (1993). Resilience: Some conceptual considerations. *Journal of Adolescent Health, 14,* 626-631.

Rutter, M., Birch, H. G., Thomas, A., & Chess, S. (1962). Temperamental characteristics in infancy and the later development of behavioral disorders. *British Journal of Psychiatry, 110,* 651-661.

Ryan, C., & Futterman, D. (2001). Lesbian and gay adolescents: Identity development. *Prevention Researcher, 8*(1), 3-5.

Ryan, R. M., Stiller, J. D., & Lynch, J. H. (1994). Representatons of relationships to teachers, parents, and friends as predictors of academic motivation and self-esteem. *Journal of Early Adolescence, 14,* 226-249.

Sadler, L. S., & Daley, A. M. (2002). A model of teen-friendly care for young women with negative pregnancy test results. *Nursing Clinics of North America, 37*(3), 523-536.

Sargent, J. D., Dalton, M. A., Beach, M. L., Mott, L. A., Tickle, J. J., Ahrens, M. B., et al. (2002). Viewing tobacco use in movies: Does it shape attitudes that mediate adolescent smoking? *American Journal of Preventive Medicine, 22,* 137-145.

Sawin, K. J., Brei, T. J., Buran, C. F., & Fastenau, P. S. (2002). Factors associated with quality of life in adolescents with spina bifida. *Journal of Holistic Nursing, 20,* 279-304.

Scaffa, M. E. (1998). Adolescents and alcohol use. In A. Henderson, S. Champlin, & W. Evashwick (Ed.), *Promoting teen health: Linking schools, health organizations, and community* (pp. 78-99). Thousand Oaks, CA: Sage.

Scales, P. C. (1999). Reducing risks and building developmental assets: Essential actions for promoting adolescent health. *Journal of School Health, 69*(3), 113-119.

Scales, P.C. (2000). Building students' developmental assets to promote health and school success. *Clearing House, 74,* 84-88.

Scales, P. C., Benson, P. L., Leffert, N., & Blyth, D. A. (2000). Contribution of developmental assets to the prediction of thriving among adolescents. *Applied Developmental Science, 4*(1), 27-46.

Scales, P. C., Blyth, D. A., Berkas, T. H., & Kielsmeier, J. C. (2000). The effects of service-learning on middle school students' social responsibility and academic success. *Journal of Early Adolescence, 20*(3), 332-358.

Scales, P. C., Leffert, N., & Vraa, R. (2003). The relation of community developmental attentiveness to adolescent health. *American Journal of Health Behavior, 27*(Suppl. 1), S22-S34.

Schuster, M. A., Bell, R. M., & Kanouse, D. E. (1996). The sexual practices of adolescent virgins: Genital sexual activities of high school students who have never had vaginal intercourse. *American Journal of Public Health, 86,* 1570-1576.

Schwartz, S. J. (2001). The evolution of Eriksonian and neo-Eriksonian identity theory and research: A review and integration. *Identity: An International Journal of Theory and Research, 1*(1), 7-58.

Schwartz, S. J. (2002). Convergent validity in objective measures of identity status: Implications for identity status theory. *Adolescence, 37,* 609-625.

Schwartz, S. J., & Dunham, R. M. (2000). Identity status formulae: Generating continuous measures of the identity statuses from measures of exploration and commitment. *Adolescence, 35,* 147-165.

Schwartz, S. J., & Montgomery, M. J. (2002). Similarities or differences in identity development? The impact of acculturation and gender on identity process and outcome. *Journal of Youth and Adolescence, 31,* 359-371.

Schwarzer, R., & Fuchs, R. (1996). Self-efficacy and health behaviours. In M. Conner & P. Norman (Eds.), *Predicting health behaviour: Research and practice with social cognition models.* Philadelphia: Open University Press.

Selye, H. (1974). *Stress without distress.* Philadelphia: J. B. Lippincott.

Selye, H. (1978). *The stress of life* (Rev. ed.). New York: McGraw-Hill.

Sevig, T. D., Highlen, P. S., & Adams, E. M. (2000). Development and validation of the self-identity inventory (SII): A multicultural identity development instrument. *Cultural Diversity and Ethnic Minority Psychology, 6,* 168-182.

Sex chromosome variations: About 47XXY. (n.d.). Retrieved March 8, 2004, from http://www.genetic.org/ks/scvs/47xxy.htm

Shandler, S. (1999). *Ophelia speaks: Adolescent girls write about their search for self.* New York: HarperPerennial.

Shane, P. G. (1996). *What about America's homeless children? Hide and seek.* Thousand Oaks, CA: Sage.

Sharma, M., Petosa, R., & Heaney, C. A. (1999). Evaluation of a brief intervention based on social cognitive theory to develop problem-solving skills among sixth-grade children. *Health Education and Behavior, 26,* 465-477.

Shepard, M. P., Orsi, A. J., Mahon, M. M., & Carroll, R. M. (2002). Mixed-methods research with vulnerable families. *Journal of Family Nursing, 8,* 334-352.

Shilling, L. S., Grey, M., & Knafl, K. (2002).The concept of self-management of type 1 diabetes in children and adolescents: An evolutionary concept analysis. *Journal of Advanced Nursing, 37*(1), 87-99.

Sinaiko, A. R., Donahue, R. P., Jacobs, D. R., & Prineas, R. J. (1999). Relation of weight and rate of increase in weight during childhood and adolescence to body size, blood pressure, fasting insulin, and lipids in young adults. *Circulation, 99,* 1471-1476.

Siqueira, L., Diab, M., Bodian, C., & Rolnitzky, L. (2000). Adolescents becoming smokers: The roles of stress and coping methods. *Journal of Adolescent Health, 27,* 399-408.

Slovic, P. (2003). Affect, analysis, adolescence, and risk. In D. Romer (Ed.), *Reducing adolescent risk: Toward an integrated approach* (pp. 44-48). Thousand Oaks, CA: Sage.

Slusher, I. L. (1999). Self-care agency and self-care practice of adolescents. *Issues in Comprehensive Pediatric Nursing, 22,* 49-58.

Small, S. P., Brennan-Hunter, A. L., Best, D. G., & Solberg, S. M. (2002). Struggling to understand: The experience of nonsmoking parents with adolescents who smoke. *Qualitative Health Research, 12,* 1202-1219.

Smith, D. W., Colwell, B., Zhang, J. J., Brimer, J., McMillan, C., & Stevens, S. (2002). Theory-based development and testing of an adolescent tobacco-use awareness program. *American Journal of Health Behavior, 26,* 137-144.

Smith, K. W., McGraw, S. A., Costa, L. A., & McKinlay, J. B. (1996). A self-efficacy scale for HIV risk behaviors: Development and evaluation. *AIDS Education and Prevention, 8*(2), 97-105.

Smith, M. C. (2002). Health, healing, and myth of the hero journey. *Advances in Nursing Science, 24*(4), 1-13.

Smith, P., Flay, B. R., Bell, C. C., & Weissberg, R. P. (2001). The protective influence of parents and peers in violence avoidance among African-American youth. *Maternal and Child Health Journal, 5,* 245-252.

Snell, W. E. (1998). The Multidimensional Sexual Self-Concept Questionnaire. In C. M. Davis, W. L. Yarber, R. Bauserman, G. Schreer, & S. L. Davis (Eds.), *Handbook of sexuality-related measures* (pp. 521-524). Thousand Oaks, CA: Sage.

Sobo, E. J., Zimet, H. F., Zimmerman, T., & Celcil, H. (1997). Doubting the experts: AIDS misconceptions among runaway adolescents. *Human Organization, 56*(3), 311-320.

Sohng, S. S. L. (2003). Participatory research and community organizing. *New Social Movement Network.* Retrieved April 6, 2004, from http://www.interweb-tech.com/nsmnet/docs/sohng.htm

Soubhi, H., & Potvin, L. (2000). Homes and families as health promotion settings. In B. D. Poland, L. W. Green, & I. Rootman (Eds.), *Settings for health promotion: Linking theory and practice* (pp. 44-67). Thousand Oaks, CA: Sage.

Spaccarelli, S., & Kim, S. (1995). Resilience criteria and factors associated with resilience in sexually abused girls. *Child Abuse and Neglect, 19*(9), 1171-1182.

Spielberger, C. D. (1983). *State-trait anxiety inventory.* Palo Alto, CA: Consulting Psychologists Press, Inc.

Stake, R. E. (1998). Case studies. In N. K. Denzin & Y. S. Lincoln (Eds.), *Strategies of qualitative inquiry* (pp. 86-109). Thousand Oaks, CA: Sage.

Stanton, B. F., Li, X., Galbraith, J., Cornick, G., Feigelman, S., Kaljee, L., et al. (2000). Parental underestimates of adolescent risk behavior: A randomized, controlled trial of a parental monitoring intervention. *Journal of Adolescent Health, 26*(1), 18-26.

Stein, K. F., Roeser, R., & Markus, H. R. (1998). Self-schemas and possible selves as predictors and outcomes of risky behaviors in adolescents. *Nursing Research, 47,* 96-106.

Steinberg, L. (1996). *Adolescence* (4th ed.). New York: McGraw-Hill.

Steinberg, L. (2003). Is decision making the right framework for research on adolescent risk taking? In D. Romer (Ed.), *Reducing adolescent risk: Toward an integrated approach* (pp. 18-24). Thousand Oaks, CA: Sage.

Steiner, H., Erickson, S. J., Hernandez, N. L., & Pavelski, R. (2002). Coping styles as correlates of health in high school students. *Journal of Adolescent Health, 30,* 326-335.

Steiner, H., Ryst, E., Berkowitz, J., Gschwendt, M. A., & Koopman, C. (2002). Boys' and girls' responses to stress: Affect and heart rate during a speech task. *Journal of Adolescent Health, 30*(4, Suppl.), 14-21.

Stephen, J. E., Fraser, E., & Marcia, J. E. (1992). Lifespan identity development: Variables related to moratorium-achievement (MAMA) cycles. *Journal of Adolescence, 15,* 283-300.

Stevens, S. J., Murphy, B. S., & McKnight, K. (2003). Traumatic stress and gender differences in relationship to substance abuse, mental health, physical health, and HIV risk behavior in a sample of adolescents enrolled in drug treatment. *Child Maltreatment, 8*(1), 46-57.

Stewart, C. (2001). The influence of spirituality on substance use of college students. *Journal of Drug Education, 31,* 343-351.

Stewart, J. B., Hardin, S. B., Weinrich, S., McGeorge, S., Lopez, J., & Pesut, D. (1992). Group protocol to mitigate disaster stress and enhance social support in adolescents exposed to Hurricane Hugo. *Issues in Mental Health Nursing, 13,* 105-119.

Stewart, M., Reid, G., & Mangham, C. (1997). Fostering children's resistance. *Journal of Pediatric Nursing, 12*(1), 21-31.

St. Lawrence, J. S., Brasfield, T. L., & Jefferson, K. W. (1995). Cognitive-behavioral intervention to reduce African American adolescents' risk for HIV infection. *Journal of Consulting and Clinical Psychology, 63,* 221-237.

Stouthamer-Loeber, M., Loeber, R., Farringon, D. P., Zhang, Q., van Kammen, W., & Maguin, E. (1993). The double edge of protective and risk factors for delinquency: Interrelations and developmental patterns. *Development and Psychopathology, 5,* 683-701.

Straughn, H. K. (2003). *My interview with James W. Fowler on the stages of faith.* Retrieved April 6, 2004, from http://www.lifespirals.com/TheMindSpiral/Fowler/fowler.html

Strauss, A., & Corbin, J. (1998). Grounded theory methodology: An overview. In N. K. Denzin & Y. S. Lincoln (Eds.), *Strategies of qualitative inquiry* (pp. 158-183). Thousand Oaks, CA: Sage.

Strauss, R. S., Rodzilsky, D., Burack, G., & Colin, M. (2001). Psychosocial correlates of physical activity in healthy children. *Archives of Pediatrics and Adolescent Medicine, 155,* 897-902.

Strecher, V. J., DeVellis, B. M., Becker, M. H., & Rosenstock, I. M. (1986). The role of self-efficacy in achieving health behavior change. *Health Education Quarterly, 13*(1), 73-91.

Strecher, V. J., & Rosenstock, I. M. (1997). The health belief model. In K. Glanz, F. M. Lewis, & B. K. Rimer (Eds.), *Health behavior and health education: Theory, research, and practice* (2nd ed., pp. 41-59). San Francisco: Jossey-Bass.

Suarez, L., & Ramirez, A. G. (1999). Hispanic/Latino health and disease: An overview. In R. M. Huff & M. V. Kline (Eds.), *Promoting health in multicultural populations: A handbook for practitioners* (pp. 115-136). Thousand Oaks, CA: Sage.

Sue, D. W., & Sue, D. (1990). *Counseling the culturally different: Theory and practice* (2nd ed.). New York: John Wiley.

Sullivan, M., & Wodarski, J. S. (2002). Social alienation in gay youth. *Journal of Human Behavior in the Social Environment, 5*(1), 1-17.

Susman, E. J., Reiter, E. O., Ford, C., & Dorn, L. D. (2002). Developing models of healthy adolescent physical development. *Journal of Adolescent Health, 31*(6S), 171-174.

Sutton, S. (2000). A critical review of the transtheoretical model applied to smoking cessation. In P. Norman, C. Abraham, & M. Conner (Eds.), *Understanding and changing health behaviour: From health beliefs to self-regulation* (pp. 207-225). Amsterdam, The Netherlands: Harwood Academic.

Svetaz, M. V., Ireland, M., & Blum, R. (2000). Adolescents with learning disabilities: Risk and protective factors associated with emotional well-being: Findings from the National Longitudinal Study of Adolescent Health. *Journal of Adolescent Health, 27,* 340-348.

Swaim, R. C., Bates, S. C., & Chavez, E. L. (1998). Structural equation socialization model of substance use among Mexican-American and White non-Hispanic school dropouts. *Journal of Adolescent Health, 23,* 128-138.

Tanner, J. M. (1962). *Growth at adolescence* (2nd ed.) Springfield, IL: Charles C Thomas.

Tapert, S. F., Aarons, G. A., Sedlar, G. R., & Brown, S. A. (2001). Adolescent substance use and sexual risk-taking behavior. *Journal of Adolescent Health, 28,* 181-189.

Taussig, H. N. (2002). Risk behaviors in maltreated youth placed in foster care: A longitudinal study of protective and vulnerability factors. *Child Abuse and Neglect, 26,* 1179-1199.

Taylor, V. (1994). Medical community involvement in a breast cancer screening promotional project. *Public Health Reports, 109,* 491-500.

Tencati, E., Kole, S. L., Feighery, E. H., Winkleby, M., & Altman, D. G. (2002). Teens as advocates for substance use prevention: Strategies for implementation. *Health Promotion Practice, 3*(1), 18-29.

Thatcher, W. G., Reininger, B. M., & Drance, J. W. (2002). Using path analysis to examine adolescent suicide attempts, life satisfaction, and health risk behavior. *Journal of School Health, 72*(1), 71-77.

Thato, S., Charron-Prochownik, D., Dorn, L. D., Albrecht, S. A., & Stone, C. A. (2003). Predictors of condom use among adolescent Thai vocational students. *Journal of Nursing Scholarship, 35,* 157-163.

Thoits, P. A. (1991). Gender differences in coping with emotional distress. In J. Eckenrode (Ed.), *The social context of coping* (pp. 107-138). New York: Plenum.

Tigges, B. B. (2001). Affiliative preferences, self-change, and adolescent condom use. *Journal of Nursing Scholarship, 33,* 231-237.

Troiden, R. R. (1989). The formation of homosexual identities. *Journal of Homosexuality, 17,* 43-73.

Turner, R. J., & Lloyd, D. A. (1995). Lifetime traumas and mental health: The significance of cumulative adversity. *Journal of Health and Social Behavior, 36,* 360-376.

Udry, J. R., & Bearman, P. S. (1998). New methods for new research on adolescent sexual behavior. In R. Jessor (Ed.), *New perspectives on adolescent risk behavior* (pp. 241-269). Cambridge, England: Cambridge University Press.

U.S. Department of Health and Human Services. (1992a). *Healthy children 2000.* Boston: Jones and Bartlett.

U.S. Department of Health and Human Services. (1992b). *Healthy People 2000. National health promotion and disease prevention objectives.* Washington, DC: U.S. Government Printing Office [DHHS Publication No. (PHS)91-50212].

U.S. Department of Health and Human Services. (2000). *Healthy people 2010: National health promotion and disease prevention objectives.* Sudbury, MA: Jones and Bartlett.

Utter, J., Neumark-Sztainer, D., Wall, M., & Story, M. (2003). Reading magazine articles about dieting and associated weight control behaviors among adolescents. *Journal of Adolescent Health, 32,* 78-82.

Velicer, W. F., DiClemente, C. C., Prochaska, J. O., & Brandenberg, N. (1985). A decisional balance measure for assessing and predicting smoking status. *Journal of Personality and Social Psychology, 48,* 1279-1289.

Velicer, W. F., Prochaska, J. O., Fava, J. L., Norman, G. J., & Redding, C. A. (1998). Smoking cessation and stress management: Applications of the transtheoretical model of behavior change. *Homeostasis, 38,* 216-233.

Velicer, W. F., Rossi, J. A., Prochaska, J. O., & DiClemente, C. C. (1996). A criterion measurement model for addictive behaviors. *Addictive Behaviors, 21,* 555-584.

Villarruel, A. M., & Rodriguez, D. (2003). Beyond stereotypes: Promoting safer sex behaviors among Latino adolescents. *Journal of Obstetrics, Gynecology, and Neonatal Nursing, 32,* 258-263.

Wagnild, G., & Young, H. (1993). Development and psychometric evaluation of the Resiliency Scale. *Journal of Nursing Measurement, 1*(2), 165-178.

Walker, L. O., & Avant, K. C. (2005). *Strategies for theory construction in nursing* (5th ed.). Norwalk, CT: Appleton & Lange.

Wallace, J. M., & Forman, T. A. (1998). Religion's role in promoting health and reducing risk among American youth. *Health Education and Behavior, 25,* 721-741.

Wallace, J. M., Jr., & Williams, D. R. (1998). Religion and adolescent health-compromising behavior. In J. Schulenberg, J. L. Maggs, & K. Hurrelmann (Eds.), *Health risks and developmental transitions during adolescence* (pp. 444-468). Cambridge, MA: Harvard University Press.

Walters, A. S. (1999). HIV prevention in street youth. *Journal of Adolescent Health, 25*(1), 87-198.

Wapner, S., & Demick, J. (1998). Developmental analysis: A holistic, developmental, systems-oriented perspective. In W. Damon (Ed.), *Handbook of child psychology: Vol. 1. Theoretical models of human development* (5th ed., pp. 761-805). New York: John Wiley.

Warren, J. K. (1998). Perceived self-care capabilities of abused/neglected and nonabused/non-neglected pregnant, low-socioeconomic adolescents. *Journal of Child and Adolescent Psychiatric Nursing, 11*(1), 30-37.

Waterman, A. S. (1983). The Ego Identity Interview. In J. E. Marcia, A. S. Waterman, D. R. Matteson, S. L. Archer, & J. L. Orlofsky (Eds.), *Ego identity: A handbook for psychosocial research* (pp. 156-176). New York: Springer.

Waterman, A. S., & Archer, S. L. (1983). Identity status during the adult years: Scoring criteria. In J. E. Marcia, A. S. Waterman, D. R. Matteson, S. L. Archer, & J. L. Orlofsky (Eds.), *Ego identity: A handbook for psychosocial research* (pp. 241-270). New York: Springer.

Weiler, R. M. (1997). Adolescents' perceptions of health concerns: An exploratory study among rural Midwestern youth. *Health Education and Behavior, 24,* 287-299.

Weist, M. D., Goldstein, J., Evans, S. W., Lever, N. A., Axelrod, J., Schreters, R., et al. (2003). Funding a full continuum of mental health promotion and intervention programs in the schools. *Journal of Adolescent Health, 32*(6, Suppl.), 70-78.

Weisz, J. R., Southam-Gerow, M. A., & McCarty, C. A. (2001). Control-related beliefs and depressive symptoms in clinic-referred children and adolescents: Developmental differences and model specificity. *Journal of Abnormal Psychology, 110*(1), 97-109.

Weisz, J. R., Southam-Gerow, M. A., & Sweeney, L. (1998). *The perceived control scale for children.* Los Angeles: University of California, Los Angeles.

Weitzel, M. H. (1989). A test of the health promotion model with blue collar workers. *Nursing Research, 38,* 99-104.

Werner, E. E. (1989). High-risk children in young adulthood: A longitudinal study from birth to 32 years. *American Journal of Orthopsychiatry, 59*(1), 72-81.

Werner, E. E. (2003). Vulnerability and resilience in adversity: A longitudinal perspective. *Proceedings from the 2003 Children, Youth, Families At-Risk Conference* (pp. 1-13). Retrieved April 28, 2004, from http://www.cyfernet.org/cyfar03/Werner.ppt

Werner, E. E., & Smith, R. S. (1992). *Overcoming the odds: High risk children from birth to adulthood.* Ithaca, NY: Cornell University Press.

White, J. M., & Porth, C. M. (2000). Physiological measurement of the stress response. In V. H. Rice (Ed.), *Handbook of stress, coping, and health: Implications for nursing research, theory, and practice* (pp. 69-94). Thousand Oaks, CA: Sage.

Wichstrøm, L. (2001). The impact of pubertal timing on adolescents' alcohol use. *Journal of Research on Adolescence, 11,* 131-150.

Wiesner, M., & Ittel, A. (2002). Relations of pubertal timing and depressive symptoms to substance use in early adolescence. *Journal of Early Adolescence, 22*(1), 5-23.

Williams, A. F. (1998). Risky driving behavior among adolescents. In R. Jessor (Ed.), *New perspectives on adolescent risk behavior* (pp. 221-237). Cambridge, MA: Harvard University Press.

Wills, T. A., Sandy, J. M., & Yaeger, A. M. (2002). Moderators of the relation between substance use level and problems: Test of a self-regulation model in middle adolescence. *Journal of Abnormal Psychology, 111*(1), 3-21.

Wilson, D. K., Friend, R., Teasley, N., Green, S., Reaves, I. L., & Sica, D. A. (2002). Motivational versus social cognitive interventions for promoting fruit and vegetable intake and physical activity in African American adolescents. *Annals of Behavioral Medicine, 24,* 310-319.

Wilson, K. G., Stelzer, J., Bergman, J. N., Kral, M. J., Inayatullah, M., & Elliott, C. A. (1995). Problem solving, stress, and coping adolescent suicide attempts. *Suicide and Life-Threatening Behavior, 25,* 241-252.

Wingood, G. M., DiClemente, R. J., Crosby, R., Harrington, K., Davies, S. L., & Hook, E. W., III. (2002, November). Gang involvement and the health of African American female adolescents. *Pediatrics, 110*(5), e57. Retrieved April 6, 2004, from http://www.pediatrics.org/cgi/content/full/110/5/e57

Winters, E. R., Petosa, R. L., & Charlton, T. E. (2003). Using social cognitive theory to explain discretionary, "leisure-time" physical exercise among high school students. *Journal of Adolescent Health, 32,* 436-442.

Winters, K. C., Henly, G. A., & Stinchfield, R. D. (1987). *Problem recognition questionnaire.* Minneapolis: Center for Adolescent Substance Abuse, University of Minnesota.

Wood, J., Foy, D. W., Layne, C., Pynoos, R., & James, C. B. (2002). An examination of the relationships between violence exposure, posttraumatic stress symptomatology, and delinquent activity: An "ecopathological" model of delinquent behavior among incarcerated adolescents. *Journal of Aggression, Maltreatment and Trauma, 6*(1), 127-147.

Wooten, P. (1996). Humor: An antidote for stress. *Holistic Nursing Practice, 10,* 49-56.

World Health Organization. (1946, June 19-22). *Preamble to the Constitution of the World Health Organization.* Geneva, Switzerland: Author.

World Health Organization. (1986). *Alma-alta 1978: Primary health care.* Geneva Switzerland: Author.

Wu, Y. Y., & Pender, N. (2002). Determinants of physical activity among Taiwanese adolescents: An application of the health promotion model. *Research in Nursing and Health, 25,* 25-36.

Yarcheski, A., Mahon, N. E., & Yarcheski, T. J. (1997). Alternate models of positive health practices in adolescents. *Nursing Research, 46,* 85-92.

Yeatts, K., & Shy, C. M. (2001). Prevalence and consequences of asthma and wheezing in African-American and White adolescents. *Journal of Adolescent Health, 29,* 314-319.

Zbikowski, S. M., Klesges, R. C., Robinson, L. A., & Alfano, C. M. (2002). Risk factors for smoking among adolescents with asthma. *Journal of Adolescent Health, 30,* 279-287.

Zimmerman, M. A., & Arunkumar, R. (1994). Resiliency research: Implications for schools and policy. *Social Policy Report: Society for Research in Child Development, 8*(4), 1-17.

Zimrin, H. (1986). A profile of survival. *Child Abuse and Neglect, 10,* 339-349.

Zweig, J. M., Phillips, S. D., & Lindberg, L. D. (2002). Predicting adolescent profiles of risk: Looking beyond demographics. *Journal of Adolescent Health, 31,* 343-353.

Author Index

Subject Index _____

About the Author _____

Lynn Rew is the Denton and Louise Cooley and Family Centennial Professor in Nursing at The University of Texas at Austin. Born and raised in rural Iowa, she earned her Bachelor of Science degree in nursing from the University of Hawaii, Honolulu; her master's degree in community health nursing and her Ed.D. in counselor education were earned at Northern Illinois University, DeKalb. In 1996, she completed a postdoctoral fellowship in adolescent health at the University of Minnesota School of Medicine, where Michael D. Resnick, Ph.D., served as her supervising mentor. At The University of Texas at Austin School of Nursing, she serves as Graduate Advisor and is Director of the Southwest Partnership Center for Health Disparities Research. She is currently Principal Investigator on two R01 studies funded by the National Institutes of Health that focus on adolescent health-risk behaviors. She also serves as editor of the *Journal of Holistic Nursing.*